Audiology:
The Fundamentals

Fourth Edition

Audiology:
The Fundamentals

Fourth Edition

FRED H. BESS, PhD
Professor and Chair
Department of Hearing and Speech Sciences
Vanderbilt Bill Wilkerson Center for Otolaryngology
  and Communication Sciences
Vanderbilt University Medical Center
Nashville, Tennessee

LARRY E. HUMES, PhD
Professor
Department of Speech and Hearing Sciences
Indiana University
Bloomington, Indiana

Wolters Kluwer | Lippincott Williams & Wilkins
Health

Philadelphia · Baltimore · New York · London
Buenos Aires · Hong Kong · Sydney · Tokyo

Acquisitions Editor: Pete Sabatini
Managing Editor: Andrea M. Klingler
Marketing Manager: Allison Noplock
Production Editor: Gina Aiello
Designer: Steve Druding
Compositor: International Typesetting and Composition
Printer: R. R. Donnelley Shenzhen

Fourth Edition

© 2009 by Lippincott Williams & Wilkins, a Wolters Kluwer business
530 Walnut Street
Philadelphia, PA 19106
LWW.com

First Edition, 1990
Second Edition, 1995
Third Edition, 2003

Printed in China

Library of Congress Cataloging-in-Publication Data

Bess, Fred H.
  Audiology: the fundamentals/Fred H. Bess, Larry E. Humes. — 4th
ed.
      p. ; cm.
  Includes bibliographical references and index.
  ISBN-13: 978-0-7817-6643-2
  ISBN-10: 0-7817-6643-5
  1. Audiology.   I. Humes, Larry.   II. Title.
  [DNLM: 1. Audiology.   WV 270 B557a 2008]
  RF290.B44 2008
  617.8—dc22

                                      2007038510

To purchase additional copies of this book, call our customer service department at (800) 639-3030 or fax orders to (301) 824-7390. International customers should call (301) 714-2324. Lippincott Williams & Wilkins customer service representatives are available from 8:30 am to 6:00 pm, EST, Monday through Friday, for telephone access. Visit Lippincott Williams & Wilkins on the Internet: http://www.lww.com.

10 9 8 7 6 5 4 3 2

To our wives, Susie and Marty
Our children, Danny, Amy, Rick, Andy, Liz, Lauren, and Adam
and
To the undergraduate and graduate students whom
we have had the pleasure to work with
over the past few decades

Preface

The fourth edition of *Audiology: The Fundamentals* continues to offer a contemporary treatment of the profession of audiology at the introductory level. Although audiology is a relative newcomer to the health care profession, it is a dynamic discipline that has undergone rapid change and growth since its inception during World War II. In fact, the multitude of changes that have occurred since the first edition have been impressive. Because of these transformations and space limitations, we found ourselves once again forced to make choices regarding which areas of audiology to include in this edition. As in the first three editions, we have chosen to discuss those topics considered most important to the beginning student rather than to provide a cursory review of the broad scope of the profession.

Initially, this book was written for three reasons. First, we believed that there was a need for an introductory book that provided a contemporary approach to audiology—one that strikes a balance between the traditional concepts and newer developments in the profession. Second, we believed there was a place for an introductory book that considered the type of student typically enrolled in a beginning audiology course. Our experience suggested that most students taking an introductory course in audiology were planning careers in speech-language pathology, special education, or psychology. With this in mind, we have tried to emphasize material on auditory pathology in children, especially middle ear disease, and we have included chapters on screening auditory function and education for the individual with hearing loss. It was our hope that such information would be of value to students when they began practicing their chosen profession. Finally, we wanted to share with the beginning student our enthusiasm for audiology—most important, the challenges and rewards associated with this health-related discipline. The widespread acceptance of the first three editions of this text reaffirmed our belief that a need existed for an introductory book of this type in audiology.

Organization

The book is organized into three parts. Part 1 provides background information on the profession of audiology and a basic review of the underlying principles of acoustics and the anatomy and physiology of the auditory system. A general understanding of the concepts in Part 1 is essential to the practice of the profession of audiology. Part 2 is concerned with the principles of audiologic measurement and the general application of audiologic procedures. Toward this end, Part 2 focuses on basic measurement of auditory function, auditory pathologies and their associated audiologic manifestations and screening for hearing loss, and middle ear disease. Part 3 is directed at providing a general understanding of rehabilitative approaches used with children and adults with hearing loss and the status of education of individuals with hearing loss.

Features and Items New to This Edition

This fourth edition offers many additions and updates from the previous edition and provides much greater detail in several chapters. In fact, this edition may be more suitable for advanced undergraduates or even first-year doctor of audiology students. Advanced material that was previously appended to the end of each chapter as supplemental material has now been inserted into the main body of text in each chapter. In addition, close to 50 new figures and vignettes have been added to this edition, and many of them have been redrawn and a second color has been added to improve aesthetics and to enhance readability.

Moreover, we expanded the material offered in virtually every chapter of this book. We have also tried to maintain the easy-to-read, easy-to-understand style. A new reader-friendly design has also been developed for this new edition. **Learning objectives** provide guidelines regarding material that will be discussed in each chapter. As before, **References** are intentionally omitted from the body of the book with the exception of a few direct quotations. A popular component of the previous editions was the **vignettes**. The fourth edition again uses these short, descriptive sketches designed to enhance interest, to provide illustrative examples of ideas, and to crystallize definitions of concepts that are difficult to grasp. **Chapter summaries** provide a brief recap of important information discussed in each chapter.

Ancillaries

A companion Web site (included with each book) has been developed for students to accompany this new edition of *Audiology: The Fundamentals*. Audiograms, color anatomy and pathophysiology images, case studies, and a quiz bank have been provided for use while learning and reviewing the information presented in the text. PowerPoint lecture outlines and an image bank have been created for use by instructors. Both will be available online.

F.H.B.
L.E.H.

Reviewers

Acknowledgments

The preparation of this book could not have been completed without the generous help and support of many individuals. Shelia Lewis expertly and cheerfully prepared all of the drafts as well as the final version of the book chapters. Dominic Doyle once again spent numerous hours preparing new figures and vignette images. In this fourth edition, we are grateful for the suggestions of Marjorie Grantham, Andrea Hillock, Linda Hood, Ben Hornsby, Gus Mueller, Todd Ricketts, Melanie Schuele, Christopher Spankovich, and Ross Genovese; the constructive comments of these colleagues strongly influenced the content of this book. We have also tried to incorporate the suggestions volunteered by the faculties of several universities who are using the book in their introductory courses. Pete Sabatini, Andrea Klingler, and Kevin Dietz at Lippincott Williams & Wilkins provided support and encouragement throughout the revision process. The staff and faculty of the Vanderbilt Bill Wilkerson Center, Vanderbilt University Medical Center (Department of Hearing and Speech Sciences) and Indiana University (Department of Speech and Hearing Sciences) offered continued support and facilities. To all of these individuals, we offer our sincere appreciation.

Finally, in the first edition, we took the opportunity to express our love and gratitude to our parents, Helen and Samuel H. Bess and Mary and Charles E. Humes, for their confidence, direction, and continual support. Since then, each of the authors has experienced the loss of both parents; their memories will always be with us.

F.H.B.
L.E.H.

Contents

PART 1

Introduction

CHAPTER 1

Audiology as a Profession

After completion of this chapter, the reader should be able to:

- Discuss the prevalence of hearing loss and the complications associated with hearing impairment.
- Define the profession of audiology.
- Appreciate the lineage of the profession of audiology.
- Describe the employment opportunities available to the audiologist.
- Understand the academic and clinical requirements needed to become an audiologist.
- Appreciate the essential accreditations and professional affiliations important to clinical audiology.

The purpose of this opening chapter is to offer a general discussion and review of the profession of audiology. The discussion focuses on several areas. First, statistics on the total number of cases of hearing loss, or the prevalence of hearing loss, are reviewed. The impact of hearing loss on the well-being of the individual is also briefly described. These two areas are reviewed to give the reader some sense of the magnitude of the problem, both on a national scale and as it is experienced by the affected individuals themselves. Next, the definition and historical evolution of audiology are reviewed. Various employment opportunities in this health-related discipline are surveyed. The chapter concludes with a summary of typical graduate and professional training programs in audiology, a brief discussion of accreditation/licensure, and a description of some of the professional affiliations that audiologists find worthwhile.

PREVALENCE AND IMPACT OF HEARING LOSS

Before a discussion of audiology as a profession, it is helpful to develop some understanding of the nature of hearing loss in the United States. The estimated prevalence, or total number of existing cases, of hearing loss varies according to several factors. These factors include (*a*) how hearing loss was determined (i.e., questionnaire versus hearing test), (*b*) the criterion or formula used to define the presence of a hearing loss (severe versus mild hearing loss), and (*c*) the age of the individuals in the population sampled (adults versus children). Regardless of the methods used to determine prevalence, hearing loss is known to affect a large segment of the population in the United States. Studies focusing on the population under 18 years of age estimate that approximately 56,000 children under age 6 years are living with significant hearing loss in both ears. "Significant hearing loss" means that these children exhibit a hearing deficit in both ears, with the better ear exhibiting some difficulty in hearing and understanding speech. It has also been estimated that 2 to 3 of every 1000 infants in the United States are born with a congenital hearing loss in the moderate to severe range. These data do not include children born with normal hearing who develop hearing loss later, a condition commonly referred to as progressive hearing loss. If young children with the milder forms of hearing loss are included, the prevalence rate is thought to involve significantly more children; estimates range from 120 in 1000 to 150 in 1000. Assuming a prevalence rate of 130 in 1000 and a school-age population of 46 million (kindergarten through grade 12), the number of school-age children with some degree of hearing loss is approximately 3.5 million. These data should be viewed in light of the fact that elementary school enrollment is expected to increase as the baby boomlet continues to swell the school-age ranks.

Estimates of the prevalence of hearing loss for the adult population as a whole and for various age groups are summarized in Table 1.1. This table illustrates that based on figures from 2004, the total number of persons over 18 years of age with hearing loss in the United States is slightly more than 35 million. Also note that the prevalence rate for hearing loss increases with age. For example, in the age category of 18 to 44 years, the prevalence rate is 70.7 in 1000, whereas for the age groups 65 to 74 years and 75 years and older, the prevalence rates are 310.7 in 1000 and 480.9 in 1000, respectively.

TABLE 1.1   Prevalence and Prevalence Rates According to Age for Hearing Loss in the United States (18 years and over)[a]

Age Group (y)	Prevalence	Prevalence Rate (per thousand)
All ages (Total)	35,135,000	160.3
18–44	8,459,000	70.7
45–64	12,960,000	180.5
65–74	5,800,000	310.7
75+	7,917,000	480.9

[a]Data were obtained from household interviews and reflect the prevalence of hearing loss in either one or both ears.

Adapted from Lethbridge-Cejku M, Rose D, Vickerie J. Summary Health Statistics for U.S. Adults: National Health Interview Survey. 2004 National Health Statistics, Series 10 (228), 2006.

These statistics confirm what many of us with living grandparents and great-grandparents already know: hearing loss is commonly associated with old age. This is particularly important when one considers the number of elderly persons in the United States and the projected growth rates of the aged population. The number of individuals older than 65 years exceeds 35 million, and that figure is expected to increase to more than 80 million by the year 2050. This substantial increase in longevity has stemmed in part from the medical profession's improved success in controlling infectious and chronic diseases.

The preceding paragraphs establish that many Americans of all ages have significant hearing problems. Although statistics such as these are important, they provide little insight into the devastating impact that a significant hearing loss can have on the individual. Children born with a severe or profound hearing loss experience the greatest hardship and under most circumstances exhibit a significant lag in educational progress. This is because the hearing loss interferes with the child's speech perception ability, which in turn may result in impairment of speech and language development, reduction in academic achievement, and disturbances in social and emotional development. Because the development of our language system depends heavily on auditory input, a reduction or elimination of auditory input drastically curtails the ability to learn speech and language. To illustrate, it has been noted that the average high-school graduate from a state school for the deaf has the equivalent of an eighth-grade education. Even children with hearing losses in only one ear or very mild losses in both ears may experience difficulties in speech or language development, speech recognition under adverse listening conditions (e.g., classroom noise), educational achievement, and psychosocial behavior.

Children are not the only ones affected negatively by significant hearing loss. Hearing loss in the adult can produce a number of psychosocial complications. For the elderly adult, the deterioration in hearing sensitivity and the associated problems with understanding speech are known to affect the quality of the individual's daily living. That is, the elderly who have hearing loss are more likely than those with normal hearing to have poor general health, reduced mobility, fewer excursions outside the home, fewer interpersonal contacts, more depression and anxiety, and increased tension.

Hearing loss also imposes a significant economic burden; relatively few deaf individuals are employed in professional, technical, and managerial positions. Moreover, the lifetime cost of deafness is substantial. The overall societal costs of deafness include such factors as diagnosis, periodic medical visits, audiologic evaluations, hearing aid fittings, assistive listening devices, special education, rehabilitation, and loss of potential income. As shown in Figure 1.1, the cost of deafness increases as age of onset decreases. For the child who is deaf before learning to talk, the lifetime cost exceeds $1 million, whereas lifetime cost is much less for individuals who acquire hearing loss later in life. Overall, the lifetime cost of deafness averages $297,000. Other less tangible costs borne by affected individuals and by their families derive from emotional stress, breakdowns in family communication, and isolation from peer and educational systems.

In summary, hearing loss occurs in large numbers of people and affects both children and adults. In addition, the prevalence rate of hearing loss increases markedly for the elderly population. Finally, the overall impact of hearing loss in both children and adults is significant, causing delays in the psychoeducational progress of children and producing serious psychosocial consequences for those who acquire hearing loss later in life.

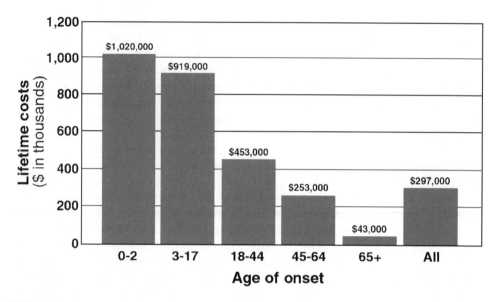

FIGURE 1.1 Bar graph illustrating the lifetime costs of deafness as a function of age of onset. (Adapted from Mohr PE, Feldman JJ, Dunbar JL. The Societal Costs of Severe to Profound Hearing Loss in the United States. Project Hope Center for Health Affairs, Policy Analysis Brief, 2000.)

AUDIOLOGY DEFINED

Audiology is a relatively new health care profession concerned with the study of both normal and disordered hearing. It evolved as a spinoff from such closely related fields as speech-language pathology, medicine, special education, psychology, and hearing aid instrumentation. In the most literal sense, the term *audiology* refers to the study of hearing. A much broader definition of audiology is *the discipline involved in the prevention, identification, and evaluation of hearing disorders, the selection and evaluation of hearing aids, and the habilitation/rehabilitation of individuals with hearing loss.* Although these definitions are commonly accepted descriptions of the profession, they in no way reflect adequately the breadth of the field or the challenges, rewards, and self-fulfillment that can result from a career in audiology. Whether your interest centers on serving people or producing new knowledge through inquiry and study, a career in audiology has much to offer.

Audiology is typically subdivided into specialties according to the nature of the population served or the setting in which the audiologist is employed (Vignette 1.1). For example, a common area of specialization is pediatric audiology, in which the focus is placed on the identification, assessment, and management of the neonate, infant, and school-age child with hearing loss. The pediatric audiologist develops special knowledge in such areas as the causes of childhood deafness, the development of audition in children, child development, the audiologic screening and evaluation of children of different age groups, and parent counseling.

Another common specialty area is medical audiology. The medical audiologist is typically employed in a medical center to assist the physician in establishing an accurate diagnosis of an auditory disorder. Toward this end, the audiologist employs highly sophisticated and specialized tests to help pinpoint the location and cause of the

VIGNETTE 1.1   Illustration of various specialty areas in audiology

Audiology is categorized into a number of specialty areas based on the population served or the employment setting. The pediatric audiologist concentrates on the audiologic management of children of all ages. The pediatric audiologist is often employed in a children's hospital or a health care facility primarily serving children. The medical audiologist works with patients of all ages and is more concerned with establishing the site and cause of a hearing problem. Medical audiologists are typically employed in hospitals as part of either a hearing and speech department or a department of otolaryngology (i.e., Ear, Nose, and Throat, or ENT). The rehabilitative or dispensing audiologist focuses on the management of children or adults with hearing loss. Rehabilitative audiologists are often seen in private practice and specialize in the direct dispensation of hearing aids. Rehabilitative audiologists are also employed by a variety of health care facilities (e.g., hospitals, nursing homes). The industrial audiologist provides consultative hearing conservation services to companies whose workers are exposed to high noise levels. The industrial audiologist may be in private practice or work on a part-time basis. Finally, the educational audiologist serves children in the schools and is employed or contracted by the educational system.

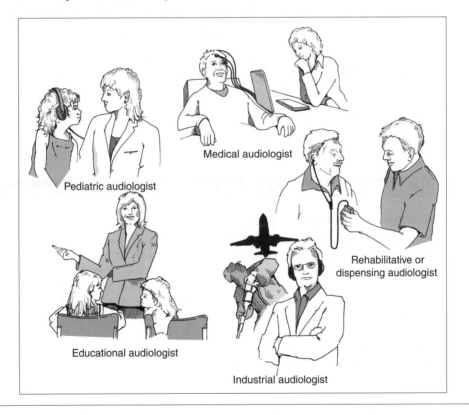

Pediatric audiologist

Medical audiologist

Rehabilitative or dispensing audiologist

Educational audiologist

Industrial audiologist

hearing problem. The medical audiologist spends much of his or her time determining whether hearing loss is caused by a problem in the middle ear, the inner ear, or the higher centers of the auditory system within the brainstem and cortex.

Rehabilitative audiology is a third area of specialization that is gaining widespread popularity and acceptance. The rehabilitative audiologist is concerned with the appropriate management of an individual with a hearing deficit. It is common for the rehabilitative audiologist to specialize even further by limiting the service population to either adults or children. The rehabilitative audiologist is interested in fitting the individual with appropriate amplification, such as a personal hearing aid, to help compensate for the hearing loss. This specialist also provides the individual with information on the use and care of the hearing aid. Other services offered might include speech reading, speech remediation, auditory training, and individual and family counseling. If the audiologist specializes in the rehabilitation of children, his or her activities might also include conducting special parent-infant training programs, teaching speech and language, counseling parents, and readying the child for school.

Some audiologists practice exclusively in an industrial setting. These audiologists are referred to as industrial audiologists. Noise is a common byproduct of our highly industrialized society. As we'll learn later, high levels of noise can produce permanent loss of hearing. Because many industries have work areas that produce high noise levels, audiologists are needed to develop programs that will protect employees from noise. Audiologists organize hearing conservation programs. These programs are designed to protect the worker from hearing loss by reducing the noise levels produced by noisy equipment, monitoring the hearing of employees, teaching employees about noise and its damaging effects, and providing ear protection to those who work in high-noise areas.

Finally, some audiologists specialize in educational audiology and are employed by public schools. Recall that the prevalence of hearing loss among school-age children is considerable. Educational audiologists are involved in identification, assessment, and monitoring of all school-age children with temporary or permanent hearing problems. The educational audiologist also selects and maintains hearing aids for children with hearing loss and assists regular teachers with educational programming.

HISTORICAL DEVELOPMENT OF AUDIOLOGY

Although instruments (audiometers) used to measure hearing date to the late 1800s, audiology as a discipline essentially evolved during World War II. During and following this war, many military personnel returned from combat with significant hearing loss resulting from exposure to the many and varied types of warfare noises. Interestingly, it was a prominent speech pathologist, Robert West, who called for his colleagues to expand their discipline to include audition. West (1936) stated: "Many workers in the field of speech correction do not realize that the time has come for those interested in this field to expand the subject so as to include . . . problems of those defective in the perception of speech. Our job should include . . . aiding the individual to hear what he ought to hear." Although a term had not yet been coined for this new field proposed by West, there was evidence that activity and interest in hearing disorders was present as early as 1936.

There has been considerable debate over who was responsible for coining the term *audiology*. Most sources credit Norton Canfield, an otolaryngologist (ear, nose, and throat physician), and Raymond Carhart, a speech-language pathologist, for coining the term independently of one another in 1945. Both of these men were intimately involved in planning and implementing programs in specialized aural rehabilitation hospitals established for military personnel during World War II. Today, Carhart is recognized by many as the Father of Audiology (Vignette 1.2).

VIGNETTE 1.2 **Raymond Carhart (1912–1975), Father of Audiology**

The contributions of Dr. Raymond Carhart to the development of audiology from its earliest origins were so numerous and so significant that many think of him today as the Father of Audiology. A young professor in the School of Speech at Northwestern University when World War II broke out, he was commissioned as a captain in the army to head the Deshon General Hospital aural rehabilitation program for war-deafened military personnel at Butler, Pennsylvania. Deshon was named as one of three army general hospitals to receive, treat, and rehabilitate soldiers who incurred hearing loss as a result of their military service. These three hospitals, together with the Philadelphia Naval Hospital, admitted and served some 16,000 enlisted personnel and officers with hearing loss during the war.

This wartime mobilization effort served as the basis for the development of the new discipline that is now audiology. In 1945, Carhart and otologist Norton Canfield were credited with coining the word *audiology* to designate the science of hearing. From the outset, Carhart recognized that the strong interprofessional relationships between audiology and otology must be maintained. The military program was modeled on this concept, which determined its direction for the future. As a leader in the American Speech Correction Association, Carhart was instrumental in changing the name to the American Speech and Hearing Association soon after the close of World War II. Moreover, over the years he was one of the ASHA's most effective liaisons between audiology and otology when potentially divisive issues arose.

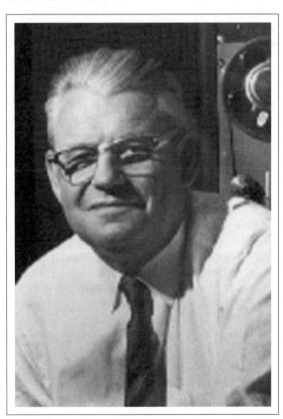

Returning to Northwestern as professor of audiology at the close of the war, Carhart set about immediately to develop a strong audiology graduate program and a clinical service center, placing Northwestern at the forefront of this field nationally. Many of his graduates became prominent in other universities across the country as teachers, research scientists, and clinical specialists. They, as well as his many professional associates in audiology and medicine, remember him for his brilliant and inquiring mind, which provided many of the research findings still undergirding the field today; for his scholarly publications; for his masterful teaching and speaking ability; and for his skill in the management of controversies within his national association, now the ASHA. But most of all, his former students and associates remember him as a warm human being and a mentor who was first of all a friend.

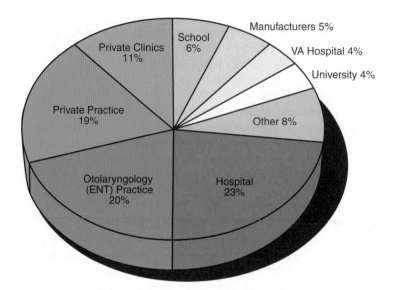

FIGURE 1.2 Distribution of employment settings for audiologists. Private practitioners are most typically seen in two employment settings, the physician's office (ENT) and the autonomous audiology office. (Adapted from American Academy of Audiology. 2005 Compensation and Benefits Report.)

PROFESSIONAL OPPORTUNITIES

As shown in Figure 1.2, the modern-day audiologist has the opportunity to work within a wide variety of employment settings. The largest numbers of audiologists are employed in community and university hospitals (23%), otolaryngology (ENT) practices (20%), private practice in audiology (19%), private clinics (11%), and schools (6%). Other work settings include manufacturing, universities, Veteran's Administration hospitals, and federal agencies. The following discussion is a more detailed presentation of some of the professional opportunities in audiology.

Community and University Hospitals

Most hospitals in the United States employ audiologists. The demand for audiologic services in hospitals, long-term care facilities, and home health agencies is increasing steadily. The increased demand for audiologists in this type of setting, especially since the mid 1980s, may be attributed to several factors. First, there is a growing trend for hospitals to develop or enhance their rehabilitation programs, because the government's reimbursement systems (e.g., Medicare) now emphasize short-term hospital stays and subsequent outpatient rehabilitative services. Audiologic services are one form of outpatient rehabilitative service. Second, there is an increased awareness of the overall value of audiology and its contributions to health care. Third, many states are now mandating universal newborn hearing screening (see Chapter 6). Audiologists typically are employed by hospitals to coordinate those newborn screening programs. Finally, as was mentioned, the number of elderly individuals in the United States is growing, with at least one-third seeking health care, including audiologic services in many cases.

Predictably, the audiologic services provided in the hospital setting tend to be medically based. These audiologic services usually focus on providing information about the identification and location of an auditory disorder. The audiologist utilizes sophisticated auditory tests to evaluate the middle ear, the inner ear, the nerve pathways to the brain, and the auditory portions of the brain. This information is then pooled with diagnostic data obtained from other disciplines, such as otology (ear specialists), neurology, pediatrics, and psychology, to obtain a final diagnosis. In the hospital setting, the audiologist often works as part of a multidisciplinary team of medical and other professionals.

Assisting the team in determining the diagnosis, however, is not the only service the audiologist provides in the hospital environment. Other services include dispensing hearing aids, managing patients with unconventional hearing devices, screening, and monitoring the hearing of patients who are treated with drugs that could damage hearing.

Audiology as a Private Practice

Certainly the fastest growing and perhaps most exciting employment setting is that of private practice. No other subgroup within the profession has shown such accelerated growth. In the 1970s, few audiologists were in private practice (Vignette 1.3). As noted

---

VIGNETTE 1.3   George S. Osborne (1940–2007), "Pioneer in Private Practice"

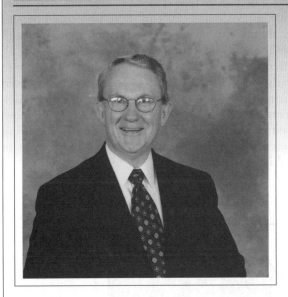

George S. Osborne, a pioneer, entrepreneur, visionary, and leader in the profession of audiology is perhaps best known for starting one of the very first successful private practices in the country. In the early 1970s there were very few audiologists in private practice—most audiologists during this time worked in universities, hospitals, and community hearing and speech centers. Dr. Osborne, an audiologist and a dentist, saw the upside potential for private practice in audiology and launched the Oak Park Speech and Hearing Center in Oak Park, Illinois. The practice grew quickly and became one of the largest practices in the nation—in fact, the practice served as a model for many other audiologists to emulate. In addition to Oak Park, Dr. Osborne started two additional private practices in audiology—one in Minnesota and one in Pennsylvania. Today, private practice is one of the most popular and fastest growing work settings in the profession of audiology.

Dr. Osborne's enthusiasm for private practice led him to become an advocate for the profession; especially regarding the role of the private practitioner in audiology. He worked steadfastly to promote audiology to ensure that audiologists would achieve recognition and parity with other health care professionals. To this end, he actively promoted the doctorate in audiology (AuD) as the entry level degree for the profession and he developed a well-recognized AuD program at the Pennsylvania College of Optometry (School of Audiology) serving as its first Dean.

earlier, 19% of today's audiologists are employed full-time in private practice. In fact, the private practice phenomenon has created an excellent market for professional opportunities in other areas of the profession. Many audiologists are leaving the traditional employment settings, attracted by the lure of a small business practice. The focus of these practices is on the sale of hearing aids, although many audiologists in private practice offer a wide array of audiologic services. Some audiologists may operate their businesses in medical clinics, hospitals, speech-language pathology offices, or otolaryngology practices; others may set up their own free-standing operation. There is, of course, a substantial risk involved in setting up a small business. The Small Business Administration estimates that about 60% of all new businesses fail during the first 5 years. Today, however, more and more successful businesses in audiology are started each year.

Why is it that private practice has become so popular, and why is it growing at such a fast pace? There are several reasons. First, small businesses provide an opportunity for financial independence and entrepreneurial expression and, perhaps most importantly, an opportunity to work for oneself. Second, private practice is growing because the opportunities it provides are becoming much more visible to those audiologists working in other settings. There is a dramatic increase in the memberships of organizations that are concerned with private practice and hearing aid dispensing and in the number of publications that serve the field. Third, the concept of franchises, or regional and national chains, in the hearing aid dispensing business has developed recently. Fourth, the sale of hearing aids has increased steadily over the past three decades (Fig. 1.3), yet, for adults, only approximately 20% of those who could benefit from hearing aids have purchased them. This suggests considerable potential and promise for future growth regarding the sale and delivery of hearing aids.

The sale of such devices remained relatively stable throughout the early and mid 1970s. From the late 1970s to the early 1990s, however, sales of hearing aids exhibited more than a threefold increase. During this same period, as noted previously, audiologists in private practice increased considerably in number. Since the early 1990s, however, hearing aid sales have increased at a much slower rate, most recently stabilizing at approximately 1.9 million instruments. Interestingly, the number of audiologists in private practice has increased over this same period.

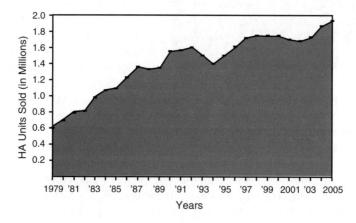

FIGURE 1.3 Annual hearing aid sales from 1979 to 2005. (Adapted from Strom KE. Rapid product changes mark the new mature digital market. Hear Rev 13(5):70–74, 2006.)

Community-Based Clinics and Rehabilitation Centers

A common setting for the practice of audiology has been the private community-based clinics. Such practices can be implemented as a freestanding hearing and speech center or as a component of a larger rehabilitation center. Today, many metropolitan communities with populations greater than about 50,000 maintain community hearing and speech centers. These facilities provide comprehensive diagnostic and rehabilitative services to individuals with disorders of hearing, speech, or language. These centers receive much of their financial support from the community through individual contributions and through organizations such as the United Way and civic clubs. It is because of this type of support that such centers are able to serve substantial numbers of low-income patients. Audiologists are typically employed by these centers to provide a wide array of hearing services, such as hearing assessment, hearing aid selection and evaluation, hearing aid orientation, and aural rehabilitation for both children and adults with hearing loss. Some of the larger community-based hearing and speech centers in the United States are also involved in conducting hearing research and in training future professionals in audiology.

Audiology in the Schools

The passage in 1975 of the Education of All Handicapped Children Act (PL 94-142), a federal law designed to ensure all handicapped children a free and appropriate public school education, resulted in an increased awareness of the need for audiologic services in the schools. In 1990, this act became known as the Individuals with Disabilities Education Act (IDEA). In 1997, President Clinton signed the bill reauthorizing, updating, and expanding IDEA; the bill became known as public law 105-17. Finally, in 2004, President Bush signed a new bill, public law 108-446, now referred to as the Individuals with Disabilities Education Improvement Act (IDEIA, 2004). In essence, IDEIA (2004) has brought unprecedented expansion of services to infants, toddlers, and preschool children with disabilities and their families. IDEIA (2004) retains the major provisions of the other federal laws, including a free and appropriate education to all children with disabilities. Part B of the law provides the rules and regulations for eligible children with disabilities aged 3 through 21. Part C helps states to develop and operate an early-intervention program for infants and toddlers with disabilities. This important bill specifies that local educational systems must provide, at no cost to the child, a wide range of audiologic services. These services included hearing evaluations, auditory training, speech reading, language training, and the selection and fitting of both personal and group amplification units. The fitting and management of cochlear implants are also covered under IDEIA (2004). Needless to say, such a mandate necessitates that audiologic services be offered in the schools. Additional factors, such as the policy of inclusion, have further increased the demand for educational audiology.

Within the context of audiology, inclusion refers to the practice of placing children with hearing loss in regular classrooms instead of in special classrooms containing only children with hearing loss. As more children with hearing loss are integrated into regular classroom settings, the need to provide these children with special audiologic assistance increases.

Another important variable has been the general recognition that many children with hearing loss in the schools are not being adequately served. It has been reported, for example, that fewer than 50% of children with hearing loss in the educational system are receiving adequate services. To be sure, the introduction of IDEIA (2004), along with inclusion and an awareness of the audiologic needs of a larger group of children, has created a market for educational audiology. It is expected that this market will continue to grow as audiology continues to demonstrate how it can contribute significantly to the needs of children with hearing loss in the schools.

The responsibilities of the school audiologist include many shared by most audiologists, such as hearing screening, hearing assessment, selection and evaluation of hearing aids, and direct provision of rehabilitative services. Additional services specific to the educational setting include maintenance of personal and group hearing aids; parent counseling; in-service education to teachers, special educators, and administrators; consulting for educational placement; and serving as a liaison to the community and other professional agencies.

Manufacturers

A growing employment opportunity for audiologists is with the manufacturers of hearing aids and audiologic equipment. In fact, virtually all hearing aid companies today employ audiologists to work in a variety of capacities. Clinical audiologists with good interpersonal communicative skills are always needed to provide expert services to audiologists who dispense a given manufacturer's hearing aid. Usually such support services are related to fitting of the manufacturer's hearing aid, programming and installation of hearing aid fitting software, and general troubleshooting. Other opportunities for clinical audiologists might include positions that focus on administration, sales and educational training, and marketing. Similar positions are available with companies that manufacture audiologic equipment. Research audiologists can play an important role for the hearing aid manufacturer in the strategic planning, implementation, and reporting of research that leads to the development and enhancement of hearing instruments. Research audiologists in industry may also contract other research laboratories to assist the company in the development of data to support a new product or product strategy.

Department of Veterans Affairs Medical Centers and Other State and Federal Agencies

Most Department of Veterans Affairs (VA) medical centers offer audiology and speech-language pathology services. In an effort to provide veterans with all of the patient services that might be needed, the VA has grouped medical centers, outpatient clinics, and community-based clinics into 21 Veterans Integrated Service Networks (VISNs) on the basis of geography, distribution of the veteran population, and availability of specialized services among medical centers in a VISN. A veteran patient may seek audiologic services in any of the approximately 130 VA settings with an audiology program; however, most veterans elect to receive services from the program nearest to where they reside.

The number of VA audiology programs has increased significantly during the past 5 years. The incidence and prevalence of hearing loss in the veteran population are greater than in the general population, probably as a result of noise exposure and the increasing age of the veteran population. Hearing loss is the most common service-related disability in the VA, and 65% of male veterans are over age 62. In addition to providing audiology and speech-language pathology services, the VA, in association with affiliated universities, provides a training program for graduate students enrolled in doctor of philosophy (PhD) and doctor of audiology (AuD) programs. Moreover, the VA conducts a variety of basic and applied research in communication sciences and disorders.

A number of other federal and state agencies also employ audiologists. At the state level, there is typically a department responsible for ensuring the hearing health care needs of young children, usually associated with the department of public health. Departments of public health employ audiologists to perform the full range of audiologic services and to serve as advocates for children with hearing loss and their parents. Similarly, state departments of education and of vocational rehabilitation often employ audiologists to meet the audiologic needs of the populations that their agencies are charged with serving. At the federal level, most opportunities for audiologists are administrative and are not concerned with direct service delivery. Their function is usually to assist the states and regions in implementing or improving programs for hearing-handicapped citizens.

Military-Based Programs

Hearing health care services are available in all branches of the armed forces (army, navy, and air force). As noted earlier, the military services played a key role in the development of audiology as a profession. In fact, immediately after World War II, the army set up and staffed three hospitals, and the navy, one; each of these hospitals was devoted entirely to the rehabilitation and care of military personnel with hearing loss or other disorders of communication acquired in the military service.

Audiologic services are still an important and growing need in the armed forces. In 1975, it was reported that as many as 50% of service personnel assigned to combat arms jobs underwent measurable noise-induced hearing loss after 10 years of military service. Such documentation led to the recognition of great need for military audiologists. In 1967, the army employed only 11 audiologists, whereas in 1985, it employed more than 70. The resulting increased awareness of hearing conservation appears to have been successful. A recent prevalence study of hearing loss among army combat arms personnel revealed that about 20% of these soldiers have measurable noise-induced hearing loss after a 20-year military career.

The most dramatic change over the past several years for the employment of audiologists in the military setting has been the rapid increase in the number of female audiologists. Presently, half of army audiology officers are women. The other branches of the military have similar percentages of female audiology officers.

Another dramatic recent change is the military audiologist's role in operational hearing conservation. Fifteen army audiologists served in Saudi Arabia during the first Gulf war, and six have served in Iraq and Afghanistan during the war on terrorism. That is, audiologists no longer work solely in clinical and research environments; today they are front-line contributors to survival and hearing health care wherever soldiers, sailors, marines, and airmen serve.

Because of the overall reduction of troop strength in the past several years, the number of active-duty officers in the military has been reduced significantly. Nevertheless, many audiologists have attained the prestigious rank of colonel and serve as commanders and administrators of large health care commands. In fact, several of today's prominent audiologists started their career in the military.

The military audiologist provides a full range of services. Typically, emphasis is placed on hearing conservation, screenings and assessments, diagnostic evaluations, hearing aid evaluations, and aural rehabilitation. Military hearing conservation programs include such components as identification of noise hazards, noise measurement analysis and noise reduction, selection and fitting of hearing protection devices, hearing health education, audiometric testing, and audiometric database management.

Finally, the military audiologist has the opportunity to participate in research in hearing conservation, auditory perception and processing, and developing technology to increase soldiers' survivability and enhance their capability.

College and University Settings

A large number of major colleges and universities offer undergraduate and/or graduate training in audiology. Many audiologists with doctoral degrees assume academic positions in the university and become involved in teaching, service, and research. To train a clinical audiologist adequately, the university must offer appropriate clinical training. Accordingly, audiologists, many without doctoral degrees, are employed by the university to service patients with hearing loss from the community and to supervise students in training for a graduate degree in audiology. Audiologists working in this setting have frequent opportunities to participate in research and to train students.

EDUCATIONAL PREPARATION FOR AUDIOLOGY

For several decades, the entry-level degree required for the practice of clinical audiology was the master's degree. In 1993, however, the American Speech-Language-Hearing Association (for historical reasons, generally referred to as the ASHA instead of ASLHA), one of the primary accrediting bodies for training programs in audiology, endorsed the doctorate as the entry-level degree required for the practice of audiology. Accordingly, almost all residential master's degree programs in audiology have now been phased out. Presently, we have two doctoral degrees available, the clinical PhD, which has been in existence for many years, and a new professional doctorate, the AuD. In 1993, the first AuD program was established in the United States. Many others have been developed since then, and as of 2007, there were 71 such programs in the United States, including both traditional residential postbaccalaureate (4-year) programs and shorter distance-learning programs for those who already have a master's degree. The first quarter of this century will be a very significant period of transition in the type of education required to practice audiology, since entry level to the field has now moved from a master's degree to the doctoral degree.

Preparation for a career in audiology should begin at the undergraduate level with basic courses that provide a strong foundation for graduate or professional study. Courses in physics, biology, statistics, mathematics, computer science, anatomy and physiology, psychology, child development, human behavior, and education can provide meaningful preparation for graduate or professional study in audiology.

Students pursuing postbaccalaureate work in audiology come from a variety of backgrounds. In a typical large doctoral program (10–15 students), it is fairly common to find students with diverse undergraduate majors, including speech-language pathology, psychology, education, and special education. Students with undergraduate majors in the basic sciences and the humanities have been encountered less frequently. With the advent of the AuD, however, it is hoped that more students will come with undergraduate degrees in basic or life sciences, much like other preparatory professional health care disciplines (e.g., preparation for medicine, dentistry, and optometry).

What is a doctoral curriculum in audiology like? Table 1.2 details a training program for an audiology student enrolled in a 4-year postbaccalaureate doctoral program. Typically, AuD students complete a minimum of 75 semester credit hours of postbaccalaureate study. In the first year of study, most of the course work focuses on basic science and background information. The practicum during this first year is

TABLE 1.2 Sample Student Program for AuD

Semester	Course 1[a]	Course 2	Course 3	Course 4	Course 5
First Year					
Fall	Acoustics, calibration, & instrumentation	Anatomy & physiology of hearing mechanisms	Hereditary hearing loss	Measurement of hearing	Introduction to CCC[b]
Spring	Auditory clinical electrophysiology	Amplification I	Neuroscience	Psychoacoustics (3 hr)	CCC
Summer	Principles of counseling (2 hr)	Assessment of vestibular disorders (3 hr)	CCC		
Second Year					
Fall	Pediatric audiology	Management of vestibular diseases	Amplification II	Pathology of auditory system	CCC
Spring	Aural rehab for children	Capstone I	Hearing loss & speech understanding	Microbiology & pharmacology for audiology	CCC
Summer	Hearing conservation	Hearing & aging	CCC		
Third Year					
Fall	Clinical research design	Professional issues & ethics (2 hr)	Child language acquisition (2 hr)	Capstone II	CCC
Spring	Cochlear implants	Business & financial management for audiologists (4 hr)	Elective	Auditory prostheses	CCC
Fourth Year					
Externship (fourth-year placement)					

[a]All courses except CCC are 3 hours unless otherwise specified.
[b]CCC, clinical case conference. All CCC courses are 1 hour.
Rehab, rehabilitation.

a mix of observation and limited participation. In the second year, introductory and intermediate applied courses are introduced, and the student becomes much more involved in practicum experience, especially in case management. During the third year, advanced clinical courses are required, and a series of short-term clinical rotations or externships are typically initiated to provide broader clinical experience. In years 2 and 3, the students take Capstone I and II. The capstone is an independent project conducted by the student under the direction of a faculty member. It may involve a traditional research project, a literature review of a particular topic, or even development of a business or marketing plan. Finally, the fourth year is essentially full-time and quasi-independent clinical practice that may take place in residence or via an offsite clinical externship. The purpose of the externship, sometimes referred to as fourth-year placement, is to help the student make the transition from academic to professional life. Hence, it is seen that the program progresses from basic to applied science and that specialization increases during the later stages of the training program. Receiving an advanced degree in audiology is just the first step toward becoming a clinical audiologist certified by the ASHA or the American Academy of Audiology (AAA). For many audiologists, certification by the ASHA is still the desired clinical credential, since such certification is built into state requirements for professional licensure. In the master's-based educational model, once the student received the master's degree, the second step toward certification was to complete an internship known as the clinical fellowship year (CFY). This meant that the student had to spend the first year of salaried practice under the supervision of an experienced and certified audiologist. Doctoral programs have essentially built this internship into the final year, so that an additional CFY will not be required. The third step toward certification by the ASHA or the AAA, which can be completed at any time, is passing a national written examination in audiology.

Some students prefer to continue their study of audiology and obtain a doctoral degree in research, the PhD. This program usually takes 2 to 3 years beyond the AuD, and the student concentrates on theoretical and research aspects of the profession. Common employment opportunities for the PhD include college and university teaching, research, and administration.

PROFESSIONAL LICENSURE AND CERTIFICATION

All professional organizations license their practitioners through minimum standards, rules, and regulations. Such a practice helps to ensure that services are being provided in a manner that meets professional standards for practice. Regulation of audiology began in the 1950s, and all but three states now regulate the AuD. Typically, the professional license is issued by a government agency and grants an individual the right to practice a given profession. Most states model their regulatory rules in audiology after the ASHA standards for the certificate of clinical competence. The ASHA certification program began in 1942 and continues as the primary certification venue for audiologists. In 1999, AAA developed its own certification program, and more and more audiologists are now using AAA for their professional certification.

PROFESSIONAL AFFILIATIONS

Like all professionals, audiologists should maintain affiliations with their professional organizations. The AAA, founded by James Jerger in 1988, is the world's largest professional organization of, by, and for audiologists (Vignette 1.4).

VIGNETTE 1.4   James Jerger (1928–), Founder of the American Academy of Audiology

Dr. James Jerger is widely recognized as the founder and driving force of the AAA. In 1987, at the ASHA convention, 5 well-known audiologists were recruited to discuss the future of audiology. During this session, Jerger noted that it was time for a new professional organization of, by, and for audiologists. Jerger's comments were met with an overwhelmingly enthusiastic response. As a follow-up to the ASHA session, Jerger invited 32 audiology leaders to Houston, Texas, in early 1988. The purpose of the study group was to establish an independent, freestanding national organization for audiologists. The group voted unanimously to develop a new organization for audiologists, to be called the American College of Audiology, and the first national office was established in Baylor College of Medicine. In addition, an ad hoc steering committee was appointed to develop bylaws.

In the few short months to follow, remarkable progress was made. Bylaws for the organization were approved, and the organization was renamed the American Academy of Audiology. The academy was incorporated, an organizational structure was established and officers elected, and dues were established. Committee assignments were made, dates for the first annual meeting were determined, and a major membership drive was launched. In 1989, the first AAA convention was held in Kiawah Island, South Carolina, and the response exceeded all expectations. Close to 600 participants attended the meeting and overflowed the conference facilities. Since 1989 the AAA has undergone significant growth in membership and development. By 1993 the AAA had reached a point in membership size and fiscal responsibilities that it became necessary to move

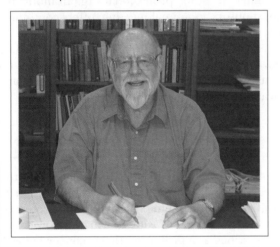

the national office to Washington, D.C., and contract staff to assist in the organization's management. Today, the AAA national office is in Reston, Virginia. Unquestionably, without the far-reaching vision and the extraordinary leadership capabilities of James Jerger, the creation of the AAA would not have been possible. Jerger will always be remembered not only for his extraordinary contributions to the research literature in audiology but also for the role that he played in furthering the cause of the profession of audiology through the development of the AAA.

The academy, with more than 10,000 members, is dedicated to providing quality hearing care of the public. It is also committed to enhancing the ability of its members to achieve career and practice objectives through professional development, education, research, increased awareness of hearing disorders, and audiologic services. The academy typically focuses on issues related to the practice of audiology, such as standards and ethics, publications, training, standardization of methods, professional meetings, and professional scope. As noted earlier, recently the AAA began to offer clinical certification to members interested in and eligible for such certification. This is separate from the clinical certification offered by the ASHA. The AAA also publishes a professional and a scientific journal, public information material, and position statements.

Another important professional organization for the audiologist is the ASHA. Similar to AAA, the ASHA decides on standards of competence for the certification of individuals in the area of audiology (also speech-language pathology). The ASHA also conducts accreditation programs for colleges and universities with degree programs in speech-language pathology and audiology and for agencies that provide clinical services to the public. Among the many services that the ASHA offers its more than 100,000 members, of whom approximately 13,000 are audiologists, is an extensive program of continuing education. This program includes an annual national convention, national and regional conferences, institutes, and workshops. The ASHA also publishes professional and scientific journals, public information material, reports and position statements, monographs, and many other special publications.

Another professional affiliation for the audiologist is the American Auditory Society, an organization encompassing numerous disciplines concerned with hearing and deafness. The membership roster includes practitioners of such professions as audiology, otolaryngology, education of those with hearing loss, pediatric medicine, and psychology, as well as members of the hearing aid industry. The society sponsors an annual convention and publishes a scientific journal.

The Academy of Doctors of Audiology (ADA), previously known as the Academy of Dispensing Audiologists, is an organization of approximately 1000 members designed to meet the professional needs of audiologists in private practice, especially those who directly dispense hearing aids. Most members of the ADA also hold membership in the AAA; in fact, the two organizations occasionally collaborate on a number of activities of mutual interest. Similar to other professional organizations, the ADA publishes a professional journal, sponsors an annual meeting, offers continuing education, and promotes public awareness of hearing loss.

Audiologists may associate with many other professional organizations depending on their areas of interest and specialization. There are professional organizations for the pediatric audiologist, the rehabilitative audiologist, the military audiologist, and the audiologist employed in the educational setting.

SUMMARY

Hearing loss affects a large segment of the population of the United States, and this figure is expected to grow over the next several years. Furthermore, hearing loss in both children and adults can be a significant handicapping condition. The profession of audiology evolved in an attempt to help individuals with hearing loss overcome these handicaps. Audiology has been described as a profession that is concerned with the prevention of hearing loss and the identification, evaluation, and rehabilitation of children and adults with hearing loss. The audiologist has numerous employment opportunities and can work in a variety of employment settings. Audiology is a young, dynamic, and challenging profession that provides a wide range of exciting opportunities for a rewarding career.

References and Suggested Readings

American Academy of Audiology. The professional doctorate. Audiology Today, August 3, 1989.
Bess FH. Prevalence of unilateral and mild hearing loss in school-age children. Workshop Proceedings: National Workshop on Mild and Unilateral Hearing Loss, Centers for Disease Control and Prevention and the Marion Downs Hearing Center, July 25–26, 2005.

Bess FH, Dodd JD, Parker RA. Children with minimal sensorineural hearing loss: Prevalence, educational performance and functional health status. Ear Hear 19:339–354, 1998.

Bess FH, Gravel JS. Foundations of Pediatric Audiology: A Book of Readings. San Diego, CA: Plural, 2006.

Bunch CC. Clinical Audiometry. St Louis: Mosby, 1943.

Hale ST, Bess FH. Professional Organizations. In Lubinski R, Golper LA, Frattali CM, eds. Professional Issues in Speech-Language Pathology and Audiology. 3rd ed. Clifton Park, NY: Thomson Delmar Learning, 2006.

Herbst KRG. Psychosocial consequences of disorders of hearing in the elderly. In Hinchcliffe R, ed. Hearing and Balance in the Elderly. Edinburgh: Churchill Livingstone, 1983.

Humes LE, Diefendorf AO. Chaos or order? Some thoughts on the transition to a professional doctorate in audiology. Am J Audiol 2:7–16, 1993.

Kochkin S, MarkeTrak III: Why 20 million in U.S. don't use hearing aids for their hearing loss. Hearing J 46(1):20–27;46(2):26–31;46(4):36–37, 1993.

Kupper L, ed. The IDEA Amendments of 1997. National Information Center for Children and Youth with Disabilities. News Digest 26, 1997.

Matkin ND. Early recognition and referral of hearing impaired children. Pediatr Rev 6:151–158, 1984.

Lethbridge-Cejku M, Rose D, Vickerie J. Summary Health Statistics for U.S. Adults: National Health Interview Survey, 2004. National Center for Health Statistics. Vital and Health Statistics Series 10(228), 2006.

Niskar AS, Kieszah SM, Holmes A, et al. Prevalence and hearing loss among children 6 to 19 years-of-age. Third National Health and Nutrition Examination Survey. JAMA 279: 1070–1075, 1988.

Northern JL, Downs MP. Hearing in Children. 5th ed. Baltimore: Lippincott Williams & Wilkins, 2001.

Strom KE. Rapid product changes mark the new mature digital market. Hear Rev 13(5):70–74, 2006.

Walden B, Prosek R, Worthington D. The Prevalence of Hearing Loss Within Selected U.S. Army Branches. Interagency No. 1A04745. Washington: Army Medical Research and Development Command, 1975.

West R. The mechanical ear. Volta Rev 38:345–346, 1936.

Web Sites

American Speech-Language-Hearing Association: www.asha.org.

American Academy of Audiology: www.audiology.org.

American Auditory Society: www.amauditorysoc.org.

Academy of Doctors of Audiology: www.audiologist.org.

PL 94–142(1975) www.ed.gov/policy/speced/leg/idea/history.html.

CHAPTER 2

The Nature of Sound

OBJECTIVES

After completion of this chapter, the reader should be able to:

- Describe the nature of a sound wave in terms of a series of events happening to air particles.
- Describe acoustic signals in terms of their amplitude, frequency, and phase.
- Understand the dual representation of acoustic signals in the time domain (waveform) and frequency domain (spectrum).
- Define the measure of sound level known as the decibel.

In this chapter, we explore some of the fundamentals of acoustics that are essential to the understanding of audiology. The chapter begins with a discussion of selected characteristics of sound waves, which is followed by a section on the representation of sound in the time domain (its waveform) and the frequency domain (its spectrum); it concludes with a brief description of the measurement of sound.

SOUND WAVES AND THEIR CHARACTERISTICS

The air we breathe is composed of millions of tiny particles. The presence of these particles makes the production of sound possible. This is made clear by the simple yet elegant experiment described in Vignette 2.1.

The aforementioned experiment demonstrates that air particles are needed for the production and transmission of sound in the atmosphere. There are approximately 400 billion air particles in every cubic inch of the atmosphere. The billions of particles

VIGNETTE 2.1   Importance of a medium for generating sound

The equipment shown in the accompanying figure can be used to demonstrate the importance of air particles, or some other medium, to the generation of sound waves. An electric buzzer is placed within the jar. The jar is filled with air. When the buzzer is connected to the battery, one hears a buzzing sound originating within the jar. Next, a vacuum is created within the jar by pumping out the air particles. When the buzzer is again connected to the battery, no sound is heard. One can see the metal components of the buzzer striking one another, yet no sound is heard. Sound waves cannot be produced without an appropriate medium, such as the air particles composing the atmosphere.

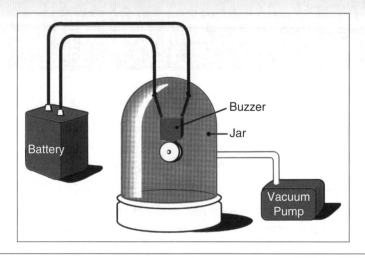

composing the atmosphere are normally moving in a random fashion. These random continual movements of air particles are what is known as Brownian motion. These random movements, however, can be ignored for the most part in our discussion of sound waves. It is sufficient to assume that each particle has an average initial or resting position.

When an object surrounded by air particles vibrates, the air particles adjacent to that object also vibrate. Thus, when a sufficient force is applied to the air particles by the moving object, the air particles will be moved or displaced in the direction of the applied force. Once the applied force is removed, a property of the air medium, known as its elasticity, returns the displaced particle to its resting state. The initial application of force sets up a chain of events in the surrounding air particles. This is depicted in Figure 2.1. The air particles immediately adjacent to the moving object (Fig. 2.1) are displaced in the direction of the applied force. They then collide with more remote air particles once they have been displaced. This collision displaces the more remote particles in the direction of the applied force. The elasticity of the air returns the air particles to their resting position. As the more remote particles are colliding with air particles still farther away from the vibrating object, force is applied to displace the object in the opposite direction. The void left by the former position of the object is filled by the adjacent air particles. This displaces the adjacent particle in the opposite direction. Note that the vibration of air particles passes on from one particle to another through this sequential series of collisions followed by a return to resting position. Thus, the displacement pattern produced by the object travels through the air particles via this chain of collisions.

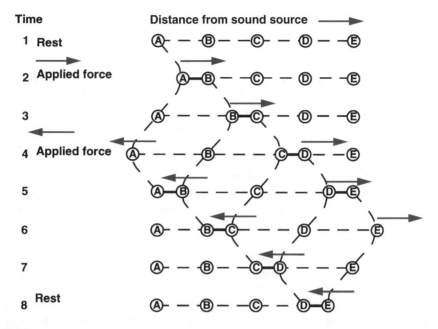

FIGURE 2.1 The movement of air particles (A through E) in response to an applied force at time = 2 and time = 4. The arrows indicate the direction of the applied force and the direction of particle displacement. Each of the particles goes through a simple back-and-forth displacement. The wave propagates through the air, so that back-and-forth vibration of particle A eventually results in a similar back-and-forth vibration of particle E.

Although we could measure this vibration in particles that are a considerable distance from the source of vibration, such as the particle labeled E in Figure 2.1, each particle in the chain of collisions has moved only a very small distance and then returned to its initial position. The air particles thus form the medium through which the vibration is carried. If the air particles adjacent to the vibrating object could actually be labeled, as is done in Figure 2.1, it would be apparent that the vibration of air particles measured away from the vibrating object at point E would not involve the particles next to the object, labeled A. Rather, the particle labeled A remains adjacent to the object at all times and simply transmits or carries the displacement from resting position to the next air particle (B). In turn, B collides with C, C with D, D with E, and so on. A sound wave, therefore, is the movement or propagation of a disturbance (the vibration) through a medium, such as air, without permanent displacement of the particles.

Propagation of a disturbance through a medium can be demonstrated easily with the help of some friends. Six to eight persons should stand in a line, with the last person facing a wall and the others lined up behind that person. Each individual should be separated by slightly less than arm's length. Each person represents an air particle in the medium. Each individual should now place both hands firmly on the shoulders of the person immediately in front of him or her. This represents the coupling of one particle to another in the medium. Another individual should now apply some force to the medium by pushing forward on the shoulders of the first person in the chain. Note that the force applied at one end of the human chain produces a disturbance or wave that travels through the chain from one person to the next until the last person is pushed forward against the wall. The people in the chain remained in place, but the disturbance was propagated from one end of the medium to the other.

Vibration consists of movement or displacement in more than one direction. Perhaps the most fundamental form of vibration is simple harmonic motion. Simple harmonic motion is illustrated by the pendulum in Figure 2.2. The pendulum swings back and forth with the maximum displacement of A. The direction of displacement is indicated by the sign (+ or −) preceding the magnitude of displacement. Thus, +A represents the maximum displacement of the pendulum to the left, 0 represents the resting position, and −A represents the maximum displacement to the right. An object that vibrates in this manner in air will establish a similar back-and-forth vibration pattern in the adjacent air particles; the surrounding air particles will also undergo simple harmonic motion.

The five illustrations of the pendulum on the left side of Figure 2.2 show the position or the displacement of the pendulum at five different instants in time ($t = 0, 1, 2, 3,$ and 4). The plot in the right-hand portion of Figure 2.2 depicts the displacement as a function of time (t). Notice, for example, that at $t = 0$ the pendulum is displaced maximally to the left, resulting in a data point (*) at +A for $t = 0$ on the graph in the right-hand portion of the figure. Similarly, at the next instant in time, $t = 1$, the pendulum returns to the resting position, or 0 displacement. This point is also plotted as an asterisk in the right-hand portion of Figure 2.2. The *solid line* connects the displacement values produced at each moment in time. If y represents the displacement, this *solid line* can be represented mathematically by the following equation: $y(t) = A \sin (2\pi f t + \varphi)$. The details regarding this equation are not of concern here. The term t in this equation refers to various instants in time. Displacement and time are related to one another in this equation via the sine function. As a result, simple harmonic motion is often also referred to as sinusoidal motion.

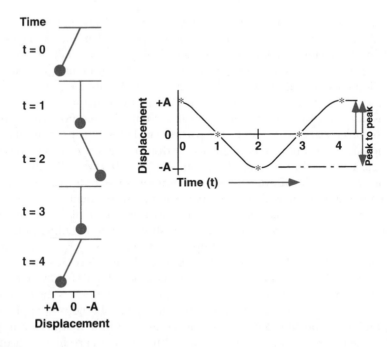

FIGURE 2.2   (Left) Illustration of the movement of a pendulum at five instants in time, $t = 0$ through $t = 4$. (Right) The simple back-and-forth vibration of the pendulum results in a sinusoidal waveform when displacement is plotted as a function of time.

Another common physical system that is used to represent simple harmonic, or sinusoidal, motion is a simple mass attached to an elastic spring. Such a system can be oriented horizontally or vertically. An example of a horizontal mass-spring system is shown in Figure 2.3. The top panel shows the mass-spring system at rest. Next, at $t = 0$, force is applied to displace the mass to the right and to stretch the spring. When

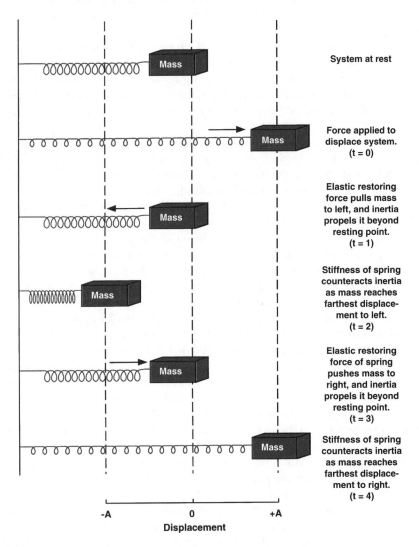

A cube (mass) attached to a spring, which is attached to a wall at its other end. The mass is sliding back and forth across a surface (such as tabletop)

FIGURE 2.3 A simple mass-spring system in horizontal orientation illustrates various stages of simple harmonic motion. The horizontal movement of the mass is depicted at five instants in time, $t = 0$ through $t = 4$. Notice that the simple back-and-forth vibration of this mass-spring system would result in a sinusoidal waveform of displacement as a function of time, just like the pendulum in Figure 2.2.

this applied force is removed, the elasticity of the spring pulls the mass toward the original resting position ($t = 1$). The inertial force associated with the moving mass, however, propels the mass beyond the resting position until it is displaced to the left of the original resting position ($t = 2$). This results in a compression of the spring. When the elastic restoring force of the spring exceeds the inertial force associated with the moving object, the motion of the object halts and then begins in the opposite direction ($t = 3$). As the moving mass reaches the original resting position, inertial forces again propel it past the resting position until it has once again been fully displaced to the right ($t = 4$). The displacement of the mass and the stretching of the spring at $t = 4$ is identical to that seen at $t = 0$. One complete cycle of back-and-forth displacement has been completed. The sinusoidal equation used previously to describe the back-and-forth motion of the pendulum can also be applied to this simple mass-spring system.

The mass-spring system, however, is often easier to relate to air particles in a medium than a pendulum system. For instance, one can think of the mass in Figure 2.3 as an air particle, with the spring representing the particle's connection to adjacent air particles. In this sense, the movement of air particles described in Figure 2.1 can be thought of as a series of simple mass-spring systems like the one shown in Figure 2.3.

All vibration, including sinusoidal vibration, can be described in terms of its amplitude (A), frequency (f), and phase (φ). This is true for both the pendulum and the mass-spring system. The primary ways of expressing the amplitude or magnitude of displacement are as follows: (*a*) peak amplitude, (*b*) peak-to-peak amplitude, and (*c*) root-mean-square (RMS) amplitude. RMS amplitude is an indicator of the average amplitude; it facilitates comparisons of the amplitudes of different types of sound waves. The peak and peak-to-peak amplitudes are shown in the right-hand portion of Figure 2.2. Peak amplitude is the magnitude of the displacement from the resting state to the maximum amplitude. Peak-to-peak amplitude is the difference between the maximum displacement in one direction and the maximum displacement in the other direction.

The period of the vibration is the time it takes for the pendulum to move from any given point and return to the same point. This describes one complete cycle of the pendulum's movement. In Figure 2.2, for example, at $t = 4$ the pendulum has returned to the same position it occupied at $t = 0$. The period in this case is the difference in time between $t = 0$ and $t = 4$. For the mass-spring system in Figure 2.3, the time taken to progress from the system's state at $t = 0$ and to return to that state at $t = 4$ is the period or time required for one full cycle of displacement. If each interval in Figure 2.2 represented one-tenth of a second (0.1 s), the period would be 0.4 s. Hence, the period may be defined as the time it takes to complete one cycle of the vibration (seconds per cycle).

The frequency of vibration is the number of cycles of vibration completed in 1 s and is measured in cycles per second. Examination of the dimensions of period (seconds per cycle) and frequency (cycles per second) reflects a reciprocal relationship between these two characteristics of sinusoidal vibrations. This relationship can be expressed mathematically as follows: $T = 1/f$, or $f = 1/T$, where T = period and f = frequency. Although the dimensions for frequency are cycles per second, a unit of measure defined as 1 cycle per second has been given the name *Hertz*, abbreviated *Hz*. Thus, a sinusoidal vibration that completed one full cycle of vibration in 0.04 s (i.e., $T = 0.04$ s) would have a frequency of 25 Hz ($f = 1/T = 1$ cycle/0.04 s).

Finally, the phase (φ) of the vibration can be used to describe the starting position of the pendulum or mass (starting phase) or the phase relationship between two

vibrating pendulums or masses. Two sinusoidal vibrations could be identical in amplitude and frequency but differ in phase, if one vibration started with the pendulum or
mass in the extreme positive position (to the left) while the other began at the
extreme negative displacement (to the right). In this case, the two pendulums or
masses would be moving in opposite directions. This is called a 180° phase relationship. The two pendulums or masses could have the same amplitude of vibration
(back-and-forth movement) and move back and forth at the same rate (same frequency) yet still have different patterns of vibration if they failed to have identical
starting phases.

Figure 2.4 contrasts the various features used to describe sinusoidal vibration. In
each panel of Figure 2.4, two separate displacement patterns or waveforms, X and Y,
are displayed. In Figure 2.4A, the two displacement patterns have identical frequencies and starting phases, but the amplitude of vibration is approximately three times
larger for wave X. The peak amplitude of the vibration pattern labeled X is A, whereas
that of pattern Y is $0.3A$. In Figure 2.4B, on the other hand, amplitude and starting
phase are equal, but the frequency of vibration for wave Y is twice as high as that for
wave X. Notice, for example, that at the instant in time labeled T in Figure 2.4B, vibration pattern X has completed one full cycle of vibration, whereas pattern Y has completed two cycles at that same instant. Interestingly, although these two functions start
in phase (both beginning at $t = 0$ with 0 displacement), their phase relationship is
very complex at other instants. At the point labeled Z in Figure 2.4B, for example, the
phase relationship is 180°. Thus, at the moment in time labeled Z, both function
X and function Y are at 0 displacement, but one is moving in a positive direction and
the other in a negative direction. Figure 2.4C illustrates two functions of identical
amplitude and frequency that differ only in their starting phase. To fully describe sinusoidal vibration as a function of time, all three parameters—amplitude, frequency, and
starting phase—must be specified.

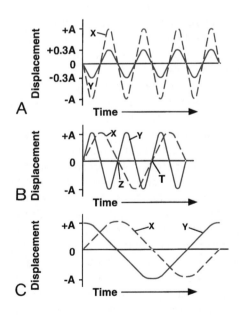

FIGURE 2.4 Sinusoidal waveforms differing only in amplitude (*A*), frequency (*B*), or starting
phase (*C*).

In the initial discussion of the vibration of air particles, a situation was described in which force was applied to an object that resulted in the object itself displacing adjacent air particles. When the force was removed, the object and the air particles returned to their resting positions. This was a case of forced vibration. Before describing the features of forced vibration in more detail, its counterpart, free vibration, deserves brief mention. In free vibration, as in the case of the pendulum or the mass-spring system, once the vibration was started by applying force, the vibration continued without additional force being required to sustain it. For free vibration, the form of the vibration is always sinusoidal, and the frequency of oscillation for a particular object is always the same. This frequency is known as the object's natural or resonant frequency (Vignette 2.2). The amplitude, moreover, can be no larger than the initial

---

VIGNETTE 2.2   Conceptual illustrations of mass, elasticity, and resonance

You will be conducting a small experiment that requires the following materials: a yardstick (or meter stick), four wooden blocks, and heavy-duty rubber bands.

Place two of the wooden blocks so that the ends of the blocks are flush with the end of the yardstick, one block on each side of the yardstick, and secure tightly with rubber bands. Hold or clamp about 6 inches of the other end of the yardstick firmly to the top of a table. Apply a downward force to the far end of the yardstick (the end with wooden blocks) to bend it down approximately 1 foot. (Don't push down too hard, or the blocks may fly off of the yardstick when released.) Now release the far end of the yardstick and count the number of complete up-and-down vibrations of the far end over a 10-second period. Repeat the measurements three times, and record the number of complete cycles of vibration during each 10-second period. This is experiment A.

Now add the other two wooden blocks to the end of the yardstick (two blocks on each side of the yardstick). Repeat the procedure and record the number of complete cycles three times. This is experiment B. If the number of complete cycles of vibration in each experiment is divided by 10 (for the 10-second measurement interval), the frequency (f) will be determined (in cycles per second). How has the system's natural or resonant frequency of vibration changed from experiment A to experiment B? Adding more blocks in experiment B increased the mass of the system. How was the system's natural or resonant frequency changed by increasing the mass of the system?

Now hold 18 inches of yardstick firmly against the table and repeat experiment B (4 wooden blocks). This is experiment C. This increases the stiffness of the system. How has the resonant frequency been affected by increasing the stiffness?

The resonant frequency of an object or a medium, such as an enclosed cavity of air, is determined largely by the mass and stiffness of the object or medium. Generally, stiffness opposes low-frequency vibrations, whereas mass opposes high-frequency vibrations. In the figure for this vignette, the solid lines show the opposition to vibration caused by mass and stiffness. The point at which these two functions cross indicates the resonant frequency of the system. The opposition to vibration caused by either mass or stiffness is lowest at this frequency. The vibration amplitude is greatest at the resonant frequency because the opposition to vibration is at its minimum value. The dashed line shows the effects of increasing the mass of the system. The resonant frequency (the crossover point of the dashed line and the solid line representing the stiffness) has been shifted to a lower frequency. The frequency of vibration in experiment B (more mass) should have been lower than that of experiment A. Similarly, if stiffness is increased, the resonant frequency increases. The frequency in experiment C should have been greater than that in experiment B.

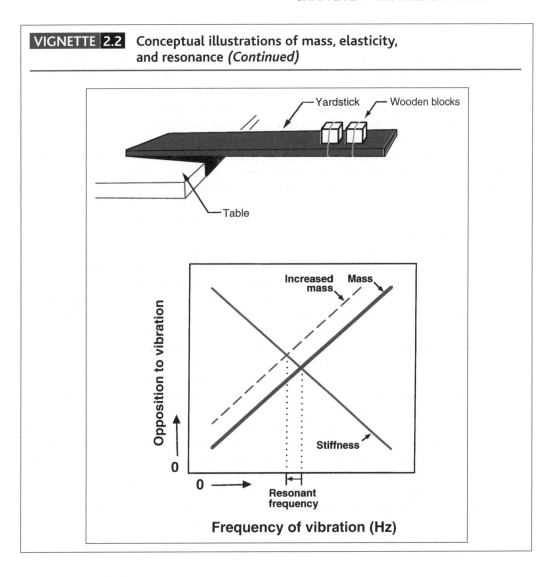

VIGNETTE **2.2** Conceptual illustrations of mass, elasticity, and resonance *(Continued)*

displacement. If there is no resistance to oppose the sinusoidal oscillation, then it will continue indefinitely. In the real world, however, this situation is never achieved. Friction opposes the vibration, which leads it to gradually decay in amplitude over time. To illustrate this, imagine that the mass depicted in the mass-spring system in Figure 2.3 is a smooth wooden cube that is sliding back and forth on a smooth glass surface. If the smooth glass surface is replaced with a sheet of coarse sandpaper, there will be greater friction to oppose the back-and-forth movement of the block. The increased friction associated with the sandpaper surface will result in a quicker decay of the back-and-forth movement of the block in comparison with the original glass surface, which offered much less resistance to the motion of the mass.

If one wanted to sustain the vibration or to force the object to vibrate at other than its resonant frequency, it would be necessary to apply additional force. This is forced vibration. The amplitude of displacement that results when an external or driving force is applied to the object depends, in part, on the amplitude and frequency of the applied force. For an applied force of constant amplitude, the vibration of the object is greatest when the frequency of vibration coincides with the resonant frequency of the object.

An object that vibrates maximally when a force is applied, with the stimulating frequency of the applied force corresponding to the resonant frequency of the object, is said to be at resonance. Perhaps one of the most familiar examples of acoustic resonance is the shattering of a wineglass by the high-pitched voice of a soprano. When the frequency of the applied force (the singer's voice) coincides with the natural frequency of the air-filled cavity formed by the wineglass, the maximal amplitude of vibration exceeds the maximum amplitude tolerable by the glass structure, resulting in its shattering.

Now that some general features of vibration have been reviewed, let us return to the discussion of sound generation and propagation. Consider the following situation. The force applied to an object surrounded by air particles is sinusoidal, resulting in a sinusoidal back-and-forth displacement of the surrounding air particles. The object displaces adjacent air particles in one direction, causing a temporary buildup or increase in density of the air particles. As the object returns to resting position because of its associated elastic restoring forces, the momentum associated with the mass of the object forces it past the resting state to its point of maximum displacement in the opposite direction. The immediately adjacent air particles attempt to fill the void left by the object, resulting in a less dense packing of air particles in this space. In doing so, the air particles surrounding the vibrating object undergo alternating periods of condensation and rarefaction. Therefore, the density of air particles is alternately increased and decreased relative to conditions at rest (no vibration). The increased concentration (density) of air particles results in an increase in air pressure according to a well-known law of physics, the gas law. Thus, as the vibration propagates through the air medium, a volume of atmosphere goes through alternating periods of increased and decreased air particle density and consequently of high and low pressure. Waves of pressure fluctuations are created and travel through the medium.

Although the pressure variations associated with sound are small compared with normal atmospheric pressure, it is these small fluctuations in pressure that are important. The pressure fluctuations can be described using the same features discussed previously to describe changes in displacement over time. A sinusoidal driving force applied to an object vibrates the object and produces sinusoidal variations in pressure. These cyclic fluctuations in pressure can be described in terms of their amplitude, frequency, and phase. Pressure is the parameter most often used to describe sound waves because most measuring devices, such as microphones, respond to changes in sound pressure.

The unit of sound pressure is the *Pascal* (abbreviated Pa). Recall that the term *Hertz*, rather than *cycles per second*, is used to describe the frequency of a sound. The use of the term *Hertz* for frequency and the term *Pascal* for sound pressure reflects the contemporary practice of naming units of measure after notable scientists (Vignette 2.3).

Unfortunately for the student, this practice often obscures the dimensions of the quantity. Pressure, however, is force per unit area and has frequently been described in units of either N/m^2 or d/cm^2 (N = newton, a unit of force named after yet another famous scientist; d = dyne, a unit of force). Vignette 2.4 explains why there are two different types of units for force, dynes versus newtons, as well as the use of various prefixes in the metric system to modify these or other physical units.

Although sound pressure is the preferred measure for depicting the amplitude of a sound wave, another commonly used measure is acoustic intensity. *Acoustic intensity* and *sound power* are used synonymously in this book. It is possible to derive the acoustic intensity corresponding to a given sound pressure. For our purposes, however, it will suffice that acoustic intensity (I) is directly proportional to sound pressure (p) squared, i.e., $I \alpha p^2$.

VIGNETTE 2.3   Units of sound named after famous scientists

The unit of frequency, the Hertz, is named in honor of Heinrich Rudolph Hertz (**A** in the figure), a German physicist born in 1857 in Hamburg. Much of his career was devoted to the theoretical study of electromagnetic waves. This theoretical work led eventually to the development of radio, an area in which frequency is very important. Hertz died in 1894.

The unit of sound pressure, the Pascal, is named in honor of Blaise Pascal (1623–1662) (**B** in the figure). Pascal was a French scientist and philosopher. He is well known for his contributions to both fields. As a scientist, he was both a physicist and a mathematician. In 1648, Pascal proved empirically that the mercury column in a barometer is affected by atmospheric pressure and not a vacuum, as was previously believed. Thus, his name is linked in history with research concerning the measurement of atmospheric pressure.

The Newton, the unit of force, is named in honor of the well-known English mathematician, physicist, and astronomer Sir Isaac Newton (1642–1727) (**C** in the figure), who spent much of his career studying various aspects of force. Of his many discoveries and theories, perhaps the two best known are his investigations of gravitational forces and his three laws of motion.

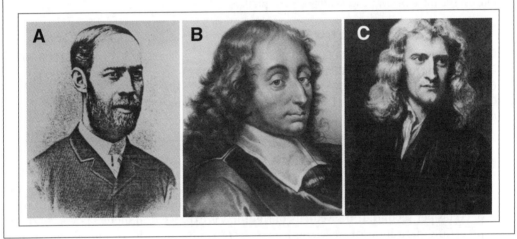

The sound wave propagates through air at a velocity or speed of approximately 330 m/s. This depends somewhat on the characteristics of the medium, including its elasticity, density, and temperature. For example, the speed of sound in air increases with temperature from 330 m/s at 0°C to a value of 343 m/s at 20°C.

Let us suppose that a vibrating object completes one cycle of vibration when the appropriate driving force is applied. As the first condensation of air particles, or local high-pressure area, is created, it travels away from the source. At the completion of one cycle, a new high-pressure area is created. By the time a second high-pressure area is completed, however, the first has traveled still farther from its point of origin. The distance between these two successive condensations, or high-pressure areas, is called the wavelength of the sound wave. If the frequency of vibration is high, the separation between successive high-pressure areas is small. Recall that a high frequency implies a short period ($f = 1/T$); that is, the time it takes to complete one cycle is short for high frequencies. Consequently, the first high-pressure area is unable to travel far from the source before the second high-pressure area arises. Thus, the wavelength (λ), the separation in distance between successive high-pressure areas, is small. The wavelength (λ), frequency (f), and speed of sound (c) are related in the following manner:

VIGNETTE **2.4**   **Review of units of measure and metric prefixes**

As mentioned in the text, one may encounter a variety of physical units for various physical quantities. For sound pressure, for example, units of Newtons per square meter or dynes per square centimeter may both be found in various sources. Although both units of pressure in this example are metric, one expresses area in meters and the other expresses area in centimeters. There are two basic measurement systems encountered in physics, the MKS system and the CGS system. The names for these two systems are derived from the units of measure within each system for the three primary physical quantities of length (meters in the MKS system and centimeters in the CGS system), mass (kilograms in the MKS system and grams in the CGS system), and time (seconds in both systems). The MKS system has been adopted as the standard international system for units of measure, so Newtons per square meter is the preferred physical description of sound pressure. As noted previously, however, these physically meaningful units of force per unit area have been supplanted by Pascals.

In the metric system, the use of standard prefixes is commonplace. It is important for a variety of auditory processes and measures to have a good grasp of many typically used prefixes. The table below provides many such prefixes.

Prefixes for Fractions of a Unit			Prefixes for Multiple Units		
10^{-9}	nano (n)	0.000000001	10^9	giga (G)	1,000,000,000
10^{-6}	micro (μ)	0.000001	10^6	mega (M)	1,000,000
10^{-3}	milli (m)	0.001	10^3	kilo (k)	1000
10^{-2}	centi (c)	0.01	10^2	hecto (h)	100
10^{-1}	deci (d)	0.1	10^1	deka (da)	10

$\lambda = c/f$. Wavelength varies inversely with frequency; the higher the frequency, the shorter the wavelength. Recall that the physical definition of frequency, f, was in units of cycles per second. If the velocity of sound, c, is expressed in meters per second, the preceding definition of wavelength ($\lambda = c/f$) results in units of meters per second being divided by units of cycles per second, which results in units of meters per cycle for wavelength. Keeping track of the units of measure for derived physical quantities, such as wavelength in this example, often helps to reinforce the definition of the quantity or measure. In this case, meters per cycle is precisely the definition of wavelength, that is, the *distance* required for one complete *cycle* of vibration.

To clarify the concept of wavelength and its inverse relationship to frequency, consider once again the human chain that represented adjacent air particles. Suppose it took 10 s for the disturbance (the push) to travel from the shoulders of the first person all the way to the end of the human chain. Let us also say that the chain had a length of 10 m. If a force was applied to the shoulders of the first person every 10 s, the frequency of vibration would be 0.1 Hz ($f = 1/T = 1/10$ s). Moreover, 10 s after the first push, the second push would be applied. Because we have stated that 10 s would be required for the disturbance to travel to the last person in the chain, when the second push is applied, the last person in the chain (10 m away) would also be pushing forward on the wall. Thus, there would be a separation of 10 m between adjacent peaks of the disturbance or forward pushes. The wavelength (λ) would be 10 m. If we double the frequency of the applied force to a value of 0.2 Hz, then the period is 5 s ($T = 1/f = 1/0.2 = 5$ s). Every 5 s, a new force will be applied to the shoulders of the first person in the chain. Because it takes 10 s for the disturbance to travel through the entire 10-m chain, after 5 s, the first disturbance will only be 5 m away as the second push is applied to the shoulders of the first person. Thus, the wavelength, or the separation between adjacent pushes in the medium, is 5 m. When the frequency of the applied force was doubled from 0.1 to 0.2 Hz, the wavelength was halved from 10 m to 5 m. Frequency and wavelength are inversely related.

Another feature of sound waves that is obvious to almost anyone with normal hearing is that the sound pressure decreases in amplitude as the distance it travels increases. It would be fruitless, for example, to attempt to yell for a taxicab a half block away with a soft whisper even on a quiet street. Because the amplitude of sound decays with increasing distance, it would probably require high vocal effort to generate enough sound amplitude at the source to be audible to the cab driver a half block away. One would have to yell "Taxi!" rather than whisper it.

Under special measurement conditions, in which sound waves are not reflected from surrounding surfaces and the sound source is a special source, known as a point source, the decrease in sound pressure with distance is well defined. Specifically, as the distance from the sound source is doubled, the sound pressure is halved. Similarly, because of the relationship between sound pressure and acoustic intensity described previously ($I \alpha p^2$), the same doubling of distance would reduce the acoustic intensity to one-fourth [or $(1/2)^2$] the initial value. This well-defined dependence of sound pressure and sound intensity on distance is known as the inverse square law.

So far, we have considered some of the characteristics or features of a single sound wave originating from one source. Moreover, we have assumed that the sound wave was propagating through a special environment in which the wave is not reflected from surrounding surfaces. This type of environment, one without reflected sound waves, is known as a free field. A diffuse field is the complement of a free field. In a diffuse field, sound is reflected from many surfaces. The inverse square law holds only for free-field conditions. In fact, in a diffuse field, sound pressure is distributed equally throughout the measurement area, so that at any distance from the sound source or anywhere in the measurement area, the sound pressure is the same. The term *sound field* is sometimes used to describe a region containing sound waves. Free fields and diffuse fields, then, are special classes of sound fields.

Interference results when multiple sound waves encounter one another. Here, we will consider only the simplest case of interaction: *two* sound waves. The two sound waves may be two independent waves arising from separate sources (e.g., two loudspeakers or two people talking) or the original wave (usually called the incident sound wave) and its reflection off a wall, ceiling, floor, or other surface. The interference that results when two sound waves encounter one another may be either constructive or destructive. In constructive interference, the two sound waves combine to yield a sound wave that is greater in amplitude than either wave alone. This is illustrated in the left-hand portion of Figure 2.5. In the case shown here, in which the waves are of equal amplitude, the maximum possible constructive interference would be a doubling of amplitude. Negative interference occurs whenever the amplitude of the sound wave resulting from the interaction is less than the amplitude of either wave alone. The extreme case of negative interference results in the complete cancellation of the sound waves, as illustrated in the right-hand portion of Figure 2.5.

In addition to the interference that results when two sound waves interact, other interference effects result when a sound wave encounters an object or structure of some kind. When a sound wave encounters an object, the outcome of this encounter is determined in large part by the dimensions and composition of the object and the

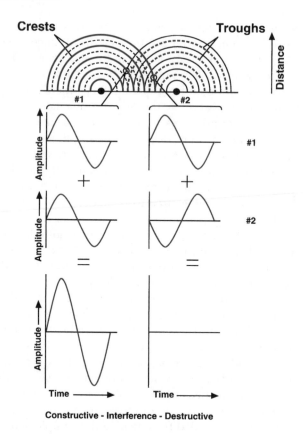

FIGURE 2.5 Constructive and destructive interference of two sound waves (#1 and #2). The origin of each wave is represented by the black circles in the upper portion of the figure. The graph at the lower left illustrates the combination of waves #1 and #2 when the crests coincide. The two waves are in phase at this point, and the resulting sound wave is greater than either wave alone. This is constructive interference. The graph at the lower right illustrates the combination of the crest of wave #1 and the trough of wave #2. The two waves are 180° out of phase, resulting in complete cancellation of the two waves. This is destructive interference. (Adapted from Durrant JD, Lovrinic JH. Bases of Hearing Science. 2nd ed. Baltimore: Williams & Wilkins, 1984:41.)

wavelength of the sound. When the dimensions of the object are large relative to the wavelength of the sound wave, a sound shadow is produced. This is analogous to the more familiar light shadow, in which an object in the path of light casts a shadow behind it. In the case of a sound shadow, the object creates an area without sound, or a dead area, immediately behind it; but not all objects cast sound shadows for all sound waves. The creation of a sound shadow depends on the dimensions of the object and the wavelength of the sound. For example, a cube having the dimensions 1 m × 1 m × 1 m will not cast a shadow for sound waves having a wavelength that is much larger than 1 m. Recall that wavelength and frequency vary inversely. In this example, a sound wave having a wavelength of 1 m has a frequency of 330 Hz ($f = c/\lambda$; $c = 330$ m/s; $\lambda = 1$ m/cycle). Thus, the object in this example would cast a sound shadow for frequencies greater than 330 Hz ($\lambda < 1$ m) (Vignette 2.5).

Finally, consider what happens when a sound wave encounters a barrier of some type. First, let us discuss the case in which a hole is present in the barrier. In this case, as was the case for the sound shadow, the results depend on the wavelength (and therefore frequency) of the incident sound wave and the dimensions of the hole. For wavelengths much greater than the dimensions of the hole, the sound wave becomes

---

VIGNETTE 2.5   Sound shadow created by the head

Sound shadow occurs whenever the dimensions of the object encountered by the sound wave are larger than the wavelength of the sound. Wavelength is inversely related to frequency, such that low frequencies have long wavelengths and high frequencies have short wavelengths. Consider the three frequencies 100, 1000, and 10,000 Hz. The corresponding wavelengths, calculated as described in the text, are 3.3, 0.33, and 0.033 m, respectively.

The human head can be grossly approximated by a sphere (or a cube for blockheads) with a diameter of approximately 0.23 m (roughly 9 inches). Therefore, when the head (preferably accompanied by the body) is placed in a sound field, it is capable of producing a sound shadow for wavelengths shorter than 0.23 m. Using the three frequencies from the preceding paragraph, the average human head would create a sound shadow for 10,000 Hz, would possibly produce one at 1000 Hz, and definitely would not produce one at 100 Hz, where the wavelength is several times greater than the diameter of the head.

The figure for this vignette illustrates how this so-called head shadow effect can be measured. In panel A, two microphones spaced approximately 9 inches apart are positioned in a free field (a sound field without any reflections) with a loudspeaker to the right of the microphones at a distance of a few meters. The loudspeaker presents a pure tone of 100 Hz, and its sound level is measured at both microphones. This is repeated for pure tones of 1000 and 10,000 Hz. All three pure tones are presented at equal levels. Because the left microphone is farther from the sound source than the right microphone, the sound level is a little lower at the left microphone, consistent with the inverse-square law described in the text. The difference for these closely spaced microphones is small enough, however, that we can ignore it here and pretend that the sound levels are identical at both the left and right microphones.

Part B of this figure shows a head with a diameter of approximately 9 inches (0.23 m) between the two microphones. When we repeat the measurements at 100, 1000, and 10,000 Hz, there is little change in sound level from panel A for 100 Hz and only a slight decrease in level at the left microphone for 1000 Hz. At 10,000 Hz, however, the sound pressure has been reduced at the left microphone to a value that is only one-tenth of what it was in panel A. In terms of sound level in decibels (described later in the text of this chapter), the sound level has been decreased at the left microphone by approximately 20 dB with the head present for the 10,000 Hz signal. The head is blocking the 10,000-Hz sound wave from reaching the left microphone. The 10,000-Hz sound would be perceived as being much louder at the ear nearest to the loudspeaker and softer at the ear farthest from the sound source.

This difference in sound level at the two ears that results from head shadow is a very strong cue for the location of a sound in the horizontal plane. The sound is generally assumed to come from the side that has the higher sound level. Given the dimensions of the human head and the wavelength of sound in air for various frequencies, the sound level difference between the two ears helps locate sounds with frequencies above 1000 Hz. Below 1000 Hz, the size of the head does not create a sound shadow, or difference in sound level, at the two ears. Cues other than the sound-level difference between the two ears are needed to locate low-frequency sounds (discussed in Chapter 3).

(continued)

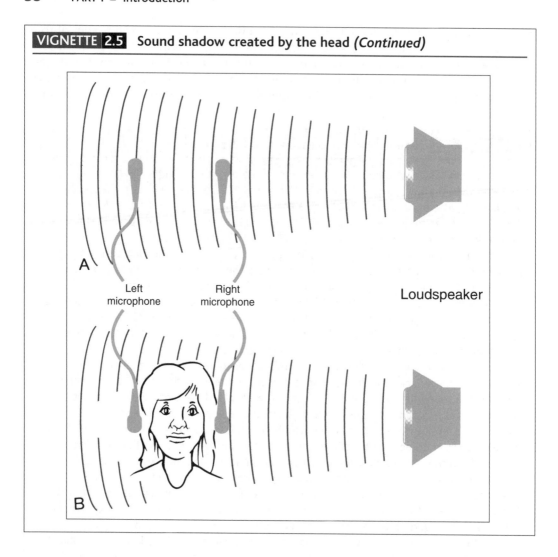

VIGNETTE 2.5 Sound shadow created by the head *(Continued)*

A

Left
microphone

Right
microphone

Loudspeaker

B

diffracted. Diffraction is a change in direction of the sound wave. Thus, under these conditions, the direction of the incident sound wave can be altered.

Next, consider what happens if the sound wave encounters a barrier that contains no holes. In this case, varying degrees of sound transmission, absorption, or reflection can occur. The proportion of the sound wave's energy reflected by the barrier and the proportion transmitted through the barrier depend on the similarity of the barrier's and the medium's impedance. Impedance may be thought of very generally as opposition to the flow of energy, in this case the advancement of the sound wave through the barrier. If the barrier and the medium have the same impedance, 100% of the energy of the sound wave will be transmitted through the barrier. If the difference in impedances, often referred to as the impedance mismatch, is large, most of the incident sound wave will be reflected and little will be transmitted across the barrier (Vignette 2.6).

Aside from being reflected or transmitted, a portion of the sound wave may also be absorbed by the barrier. In the absorption of sound energy, the acoustic energy of the impinging sound wave is changed to heat. The materials out of which the barrier is constructed determine its ability to absorb sound.

VIGNETTE 2.6 Discussion of impedance mismatch between air and water

Consider the following situation. You and a friend are out on a boat in the ocean, scuba diving. Your friend is already underwater, and you want to talk to him. He's only a few feet below the surface, yet despite your yelling, he does not respond. Why not? The sound waves carrying your voice are traveling through an air medium. When the sound waves encounter the surface of the water, a change in impedance is encountered. The impedance of ocean water is a few thousand times greater than that of air. As a consequence, only approximately 0.1% of the sound energy will be transmitted beneath the surface of the water to your friend.

Approximately 99.9% of the airborne sound wave is reflected off the surface. Thus, the impedance mismatch between the air and ocean water results in almost all of the airborne sound energy being reflected away from the surface.

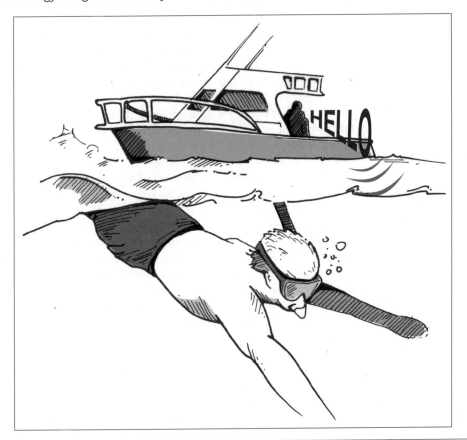

More on the Concepts of Impedance, Admittance, and Resonance

In our discussion of the vibration and displacement of objects—whether the object was a pendulum, a mass-spring system, or an air particle—mass, elasticity, and resistance (friction) have been identified repeatedly as critical factors affecting the vibration. The mass-spring system described in Figure 2.3 probably best illustrated the interplay between mass, elasticity, and resistance in the back-and-forth sinusoidal vibration of a mass. This was also illustrated in Vignette 2.2, in which a simple vibrating system is constructed from a yardstick and a cup of marbles.

Systems having mass, elasticity, and resistance can be forced to vibrate in response to applied forces of various frequencies. The frequency at which the system vibrates maximally for equal applied force is the resonant frequency of the system. The resonant frequency and the amplitude of vibration at that frequency are both determined by the impedance of the system. Impedance is the net opposition to vibration resulting from the mass, elasticity, and resistance of the system. Admittance is the reciprocal of impedance: it indicates how easily energy is admitted through a system rather than impeded by it.

Inertia is a force of opposition associated with an object having mass and one that opposes acceleration of the object (speeding up or slowing down its movement). Elastic restoring forces are associated with a system's elasticity, and they oppose the displacement of the object. When a spring is stretched, for example, its elastic restoring force opposes that displacement and attempts to restore it to its original (resting) position. Finally, friction is a form of resistance that opposes the velocity or speed at which an object is moving. The faster an object is moving, the greater the opposition to that movement as a result of friction. Frictional forces usually oppose the movement of an object by converting the kinetic energy associated with the moving object to heat. Rubbing the palms of your hands together, for example, will be opposed by frictional forces and will generate heat. The faster you rub them together, the greater the opposition caused by friction and the greater the heat generated. Again, the net sum of the inertial, elastic, and frictional forces of opposition to motion is impedance. The higher the impedance, the greater the opposition to movement or vibration of the object, and the less the object moves or vibrates.

As noted in Vignette 2.2, the opposition to vibration associated with a system's mass increases with increase in frequency, whereas the opposition associated with a system's elasticity or stiffness decreases with increases in frequency. The opposition associated with a system's mass is referred to as mass reactance (Xm), whereas that caused by a system's elasticity is referred to as elastic reactance (Xe). Frictional forces, referred to as resistance (R), do not vary with frequency; they are frequency independent. For a system with mass M, the mass reactance can be calculated from the following equation: $Xm = 2\pi f M$. For a given mass, the forces of opposition associated with that mass increase with increase in frequency, f. In addition, the greater the mass of an object, the greater the opposition to movement or vibration. For a system with elasticity E, the elastic reactance associated with that system can be calculated from this equation: $Xe = 1/(2\pi f E)$. For a given E, the opposition caused by elasticity decreases as frequency (f) increases. In addition, as elasticity increases (and stiffness decreases), the opposition caused by elasticity decreases.

Impedance, the combination of Xm, Xe, and R, is usually symbolized as Z. Impedance is a complex vector quantity, as are Xm, Xe, and R. This simply means that it is a quantity with both magnitude and direction. Wind velocity is an everyday example of a vector quantity, a quantity in which both magnitude and direction are important. For example, a weather report might cite the wind at 25 miles per hour out of the southwest, rather than simply indicating its magnitude only (25 mph). Although impedance and its constituents are vector quantities with both magnitude and direction, we will focus here on the magnitude only. The magnitude of the impedance, Z, is calculated as follows: $Z = [R^2 + (Xm - Xe)^2]^{0.5}$. That is, the size of the impedance, Z, is equal to the square root of the sum of the resistance (R) squared and the net reactance ($Xm - Xe$) squared. Increases in R, Xm, or Xe result in increases in the magnitude or size of the impedance. The greater the impedance or net opposition to vibration, the less the amount of vibration or movement.

There exists some frequency, known as the resonant frequency, for which the impedance is at a minimum. Recall that Xm varies directly with frequency, whereas Xe varies inversely with frequency. As frequency increases upward from 0 Hz, Xm is increasing and Xe is decreasing. (The resistance, R, does not vary with frequency and remains constant.) At some frequency, Xe will equal Xm. At this frequency, the net reactance ($Xm - Xe$) will equal 0. According to the equation for impedance (Z), impedance will then be equal to the square root of R^2. In other words, at the resonant frequency, the opposing forces associated with the system's mass and elasticity cancel each other, and all that remains to oppose the vibration is the resistance. At resonance, $Z = R$. This is the smallest amount of opposition to vibration possible, so the system will vibrate maximally at this frequency. At frequencies other than the resonant frequency, Xm will not cancel Xe, and the impedance will be greater than that at resonance. At resonance, how much and how long the object or system vibrates will be determined solely by R.

The reciprocal of impedance (Z) is admittance (Y). Just as impedance represented the net sum of resistance and reactance (X), admittance represents the net sum of conductance (G) and susceptance (B). Just as with reactance, a susceptance term is associated with the system's mass (Bm) and another associated with the system's elasticity (Be). Similarly, the formula for the calculation of admittance is as follows: $Y = [G^2 + (Bm - Be)^2]^{0.5}$. In general, as impedance increases, admittance decreases and vice versa. So at the resonant frequency, Z is minimum and Y is maximum. Admittance and impedance are alternative but equivalent ways of describing the flow of energy through a system. Impedance summarizes the overall opposition to vibration, whereas admittance reflects the ease with which the system is set into vibration. It's akin to having the option to describe a 12-oz glass filled with 6 oz of water as being either half full or half empty. Either description is accurate.

Although admittance-based and impedance-based descriptions of a system are equally appropriate, clinical measurement of the impedance or admittance of the middle ear system (see Chapter 4) has evolved from an initial favoring of impedance terminology to more recent consensus for admittance measures and terminology. The choice is not because one is more accurate or better than the other; it has to do with the ease with which one can be measured validly with the equipment available in the clinic.

Finally, the impedance and admittance concepts described here are for mechanical systems, although these concepts have been applied to numerous types of systems, including electrical and purely acoustical systems. Although the details change from one type of system to another, the concepts remain the same. Table 2.1 illustrates some of the parallels among mechanical, acoustical, and electrical impedance.

TABLE 2.1 Terms for Equivalent Components of Impedance (Z) for Mechanical, Electrical, and Acoustical Systems

Mechanical	Electrical	Acoustical
Mass reactance (Xm)	Inductive reactance (Xi)	Inertance (Xm)
Elastic reactance (Xe)	Capacitive reactance (Xc)	Elastic reactance (Xe)
Resistance (R)	Resistance (R)	Resistance (R)
Impedance (Zm)	Impedance (Ze)	Impedance (Za)
$Zm = [R^2 + (Xm - Xe)^2]^{0.5}$	$Ze = [R^2 + (Xi - Xc)^2]^{0.5}$	$Za = [R^2 + (Xm - Xe)^2]^{0.5}$

WAVEFORMS AND THEIR ASSOCIATED SPECTRA

Many of the important features of a sound wave, such as its amplitude, period, and frequency, can be summarized in either of two common formats. One format, the waveform, describes the acoustic signal in terms of amplitude variations as a function of time. The sinusoidal waveform described previously for simple harmonic motion is an example of a waveform or time domain representation of an acoustic signal. For every waveform, there is an associated representation of that signal in the frequency domain, called the amplitude and phase spectrum. Figure 2.6A illustrates the amplitude and phase spectrum for a simple sinusoidal waveform. the x-axis of the spectrum is frequency, whereas the y-axis is either amplitude or phase. The amplitude scale can be peak-to-peak amplitude, peak amplitude, or RMS amplitude, as described previously. The phase spectrum in this case illustrates the starting phase of the acoustic signal. Only one waveform can be associated with the amplitude and phase spectra shown in the right-hand side of Figure 2.6A. Similarly, only one set of amplitude and phase spectra is associated with the waveform in the left-hand side of Figure 2.6A. Thus, both the time domain and frequency domain representations of the acoustic stimulus uniquely summarize its features. Furthermore, knowing one, we can derive the other. Each waveform is associated with only one amplitude spectrum and phase spectrum. For every amplitude and phase spectrum there is only one possible waveform. The time domain (waveform) and frequency domain (spectrum) are simply two

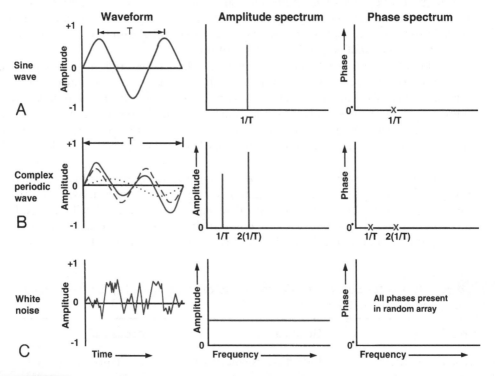

FIGURE 2.6 Waveforms and corresponding amplitude and phase spectra for a continuous sine wave **(A)**, a complex periodic wave **(B)** (solid line is complex waveform, dashed and dotted lines are the two sine waves making up the complex sound), and white noise **(C)**. All waveforms are assumed to be continuous, with only a brief snapshot of the waveform depicted here.

ways of looking at the same sound; one emphasizes moment-to-moment variations in amplitude, and the other emphasizes the frequency content of the sound. Vignette 2.7 reinforces this point.

Simple sinusoidal sounds are more the exception than the rule in everyday encounters with sound. In the 1820s, however, the mathematician Fourier determined that all complex periodic waveforms could be represented by a series of simple sinusoids. A periodic sound is one in which the waveform repeats itself every T seconds. In the left-hand portion of Figure 2.6*B*, a complex periodic waveform is illustrated by the *solid line*. The *dashed* and *dotted* waveforms illustrate the two sinusoidal signals that

---

VIGNETTE 2.7 Time domain and frequency domain representations of sound: an analogy using maps

Sound can be represented completely and equivalently in two different fashions: the time domain, or waveform, and the frequency domain, or spectrum. It is important to realize that these displays of sound just offer two different pictures of the same sound. By analogy, consider the piece of the Earth known as the state of Indiana in the United States.

As shown in this figure, there are many ways to display the features of this piece of property. The map on the left is a road map for Indiana. The map in the middle depicts the average annual rainfall in the state, and the one on the right illustrates the relative elevation of various portions of the land within the state. Each map serves a specific purpose and function, but all three represent information about the same piece of the Earth, Indiana. If the reader wanted to know the best route to take from Indianapolis, Indiana, to Fort Wayne, Indiana, for example, the road map would be the map of choice. The road map, however, conveys no information about annual rainfall or topography. If this information is of interest to the reader, the other maps would need to be consulted. This is similar to the choices available for the analysis and display of sound. If the moment-to-moment variations in the amplitude of a sound are of interest, the waveform is the most appropriate representation. Likewise, if the frequency content of the sound is of interest, the amplitude and phase spectra are the appropriate displays. In either case, the sound is the same, but the picture of that sound can be displayed in either the time domain or frequency domain.

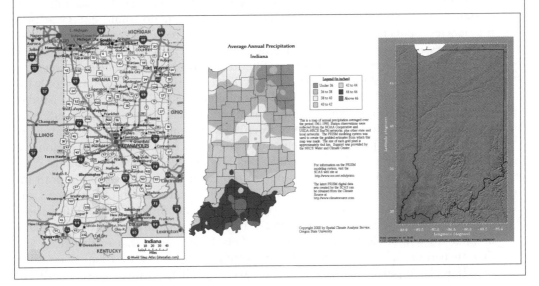

combine to yield the complex sound. The spectrum of the complex sound can be represented by the sum of the spectra of both sinusoidal components, as illustrated in the right-hand portion of Figure 2.6B. Complex periodic sounds, such as that shown in Figure 2.6B, have a special type of amplitude spectrum known as line spectra. The amplitude spectrum consists of a series of discrete lines located at various frequencies and having specified amplitudes. Each line represents a separate sinusoidal component of the complex sound. The component having the lowest frequency is called the fundamental frequency. The fundamental frequency corresponds to $1/T$, where T is the period of the complex sound. Additional components at frequencies corresponding to integer multiples of the fundamental frequency are referred to as harmonics of the fundamental. If the fundamental frequency is 200 Hz, for example, the second and third harmonics of 200 Hz are 400 Hz (2×200 Hz) and 600 Hz (3×200 Hz), respectively. The first harmonic corresponds to the fundamental frequency. Additionally, the *octave* is a range in which the frequency doubles. Continuing the same example, 400 Hz would be one octave above the fundamental frequency (200 Hz), and 800 Hz would be two octaves (another doubling) above the fundamental frequency.

Many acoustic signals in our environment are not periodic. Noise is probably the most common example. Noise is said to be an aperiodic signal, because it fails to repeat itself at regular intervals. Rather, the waveform for noise shows amplitude varying randomly over time. This is illustrated in the left-hand portion of Figure 2.6C. The case shown here is an example of a special type of noise called white noise. White noise is characterized by an average amplitude spectrum that has uniform amplitude across frequency; in other words, there is equal sound energy at all frequencies. (The term *white noise* derives its name from white light—light that is composed of all wavelengths of light at equal amplitudes.) This is depicted in the right-hand portion of Figure 2.6C. The amplitude spectrum no longer consists of a series of lines. Rather, a continuous function is drawn that reflects equal amplitude at all frequencies. Aperiodic waveforms, such as noise, have continuous amplitude spectra, not discrete line spectra.

A variety of noises can be obtained from white noise using devices known as filters. Filters are typically electronic devices that selectively pass energy in some frequency regions and block the passage of energy at other frequencies. If we begin with white noise, an acoustic signal having energy at all frequencies, and send that noise through low-pass filter, which passes only the low frequencies, the result is a low-pass noise that contains equal amplitude at low frequencies and little or no sound energy at high frequencies. Similarly, other noises, such as high-pass noise (sound energy at high frequencies only), can be generated. If a noise is sent through both a low-pass filter and a high-pass filter, the result is a band-pass filter that only passes frequencies between the two filters. For example, if a noise is low-pass filtered at 1000 Hz, so as to pass only frequencies lower than 1000 Hz, then high-pass filtered at 500 Hz, the result is a band of noise from 500 to 1000 Hz with no energy at other frequencies (assuming the edges, or rejection rates, of the filters are very steep). Filters can be applied to a variety of acoustic signals, not just noise, to eliminate energy in certain frequency regions, to shape the spectra of sounds, or to analyze the frequency composition of sounds.

As previously indicated, it is possible to represent an acoustic signal in both the frequency domain and the time domain. So far in our discussion of waveforms and spectra, we have assumed that the acoustic signals are continuous (≥ 1 s). Often, however, this is not the case. As a general rule, the shorter the duration of the signal, the broader the amplitude spectrum. Thus, a 1000-Hz pure tone that is turned on and then turned off 0.1 second later will have sound energy at several frequencies other than 1000 Hz. Approximately 90% of the sound energy will fall between 990 and 1010 Hz. If the duration of the pure tone is decreased further to 0.01 second, then 90% of the sound energy will be distributed from 900 through 1100 Hz. Hence, as the duration decreases, the spread of sound energy to other frequencies increases. The limit to the decrease in duration is an infinitely short pulse or clicklike sound. For this hypothetical sound, energy would spread equally to all frequencies.

Such short-duration sounds, or transients, are increasingly common in clinical audiology, typically consisting of either brief bursts of a pure tone or clicks. As noted, as the duration of a sound decreases, its amplitude spectrum becomes broader. Because of the increasingly common use of transient acoustic signals in audiology, this tradeoff in the time and frequency domains is examined in more detail here.

Figure 2.7A illustrates the waveform and amplitude spectrum for a continuous pure tone with a peak amplitude of A, starting phase of 0°, and a frequency of 1000 Hz. In principle, a continuous signal is one that is infinitely long. For practical purposes, however, acoustic signals having a duration, D, of 1 s or longer will be considered continuous. The 1000-Hz waveform in this panel has a period, T, of 0.001 s, or 1 ms. The

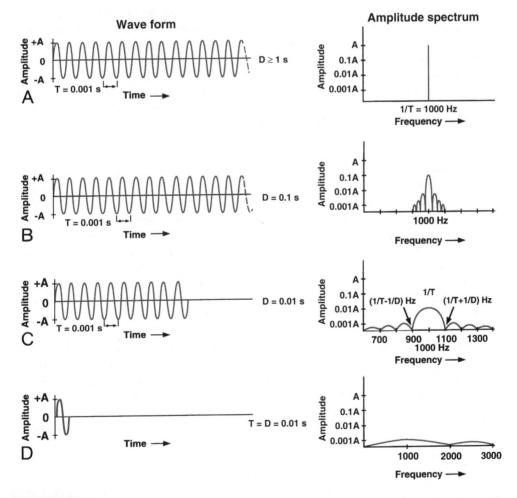

FIGURE 2.7 Trading relation between representations of an acoustic stimulus in the time and frequency domains. The left column shows the waveforms for a 1000-Hz pure tone of various durations; the right column depicts the corresponding amplitude spectra. Duration of the 1000-Hz tone is infinite (continuous) in **A**, 0.1 s in **B**, 0.01 s in **C**, and 0.001 s in **D**. As the duration decreases from A to D, the amplitude spectrum becomes flatter and broader.

amplitude spectrum plotting peak amplitude as a function of frequency therefore consists of a line with amplitude A at 1000 Hz ($f = 1/T$).

In Figure 2.7B, the 1000-Hz pure tone has been abruptly turned on and off for a total duration, D, of 0.1 s, or 100 ms. It is no longer considered a continuous periodic sound. Rather, it is a transient sound, one that occurs only once and for a duration of less than 1 s. Because it is an aperiodic transient sound, its corresponding amplitude spectrum no longer consists of lines but is a continuous function of frequency. The spectrum of this 100-ms, 1000-Hz tone burst has several key features, as shown in the right-hand portion of Figure 2.7B. First, the spectrum is broader than it was for the continuous 1000-Hz pure tone shown in the top panel (Fig. 2.7A). Acoustic energy is present at frequencies other than 1000 Hz for the tone burst, whereas this was not the case for the continuous pure tone. Second, although the peak in the amplitude spectrum is still at 1000 Hz, the amplitude at that frequency has been decreased. In fact, the amplitude is now equal to the peak amplitude of the waveform (A) multiplied by the duration of the signal (D) in seconds (0.1), or 0.1 A. Reduction in the energy present at 1000 Hz, however, is accompanied by a broader distribution of that energy across other frequencies, as noted earlier. Finally, the amplitude spectrum has several points at which the amplitude is 0, and these zero-amplitude regions occur at regular intervals above and below 1000 Hz.

These points of zero amplitude are called nodes in the amplitude spectrum. They occur at frequencies above and below the pure-tone frequency and can be determined according to the following formula: $n(1/D)$ and $-n(1/D)$, where n is 1, 2, 3, and so on. In the example shown in Figure 2.7B, $D = 0.1$ s; therefore, $1/D = 10$ Hz. The nodes or points of zero amplitude occur at $1000 + 10$ Hz, $1000 - 10$ Hz, $1000 + 20$ Hz, $1000 - 20$ Hz, $1000 + 30$ Hz, $1000 - 30$ Hz, and so on, as shown in Figure 2.7B. The frequency region between the first positive node (1010 Hz in Fig. 2.7B) and the first negative node (990 Hz) is referred to as the main lobe of the amplitude spectrum. The adjacent regions between successive nodes are referred to as side lobes. When the pure tone is instantly turned on and off, as in these examples, 90% of the signal energy is contained in the main lobe; the remaining 10% is contained in the side lobes. As we've progressed from a continuous pure tone in Figure 2.7A to one lasting only 0.1 second in Figure 2.7B, the amplitude spectrum has started to broaden such that we've progressed from 100% of the acoustic energy at 1000 Hz to 90% spread from 990 to 1010 Hz.

In Figure 2.7C, the duration of the 1000-Hz pure tone has been decreased still further ($D = 0.01$ s, or 10 ms). The main lobe of the amplitude spectrum now stretches from 900 to 1100 Hz because $1/D$ is now $1/(0.01)$, or 100 Hz. Thus, the first positive node occurs at $1000 + 100$ Hz, and the first negative node occurs at $1000 - 100$ Hz. In addition, the peak amplitude at 1000 Hz has been reduced still further to 0.01 A ($D \times A$), and 90% of the signal energy in the main lobe of the amplitude spectrum for this brief tone burst is now spread over a range of 200 Hz.

If the duration of the 1000-Hz pure tone is shortened by another factor of 10, as in Figure 2.7D, the corresponding amplitude spectrum continues to flatten and broaden. In this case, the duration of the pure tone is 0.001 s, or 1 ms, which corresponds to a single cycle of the 1000-Hz pure tone. Now the main lobe containing 90% of the signal energy spans from 0 to 2000 Hz, a signal that is very brief or compact in the time domain (short waveform) but very broad or spread out in the frequency domain (broad amplitude spectrum). Just the opposite was true for the continuous pure tone described in the top panel of this figure (Fig. 2.7A). For the continuous pure tone, the signal was widely spread in the time domain (a continuous waveform of ≥1 s) but very compact in the frequency domain (all of the amplitude at just one frequency).

This broadening of the spectrum with decrease in signal duration is apparent perceptually as well. As the listener is presented with each of the pure tones in Figure 2.7 in succession, the perception begins with that of a clear tonal sensation and progressively sounds more and more like a click. In fact, the amplitude spectrum for an ideal click (one that is infinitely short) is flat throughout the entire spectrum. The spectrum of the shortest duration tone burst (Fig. 2.7D) is beginning to look more like that associated with a click than that associated with the continuous pure tone (Fig. 2.7A).

In summary, the amplitude spectrum of a pure tone varies with its duration such that the shorter the tone, the broader the spectrum. In general, the amplitude spectrum for pure tones less than 1 s in duration having a period of T seconds, a peak amplitude of A, and turned on and off abruptly for a duration of D seconds, will have a peak amplitude at $1/T$ Hz of $A \times D$ and a main lobe containing 90% of the signal's energy between the frequencies $1/T - 1/D$ and $1/T + 1/D$ Hz. In Figure 2.7, T was 0.001 second, which resulted in all the spectra being centered at 1000 Hz ($1/T$), but these general formulas allow this same analysis to be applied to pure tones of any frequency.

In addition to these effects of duration, sound energy can spread to other frequencies by turning the sound on and off, rather than doing this abruptly (instantaneously) as in this example. Adding a gradual onset and offset of the tone is referred to as the sound's rise and fall time. If a short transient sound is desired for a particular clinical application, however, adding a brief rise and fall time will reduce but not eliminate the spread of energy to other frequencies. So in general, even with appropriate rise and fall times for a transient sound, the shorter the sound, the broader the spread of energy to other frequencies.

SOUND MEASUREMENT

As mentioned previously, the amplitude of a sound wave is typically expressed as sound pressure (p) in pascal units (Pa). Recall that one of the major reasons for this was that most measuring devices are pressure detectors. Devices such as microphones are sensitive to variations in air pressure and convert these pressure variations to variations in electrical voltage. In more general terms, the microphone can be referred to as an acousticoelectrical transducer. A transducer is any device that changes energy from one form to another. In this case, the conversion is from acoustical to electrical energy. (Usually, though, microphones are referred to as electroacoustical, rather than acousticoelectrical, transducers.)

Although the overall amplitude of sound waves is best expressed in terms of RMS pressure, the use of the actual physical units to describe the level of sound is cumbersome. In humans, the ratio of the highest tolerable sound pressure to the sound pressure that can just be heard exceeds 10 million to 1! Moreover, the units dictate that one would be dealing frequently with numbers much smaller than 1. The lowest sound pressure that can just be heard by an average young adult with normal hearing is approximately 0.00002 Pa (2×10^{-5} Pa), or 20 μPa.

Rather than deal with this cumbersome system based on the physical units of pressure, scientists devised a scale known as the decibel scale. The decibel scale quantifies the sound level by taking the logarithm (base 10) of the ratio of two sound pressures and multiplying it by 20. The following formula is used to calculate the sound level in decibels (dB) from the ratio of two sound pressures (p_1 and p_2): $20 \log_{10} (p_1/p_2)$. Let's use the range of sound pressures from maximum tolerable (200 million μPa) to just audible (20 μPa) to see how this range is represented in decibels. To do this, we begin by substituting 200 million µPa /20 µPa for p_1/p_2, which reduces to a ratio of 10 million to 1. The $\log_{10}$ of 10 million (or 10^7) is 7. When 7 is multiplied by 20, the result is 140 dB. This represents the maximum tolerable sound level. Now, for the just-audible sound pressure of 20 µPa, the ratio of p_1/p_2 is 20 µPa/20 µPa, or 1. The log of 1 is 0, and 20×0 is 0. Thus, the just-audible sound pressure is represented by a sound level of 0 dB. We have taken a scale represented by a range of physical sound pressures from 200 million µPa to 20 µPa and compressed it to a much more manageable range of 140 dB to 0 dB. The greatest sound pressure level that can be tolerated is 140 dB greater than the sound pressure level that can barely be heard (Vignette 2.8).

VIGNETTE 2.8   Compressing effect of logarithms

As noted in the text, one of the primary purposes of the decibel scale of sound level is to make the usable range of sound pressures more manageable. It would be inconvenient, and incomprehensible for many individuals, to use physical units of sound pressure to describe the range of sound amplitudes encountered in many everyday and clinical applications. For example, optimal hearing sensitivity of 0.00002 Pa can be more easily expressed as 0 dB, and painfully loud sounds of 200 Pa can be expressed as 140 dB using the same decibel scale of sound level.

Scientists frequently create different scales of measure to make working with the units more convenient. A common example can be found in the various scales of temperature (Celsius, Fahrenheit, Kelvin). The Kelvin scale was designed to make it easier to work with low temperatures, which are cumbersome in the Fahrenheit and Celsius scales: 0° in the Kelvin scale corresponds to −273.15° in the Celsius scale.

Societies and cultures have also attempted to make units of measure more practical and useful. Often this has involved a system of conversion from one type of unit to another. The English system of length, for example, expresses length in units of inches when the lengths are small, feet when the lengths are intermediate, yards for still longer distances, and miles for very long distances.

Now, imagine that by imperial decree, everyone on planet Earth is required to express length in units of inches only. All other units of length have been abolished. Expressing the length of small objects in inches presents no major difficulty in everyday applications. Even the diameter of something as small as the period at the end of this sentence could be comfortably expressed as 0.01 inches. But what about the length of the playing surface on a football field (3600 inches), a 20-mile trip to grandma's house (1,267,200 inches), or a trip around the world (1584 million inches)?!

If we were, in fact, confined to using inches as our sole unit of length, we could try to make the numbers more manageable by using logarithms. Logarithms essentially compress or squeeze a wide range of numbers into a smaller scale. Every 10-fold change in physical units would result in an increment or decrement on the log scale of just one unit.

Let's see what happens when we compress our length scale by applying the logarithm to the set of length measurements from the preceding paragraph. We will arbitrarily refer to this new scale of length based on the logarithm of length in inches as the login scale. The period with a diameter of 0.01 inches would have a new value of −2.0 logins ($\log_{10}$ of 0.01). The length of the football field would be 3.5 logins. The trip to grandma's house would be 6.1 logins, and the trip around the world would be 9.2 logins.

Wow! The logarithm function has really squeezed things together. The period at the end of this sentence has a diameter of −2.0 logins, and a trip around the world (25,000 miles) is just

---

VIGNETTE 2.8 **Compressing effect of logarithms** *(Continued)*

11.2 logins greater, or 9.2 logins! Now, if we were fairly certain that the diameter of this period was close to the smallest object we'd be interested in measuring, we could eliminate all negative numbers by taking the logarithm of ratios in which the denominator of the ratio is always 0.01 inches. This is just a way to make the zero point of the scale correspond to the smallest measurement that is likely to be made. In this new login scale, all values calculated previously simply increase by 2.0. Thus, our login values in this example range from 0.0 (period) ($\log_{10}$ of 0.01/0.01) to 11.2 (trip around the world).

Perhaps we've gotten a little carried away and have compressed our system of length measurement too much. We could decompress it by multiplying the logins by a factor of 10 (decilogins), 100 (centilogins), or 1000 (millilogins). In decilogins, our range of lengths would span from 0.0 decilogins (period) to 112 decilogins (trip around the world). (See Vignette 2.4 for a description of various metric prefixes, such as deci, centi, and milli.)

The preceding material should give you a better idea as to what transpires in the conversion from sound pressure in physical units of Pascals to sound level in decibels and why this system was developed. The use of logarithms compresses an unmanageable range of sound pressures into a more reasonable scale of numbers that is then expanded slightly through multiplication by a factor of 10 (or 20). The logarithm function, however, was not chosen arbitrarily to perform this compression of the sound pressure scale. It was chosen both for its mathematical compression capabilities and because a similar type of compression was believed to be performed by the auditory system when presented with sounds covering a wide range of sound pressures.

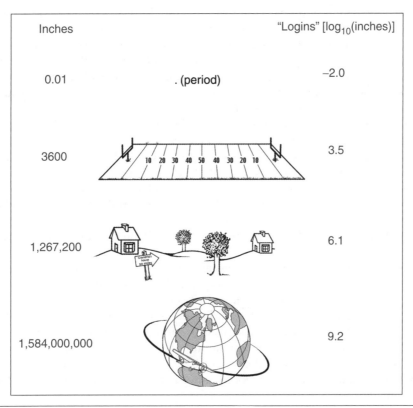

Inches		"Logins" [$\log_{10}$(inches)]
0.01	. (period)	−2.0
3600		3.5
1,267,200		6.1
1,584,000,000		9.2

A 140-dB range from softest heard to maximum tolerable sound pressure levels only indicates that the sound pressure that is just tolerable is 140 dB above that which can just be heard, but it does not indicate what either of those sound pressures is in pascal units. This is because a ratio of two sound pressures has been used in the calculation of decibels, and ratios are dimensionless quantities. Thus, we are calculating the decibel increase of one sound relative to another. Sometimes all we are interested in is a relative change in sound pressure. Recall from the discussion of the inverse square law, for example, that as the distance from the sound source doubled, the sound pressure decreased to half its original value. The corresponding change in decibels associated with this halving of sound pressure can be calculated by using a ratio of 0.5/1. The $\log_{10}$ of 0.5 is -0.301, which, when multiplied by 20, yields a change in sound pressure of approximately -6 dB. We can restate the inverse square law by indicating that as the distance from the sound source doubles, the sound pressure decreases by 6 dB. Again, this does not indicate the values of the two sound pressures involved in this change. The sound pressure may begin at 10 Pa and be halved to 5 Pa or may start at 10,000 Pa and decrease to 5000 Pa. Either of these cases corresponds to a halving of the initial sound pressure, which corresponds to a 6-dB decrease.

Often, an indication of the sound pressure level that provides an absolute rather than a relative indication of the sound level is needed. To accomplish this, all sound pressures relative to the same reference sound pressure must be evaluated. Thus, the denominator of the decibel equation becomes a fixed value called the reference sound pressure. The reference sound pressure for a scale known as the sound pressure level (SPL) scale is 2×10^{-5} Pa, or 20 μPa (20 micropascals). As noted earlier, this corresponds to the softest sound pressure that can be heard by humans under ideal conditions. Calculation of the SPL for a specific sound pressure (p_1) can be accomplished by solving the following equation: SPL in decibels = $20 \log [p_1/(2 \times 10^{-5}$ Pa$)]$. Perhaps the simplest case to consider is the lowest sound pressure that can just be heard, 2×10^{-5} Pa. If $p_1 = 2 \times 10^{-5}$ Pa, the ratio formed by the two sound pressures is $(2 \times 10^{-5}$ Pa$)/(2 \times 10^{-5}$ Pa$)$, or 1. The log of 1 is 0, which, when multiplied by 20, yields a sound level of 0 dB SPL. Consequently, 0 dB SPL does not mean absence of sound. Rather, it simply corresponds to a sound with a sound pressure of 2×10^{-5} Pa. Sound pressures lower than this value will yield negative decibel SPL values, whereas sound pressures greater than this yield positive values.

Consider another example. A sound pressure of 1 Pa corresponds to how many decibels SPL? This can be restated by solving the following equation: SPL in decibels = $20 \log [1.0$ Pa$/(2 \times 10^{-5}$ Pa$)]$. We begin by first reducing $1.0/(2 \times 10^{-5}$ Pa$)$ to 5×10^4. The log of 5×10^4 is approximately 4.7, which, when multiplied by 20, yields a sound pressure level of 94 dB. Thus, a sound pressure of 1 Pa yields a sound pressure level of 94 dB SPL. This sound level is within the range of typical noise levels encountered in many factories.

Fortunately, laborious calculations are not required every time measurements of SPL are required. Rather, simple devices have been constructed to measure the level of various acoustic signals in decibels SPL. These devices, known as sound level meters, use a microphone to change the sound pressure variations to electrical voltage variations. The RMS amplitude of these voltage variations is then determined within the electronic circuitry of the meter, and an indicator (e.g., needle, pointer, or digital display) responds accordingly. In the case of 1 Pa RMS sound pressure input to the microphone, for example, the meter would either point to or display a value of 94 dB SPL (Vignette 2.9).

VIGNETTE 2.9 Decibel values of common sounds

Sound level	Common sound at this dB level	
0 dB SPL	Softest sound level heard by average human listener	
20 dB SPL	Leaves rustling in a breeze	
40 dB SPL	Whispered speech measured 1m away	Pssst
60 dB SPL	Average coversational speech measured 1m away	Hello
80 dB SPL	Loud, shouting voice measured 1m away	HEY YOU!
100 dB SPL	City subway, nearby thunder	
120 dB SPL	Typical level at a rock concert for audience	
140 dB SPL	Jet engine at takeoff	

Other devices may be used to measure other features of the sound waves. Filters, for example, can be used in conjunction with the sound level meter to determine the amplitude of various frequencies contained in a sound. One can get at least a gross estimate of the amplitude spectrum of an acoustic signal by successively examining adjacent frequency regions of the signal. This can be accomplished with filters. For example, the filter might first be set to pass only low frequencies and the sound pressure level measured with the sound level meter. The filter could then be adjusted so as to pass only intermediate frequencies, then high frequencies, and so forth. This would provide a gross indication of how much sound energy was contained in various frequency regions. Very detailed and fine descriptions of the amplitude spectrum could be obtained by using either narrow filters or a spectrum analyzer. This device essentially plots the amplitude spectrum associated with the waveform. The waveform itself may be examined in detail with an oscilloscope, which displays the waveform of the sound impinging on the microphone. Various means can be used either to freeze or to store the waveform until all of its details (e.g., amplitude, period, phase) have been quantified.

Microphones, sound level meters, electronic filters, spectrum analyzers, and oscilloscopes are just a few of the basic tools used by scientists and clinicians in the measurement of sound. The audiologist frequently uses these tools to check the equipment used in the testing of hearing. This equipment must be checked frequently to ensure that the results obtained with the equipment are accurate and that other clinics could obtain the same findings from a given patient.

SUMMARY

The fundamentals of acoustics are reviewed in this chapter. Simple harmonic motion, or sinusoidal vibration, is discussed. The effects of varying the amplitude, frequency, and starting phase of the sinusoidal waveform are examined. The relation between the representations of sound in the time domain, the waveform, and sound in the frequency domain, the amplitude and phase spectra, are reviewed. Resonance and its relation to impedance are also discussed. Finally, the measurement of sound levels in decibels is reviewed.

References and Suggested Readings

Beranek LL. Acoustics. New York: McGraw-Hill, 1954.

Berlin CI. Programmed Instruction on the Decibel. New Orleans: Kresge Hearing Research Laboratory of the South, Louisiana State University School of Medicine, 1970.

Cudahy E. Introduction to Instrumentation in Speech and Hearing. Baltimore: Williams & Wilkins, 1988.

Denes PB, Pinson EN. The Speech Chain. New York: WH Freeman, 1993.

Durrant JD, Lovrinic JH. Bases of Hearing Science. 3rd ed. Baltimore: Williams & Wilkins, 1995.

Small AM. Elements of Hearing Science: A Programmed Text. New York: Wiley, 1978.

Speaks C. Introduction to Sound: Acoustics for the Hearing and Speech Sciences. 3rd ed. San Diego: Singular, 1999.

Yost WA. Fundamentals of Hearing: An Introduction. 4th ed. New York: Academic, 2000.

Structure and Function of the Auditory System

OBJECTIVES

After completion of this chapter, the reader should be able to:

- Recognize and identify some key anatomic features or landmarks of the auditory system.
- Understand the functional roles of the outer ear and middle ear.
- Understand the mapping of frequency to place (tonotopic organization) that occurs throughout the auditory system.
- Recognize the ability of the peripheral auditory system to code information in both a time domain and a frequency domain.
- Appreciate some basic auditory perceptual phenomena, such as loudness and masking.

This chapter is divided into three main sections. The first two deal with the anatomy, physiology, and functional significance of the peripheral and central sections of the auditory system. The peripheral portion of the auditory system is defined here as the structures from the outer ear through the auditory nerve. The central auditory nervous system begins at the cochlear nucleus and is bounded at the other end by the auditory centers of the cortex. The third section of this chapter details some fundamental aspects of the perception of sound.

PERIPHERAL AUDITORY SYSTEM

Figure 3.1 shows a cross-section of the peripheral portion of the auditory system. This portion of the auditory system is usually further subdivided into the outer ear, middle ear, and inner ear.

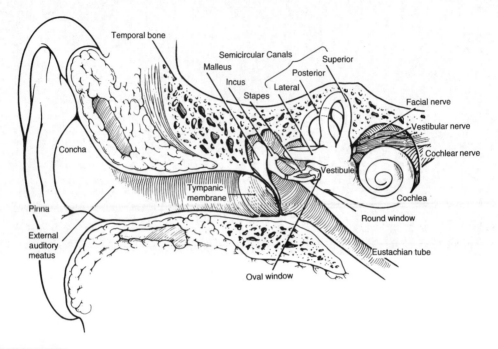

FIGURE **3.1** A cross-section of the peripheral portion of the auditory system revealing some of the anatomic details of the outer, middle, and inner ear. (Adapted from Kessel RG, Kardon RH. Tissues and Organs: A Text-Atlas of Scanning Electron Microscopy. San Francisco: Freeman, 1979.)

Outer Ear

The outer ear consists of two primary components: the pinna and the ear canal. The pinna, the most visible portion of the ear, extends laterally from the side of the head. It is composed of cartilage and skin. The ear canal is the long, narrow canal leading to the eardrum. The entrance to this canal is called the external auditory meatus. The deep bowl-like portion of the pinna adjacent to the external auditory meatus is known as the concha.

Figure 3.2 is a detailed drawing of the right pinna of a normal adult. This cartilaginous structure has several noteworthy anatomic landmarks. First, the bowl-shaped

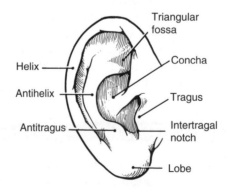

FIGURE **3.2** Detailed drawing of the right pinna showing various anatomic landmarks.

depression in the middle is the concha, which terminates at its medial end at the entrance to the ear canal (the external auditory meatus). Along the anterior inferior (front lower) portion of the concha are two cartilaginous protuberances known as the tragus and antitragus, which are separated, as shown in the figure, by the intertragal notch. The posterior and superior (rear and upper) borders of the concha are formed by a cartilaginous ridge known as the antihelix, which is closely paralleled along the posterior edge of the pinna by the helix. The helix and antihelix diverge in the superior portion of the pinna and then converge as they progress anteriorly and inferiorly. The slight depression formed between the helix and antihelix in the anterior superior portion of the pinna is the triangular fossa.

Medial to the external auditory meatus is the ear canal. The lateral two-thirds of the ear canal are cartilaginous, with the medial third composed of bone (osseous portion). An epithelium (skin) covering over the cartilaginous and osseous portions of the ear canal is contiguous with the tympanic membrane, or eardrum. That is, the lateralmost portion of the tympanic membrane is a layer of epithelium that is a part of the skin lining the ear canal.

The outer ear serves a variety of functions. First, the long (2.5 cm), narrow (5 to 7 mm) canal makes the more delicate middle and inner ear relatively inaccessible to foreign bodies. The outer third of the canal, moreover, is composed of skin and cartilage lined with glands and hairs. These glands, known as ceruminous glands, secrete a substance that potential intruders, such as insects, find terribly noxious. So both the long, narrow, tortuous path of the canal and the secretions of these glands serve to protect the remaining portions of the peripheral auditory system.

Second, the various air-filled cavities composing the outer ear, the two most prominent being the concha and the ear canal, have a natural or resonant frequency to which they respond best. This is true of all air-filled cavities. For an adult, the resonant frequency of the ear canal is approximately 2500 Hz, whereas that of the concha is roughly 5000 Hz. The resonance of each of these cavities is such that each structure increases the sound pressure at its resonant frequency by approximately 10 to 12 dB. This gain or increase in sound pressure provided by the outer ear can best be illustrated by considering the following hypothetical experiment.

Let us begin the experiment by using two tiny microphones. One microphone will be placed just outside (lateral to) the concha, and the other will be positioned very carefully inside the ear canal to rest alongside the eardrum. Now if we present a series of sinusoidal sound waves, or pure tones, of different frequencies, which all measure 70 dB SPL, at the microphone just outside the concha, and if we read the sound pressure levels measured with the other microphone near the eardrum, we will obtain results like those shown by the *solid line* in Figure 3.3. At frequencies less than approximately 1400 Hz, the microphone near the eardrum measures sound levels of approximately 73 dB sound pressure level (SPL). This is only 3 dB higher than the sound level just outside the outer ear. Consequently, the outer ear exerts little effect on the intensity of low-frequency sound. The intensity of the sound measured at the eardrum increases to levels considerably above 70 dB SPL, however, as the frequency of the sound increases. The maximum sound level at the eardrum is reached at approximately 2500 Hz, which corresponds to a value of approximately 87 dB SPL. Thus, when a sound wave having a frequency of 2500 Hz enters the outer ear, its sound pressure is increased by 17 dB by the time it strikes the eardrum. The function drawn with a *solid line* in Figure 3.3 illustrates the role that the entire outer ear serves as a resonator or amplifier of high-frequency sounds. Experiments similar to this one can be conducted to isolate the contribution of various cavities to the resonance of the total outer ear

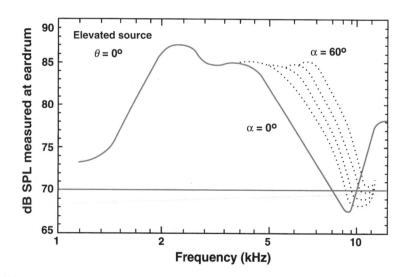

FIGURE 3.3 The response of the head, outer ear, and ear canal for various angles of elevation (α) of the sound source. Zero degrees corresponds to a sound source at eye level and straight ahead (0° azimuth, 0° elevation), whereas 60° represents a source straight ahead but at a higher elevation. If the listener's head and outer ear had no influence on the sound level measured at the eardrum, a flat line at 70 dB SPL would result. This figure illustrates the amplification of high-frequency sound by the outer ear and the way this amplification pattern changes with elevation of the sound source. (Adapted from Shaw EAG. The external ear. In: Keidel WD, Neff WD, eds. Handbook of Sensory Physiology, vol 1. New York: Springer Verlag, 1974:463.)

system. Again, the results of such experiments suggest that the two primary structures contributing to the resonance of the outer ear are the concha and the ear canal.

The resonance of the outer ear, which is represented by the *solid line* in Figure 3.3, was obtained with a sound source directly in front of the subject at eye level. If the sound source is elevated by various amounts, a different resonance curve is obtained. Specifically, the notch or dip in the solid function at 10 kHz in Figure 3.3 moves to a higher frequency, and the peak of the resonant curve broadens to encompass a wider range of frequencies as the elevation of the sound source rises. This is illustrated in Figure 3.3 by the *dotted lines*. Each dotted line represents a different angle of elevation. An elevation of 0° corresponds to eye level, whereas a 90° elevation would position the sound source directly overhead. The response of the outer ear changes as the elevation of the sound source changes. This results from the angle at which the incident sound wave strikes the various cavities of the outer ear. The result is that a code for sound elevation is provided by the outer ear. This code is the amplitude spectrum of the sound, especially above 3000 Hz, that strikes the eardrum. Thus, the outer ear plays an important role in the perception of the elevation of a sound source.

Finally, the outer ear assists in another aspect of the localization of a sound source. The orientation of the pinnae is such that the pinnae collect sound more efficiently from sources in front of the listener than from sources behind the listener. The attenuation of sound waves originating from behind the listener assists in the front/back localization of sound. This is true especially for high-frequency sounds (i.e., sounds with short wavelengths).

In summary, the outer ear serves four primary functions. First, it protects the more delicate middle and inner ears from foreign bodies. Second, it boosts or amplifies high-frequency sounds. Third, it provides the primary cue for the determination of the elevation of a sound's source. Fourth, it assists in distinguishing sounds that arise from in front of the listener from those that arise from behind the listener.

Middle Ear

The tympanic membrane forms the anatomic boundary between the outer and middle ears. The tympanic membrane itself is a multilayered structure. Approximately 85% of the surface area of the tympanic membrane is composed of three types of layers: a lateral epithelial layer, a medial membranous layer that is contiguous with the lining of the middle-ear cavity, and a fibrous layer sandwiched in between the epithelial and membranous layers. The fibrous layer actually contains two sets of fibers: one that is oriented like a series of concentric circles (as in a bull's-eye target) and another that is oriented in a radial fashion (like spokes on a bicycle wheel with the bull's-eye as the hub of the wheel). These fibrous layers give the tympanic membrane considerable strength while maintaining elasticity.

For a small portion of the tympanic membrane, an area in the superior anterior portion that represents approximately 15% of the total eardrum surface area, the two sets of fibers between the epithelial and membranous layers of the eardrum are missing. This portion of the eardrum is known as the *pars flaccida* (*pars*, part, and *flaccida*, flaccid or loose). The portion of the tympanic membrane that contains all three types of layers and constitutes the majority (85%) of the eardrum is the *pars tensa*.

As previously mentioned, the most medial layer of the eardrum is a membranous layer that is contiguous with the membranous lining of the middle ear cavity. The middle ear consists of a small (2 cm^3) air-filled cavity lined with a mucous membrane. It forms the link between the air-filled outer ear and the fluid-filled inner ear (Fig. 3.1). This link is accomplished mechanically via three tiny bones, the ossicles. The lateralmost ossicle is the malleus. The malleus is in contact with the eardrum, or tympanic membrane. At the other end of the outer ear–inner ear link is the smallest, medialmost ossicle, the stapes. The broad base of the stapes, known as the footplate, rests in a membranous covering of the fluid-filled inner ear referred to as the oval window. The middle ossicle in the link, sandwiched between the malleus and stapes, is the incus. The ossicles are suspended loosely within the middle ear by ligaments, known as the axial ligaments, extending from the anterior and posterior walls of the cavity. There are other connections between the surrounding walls of the middle ear cavity and the ossicles. Two connections are formed by the small middle ear muscles, known as the tensor tympani and the stapedius. The tensor tympani originates from the anterior (front) wall of the cavity and attaches to a region of the malleus called the neck, whereas the stapedius has its origin in the posterior (back) wall of the tympanic cavity and inserts near the neck of the stapes.

We have mentioned that the middle ear cavity is air-filled. The air filling the cavity is supplied via a tube that connects the middle ear to the upper part of the throat, or the nasopharynx. This tube, known as the auditory tube or the eustachian tube, has one opening along the bottom of the anterior wall of the middle ear cavity. The tube is normally closed but can be readily opened by yawning or swallowing. In adults, the eustachian tube assumes a slight downward orientation. This facilitates drainage of fluids from the middle ear cavity into the nasopharynx. Thus, the eustachian tube serves two primary purposes. First, it supplies air to the middle ear cavity and thereby enables equalization of the air pressure on both sides of the eardrum. This is desirable for efficient vibration of the eardrum. Second, the eustachian tube allows fluids that accumulate in the middle ear to drain into the nasopharynx.

Although the bones and muscles within the middle ear are key structural components, the middle ear cavity itself has several additional noteworthy anatomic landmarks. To review these landmarks and orient you to their location within this tiny cavity, imagine that we've surgically removed the three ossicles while leaving everything else intact and that you've been struck by a shrink ray that has reduced you in size so that you can stand on the floor of the middle-ear cavity after being inserted through a tiny surgical slit in the right eardrum ("Honey, I've shrunk the reader!"). As shown in Figure 3.4, you would find yourself standing on a mucus-covered membranous lining not unlike that which lines the inside of your nose and throat. A bulge running through the floor underneath your feet represents the tunnel, or fossa, for the jugular vein, one of the main blood vessels carrying blood to the brain.

As you gazed straight ahead, you would notice a small opening in the lower portion of the front wall and some ligaments and a tendon dangling loosely from the upper right portion of the wall. The opening is the entrance, or orifice, for the eustachian tube; the ligaments are those previously attached to the anterior process of the malleus, the lateralmost of the three middle ear ossicles; and the tendon is protruding from a bony structure that houses one of the two middle ear muscles, the tensor tympani. This muscle would normally be connected via the tendon to the neck of the malleus.

As you looked above you, you would notice a partial ceiling that appears to be constructed of bone, although covered, like all of the cavity surfaces, with a mucous membrane. This is the tegmen tympany. The unfinished portion of the ceiling, or hole in the ceiling above you, is the aditus. It opens up into an "attic" known as the epitympanic

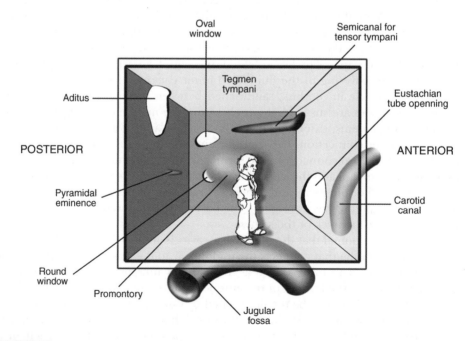

FIGURE 3.4 "Shrunken reader" in the center of the right middle ear with the ossicles removed.

recess, which leads to a series of air-filled caverns that penetrate the surrounding bone of the skull. The air-filled caverns and pockets are the mastoid air cells.

Directing your gaze to the rear or posterior wall, you would observe two primary landmarks. One is the pyramidal eminence, a bony pyramid-shaped structure in the medial superior portion of this wall. It houses the other muscle of the middle ear, the stapedius, which connects via tendon to the stapes. The other landmark, on the lateral superior portion of the wall, is the posterior portion of the axial ligaments that attaches to the incus. The axial ligaments, one attaching to the malleus from the anterior wall and the other attaching to the incus from the posterior wall, hold the ossicles in place and help to form the primary axis of rotation for the ossicular chain when it is vibrated by a sound wave striking the eardrum.

Now, as you returned to your original position facing the anterior wall, to your right along the lateral wall of the middle ear cavity you would observe the membranous layer of the eardrum; to your left, along the medial wall, you would find the oval window and round window. (Remember, you are in the *right* middle ear cavity, not the left.) A bulge running most of the way across the medial wall would also be apparent. This bulge is the promontory. It is formed by the large basal turn of the adjacent cochlea, the hearing portion of the inner ear.

These are some of the highlights of the many anatomic landmarks found in this tiny middle ear cavity. There are certainly others, such as various nerve fibers and blood vessels, but the effects of the shrink ray are starting to wear off, and we don't want to leave you trapped in here! ("Phew! Honey, it's okay. I've unshrunk the reader!")

What is the purpose of the elaborate link between the air-filled outer ear and the fluid-filled inner ear formed by the three ossicles? Recall from the example in Chapter 2 in which two people attempted to communicate, one underwater and one above the water, that the barrier formed by the interface between the media of air and sea water resulted in a "loss" of approximately 99.9% of the sound energy. That is, 99.9% of the energy in the impinging sound wave was reflected away, and only 0.1% was transmitted into the water. This loss amounts to a decrease in sound energy of approximately 30 dB. If the middle ear did not exist and the membranous entrance of the fluid-filled inner ear (oval window) replaced the eardrum, sound waves carried in air would impinge directly on the fluid-filled inner ear. This barrier is analogous to the air-to-water interface described in Chapter 2. Consequently, if such an arrangement existed, there would be a considerable loss of sound energy.

The middle ear compensates for this loss of sound energy when going from air to a fluid medium through two primary mechanisms. The first of these, the areal ratio (ratio of the areas) of the tympanic membrane to the footplate of the stapes, accounts for the largest portion of the compensation. The effective area of the tympanic membrane (i.e., the area involved directly in the mechanical link between the outer ear and inner ear) is approximately 55 mm^2. The corresponding area of the stapes footplate is 3.2 mm^2. Pressure (p) may be defined in terms of force (F) per unit area (A) ($p = F/A$). If the force applied at the eardrum is the same as that reaching the stapes footplate, the pressure at the smaller footplate must be greater than that at the larger eardrum. As an analogy, consider water being forced through a hose. If the area of the opening at the far end of the hose is the same as that of the faucet to which it is connected, the water will exit the hose under the same water pressure as it would at the faucet. If a nozzle is attached to the far end of the hose and it is adjusted to decrease the size of the opening at that end of the hose, the water pressure at that end will be increased in proportion to the degree of constriction produced by the nozzle. The smaller the opening, the greater the water pressure at the nozzle (and the farther the water will be ejected from the nozzle). Applying the same force that exists at the faucet to push the water through a smaller opening created by the nozzle has increased the water pressure at the nozzle. Another analogy explaining the pressure gain associated with areal ratios is one that explains why carpentry nails have a broad head and sharp, narrow point (Vignette 3.1).

For the middle ear, given application of equal force at the tympanic membrane and the stapes footplate ($F_1 = F_2$), the pressure at the smaller footplate ($F_1/3.2$) is greater than that at the larger tympanic membrane ($F_2/55$). The ratio of these two

---

VIGNETTE 3.1   An analogy for pressure amplification

The common carpentry nail illustrates the pressure amplification that occurs when the same force is applied over smaller versus a larger surface area. As shown, the head of the nail has more surface area than the point. When force is applied to the head of the nail with a hammer, that force is channeled through to the point. However, because the area of the point is approximately one-tenth the area at the head of the nail, the pressure applied at the point is 10 times greater. (Pressure is equal to force per unit of area: pressure = force/area.) The increased pressure at the point of the nail helps it to penetrate the material (wood, for example) into which it is being driven. Of course, other practical factors affect the design of the common carpentry nail (for example, the broader head also makes it easier to strike and to remove), but the pressure amplification is one of the key elements in the design. Also, it supplies a nice analogy to the pressure amplification achieved by the areal ratio of the tympanic membrane and stapes footplate in the middle ear.

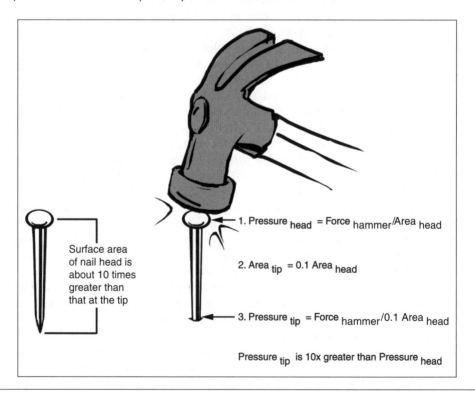

Surface area of nail head is about 10 times greater than that at the tip

1. Pressure $_{head}$ = Force $_{hammer}$/Area $_{head}$

2. Area $_{tip}$ = 0.1 Area $_{head}$

3. Pressure $_{tip}$ = Force $_{hammer}$/0.1 Area $_{head}$

Pressure $_{tip}$ is 10x greater than Pressure $_{head}$

areas is 55/3.2, or 17. Consequently, the pressure at the oval window is 17 times that at the tympanic membrane for a given driving force simply because of their difference in area. An increase in sound pressure by a factor of 17 corresponds to an increase of 24.6 dB. Thus, of approximately 30 dB that would be lost if the air-filled outer ear were linked directly to the fluid-filled inner ear, almost 25 dB is recovered solely because of the areal ratio of the eardrum to the stapes footplate.

The other primary mechanism that might contribute to compensation for the existing impedance mismatch has to do with a complex lever system presumed to exist within the ossicles. The lever is created by the difference in length between the malleus and a portion of the incus known as the long process. This lever factor recovers only approximately 2 dB of the loss caused by the impedance mismatch. The assumptions underlying the operation of this lever mechanism, moreover, are not firmly established.

The middle ear system, therefore, compensates for much of the loss of sound energy that would result if the airborne sound waves impinged directly on the fluid-filled inner ear. The middle ear compensates for approximately 25 to 27 dB of the estimated 30-dB impedance mismatch. The ability of the middle ear system to amplify or boost the sound pressure depends on signal frequency. Specifically, little pressure amplification occurs for frequencies below 100 Hz or above 2000 to 2500 Hz. Recall, however, that the outer ear amplified sound energy by 20 dB for frequencies from 2000 to 5000 Hz. Thus, taken together, the portion of the auditory system peripheral to the stapes footplate increases sound pressure by 20 to 25 dB in a range of approximately 100 to 5000 Hz. This range of frequencies happens to correspond to the range of frequencies in human speech that are most important for communication.

Another less obvious function of the middle ear also involves the outer ear–inner ear link formed by the ossicles. Because of the presence of this mechanical link, the preferred pathway for sound vibrations striking the eardrum will be along the chain formed by the three ossicles. Sound energy, therefore, will be routed directly to the oval window. Another membranous window of the inner ear also lies along the inner or medial wall of the middle ear cavity. This structure is known as the round window (Fig. 3.1). For the inner ear to be stimulated appropriately by the vibrations of the sound waves, the oval window and round window must not be displaced in the same direction simultaneously. This situation would arise frequently, however, if the sound wave impinged directly on the medial wall of the middle ear cavity where both the oval window and the round window are located. Thus, routing the vibrations of the eardrum directly to the oval window via the ossicles ensures appropriate stimulation of the inner ear.

Finally, we mentioned previously that two tiny muscles within the middle ear make contact with the ossicular chain. These muscles can be made to contract in a variety of situations. Some individuals can contract these muscles voluntarily. For most individuals, however, the contraction is an involuntary reflex arising either from loud acoustic stimuli or from nonacoustic stimuli (such as a puff of air applied to the eyes or scratching the skin on the face just in front of the external auditory meatus) or accompanying voluntary movements of the oral musculature, as in chewing, swallowing, or yawning. For acoustic activation, sound levels must generally exceed 85 dB SPL to elicit a reflexive contraction of the middle ear muscles.

The result of middle ear muscle contraction is to compress or stiffen the ossicular chain and essentially to pull the ossicular chain away from the two structures it links, the outer ear and inner ear. This results in an attenuation or decrease of sound pressure reaching the inner ear. The attenuation, amounting to 15 to 20 dB, depends on frequency. Recall from Chapter 2 that increases in a system's stiffness have the greatest effect on low-frequency vibrations. Consequently, the attenuation produced by the middle ear muscles contracting and increasing the stiffness of the ossicles exists only for frequencies below 2000 Hz. The attenuation measured for acoustically elicited contractions, moreover, appears to apply only to stimuli of high intensities. Low-level signals, such as those near threshold, are not attenuated when middle ear muscle contraction is elicited, but high-level signals (≥80 dB SPL) may be attenuated by as much as 15 to 20 dB. The middle ear reflex is known as a consensual reflex, meaning that when either ear is appropriately stimulated, the muscles contract in both ears.

Inner Ear

The inner ear is a complex structure that resides deep within a very dense portion of the skull known as the petrous portion of the temporal bone. Because of the complexity of this structure, it is often referred to as a labyrinth. The inner ear consists of a bony outer casing, the osseous labyrinth. Within this bony structure is the membranous labyrinth. The osseous labyrinth, as shown in Figure 3.5, can be divided into three major sections: the *semicircular canals* (*superior*, *lateral*, and *posterior*), the *vestibule*, and the *cochlea*. The first two sections house the sensory organs for the vestibular system. The vestibular system assists in maintaining balance and posture. The focus here, however, is on the remaining portion of the osseous inner ear, the cochlea. It is the cochlea that contains the sensory organ for hearing. The coiled, snail-shaped cochlea has approximately $2\frac{3}{4}$ turns in human beings. The largest turn is called the basal turn, and the smallest turn, at the top of the cochlea, is referred to as the apical turn. Two additional anatomic landmarks of the inner ear depicted in Figure 3.5 are the *oval window* and the *round window*. Recall that the footplate of the stapes, the medialmost bone of the three ossicles in the middle ear, is attached to the oval window.

The cochlea is cut in cross-section from top (apex) to bottom (base) in Figure 3.6. The winding channel running throughout the bony snail-shaped structure is further

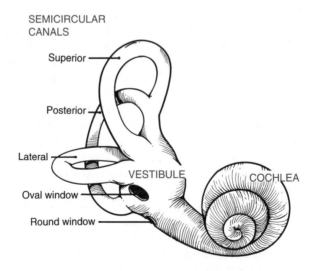

FIGURE 3.5 The osseous labyrinth and its landmarks. (Adapted from Durrant JD, Lovrinic JH. Bases of Hearing Science. 2nd ed. Baltimore: Williams & Wilkins, 1984:98.)

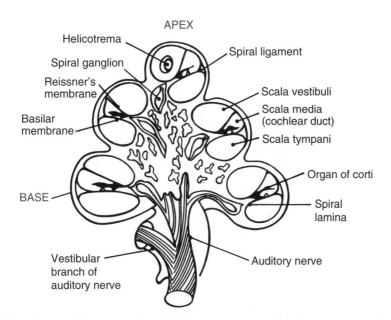

FIGURE 3.6 Modiolar cross-section of the cochlea illustrating the scalae through each of the turns. (Adapted from Zemlin WR. Speech and Hearing Science: Anatomy and Physiology. 2nd ed. Englewood Cliffs, NJ: Prentice-Hall, 1988:464.)

subdivided into three compartments. The compartment sandwiched between the other two is a cross-section of the membranous labyrinth that runs throughout the osseous labyrinth. All three compartments are filled with fluid. The middle compartment, known as the *scala media*, is filled with a fluid called endolymph. The two adjacent compartments, the *scala vestibuli* and *scala tympani*, contain a different fluid, called perilymph. At the apex of the cochlea is a small hole called the *helicotrema* that connects the two compartments filled with perilymph, the scala tympani and scala vestibuli. The oval window forms an interface between the ossicular chain of the middle ear and the fluid-filled scala vestibuli of the inner ear. When the oval window vibrates as a consequence of vibration of the ossicular chain, a wave is established within the scala vestibuli. Because the fluid-filled compartments are essentially sealed within the osseous labyrinth, the inward displacement of the cochlear fluids at the oval window must be matched by an outward displacement elsewhere. This is accomplished via the round window, which communicates directly with the scala tympani. When the oval window is pushed inward by the stapes, the round window is pushed outward by the increased pressure in the inner ear fluid.

When the stapes footplate rocks back and forth in the oval window, it generates a wave within the cochlear fluids. This wave displaces the scala media in a wavelike manner. This displacement pattern is usually simplified by considering the motion of just one of the partitions forming the scala media, the *basilar membrane*. The motion depicted for the basilar membrane also occurs for the opposite partition of the scala media, *Reissner's membrane* (Fig. 3.6). Although we will be depicting the displacement pattern of the basilar membrane, the reader should bear in mind that the entire fluid-filled scala media is undergoing similar displacement.

Figure 3.7 illustrates the displacement pattern of the basilar membrane at four successive points in time. When this displacement pattern is visualized directly, the

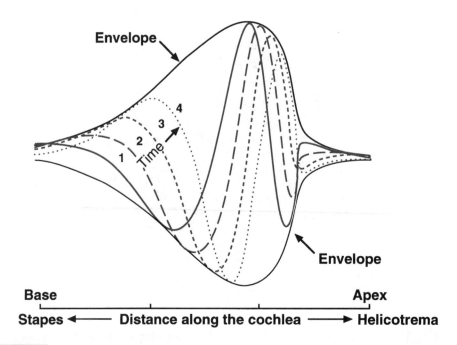

wave established along the basilar membrane is seen to travel from the base to the apex. The displacement pattern increases gradually in amplitude as it progresses from the base toward the apex until it reaches a point of maximum displacement. At that point, the amplitude of displacement decreases abruptly. The *thin solid black line* connecting the amplitude peaks at various locations for these four points in time describes the displacement envelope. The envelope pattern is symmetrical in that the same pattern superimposed on the positive peaks can be flipped upside down and used to describe the negative peaks. As a result, only the positive, or upper, half of the envelope describing maximum displacement is usually displayed.

Figure 3.8 displays the envelopes of the displacement pattern of the basilar membrane that have been observed for different stimulus frequencies. As the frequency of the stimulus increases, the peak of the displacement pattern moves in a basal direction closer to the stapes footplate. At low frequencies, virtually the entire membrane undergoes some degree of displacement. As stimulus frequency increases, a more restricted region of the basilar membrane undergoes displacement. Thus, the cochlea is performing a crude frequency analysis of the incoming sound. In general, for all but the very low frequencies (50 Hz), the place of maximum displacement within the cochlea is associated with the frequency of an acoustic stimulus. The frequency of the acoustic stimulus striking the eardrum and displacing the stapes footplate will be analyzed or distinguished from sounds of different frequency by the location of the displacement pattern along the basilar membrane.

Because the pressure wave created within the cochlear fluids originates near the base of the cochlea at the oval window, one might think that this is the reason the

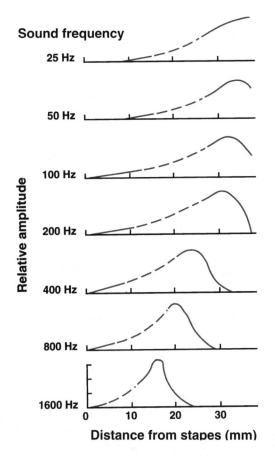

FIGURE 3.8 Envelopes of traveling wave displacement patterns for various stimulus frequencies. Low frequencies (top) produce a maximum displacement of the basilar membrane in the apex (farthest distance from the stapes), whereas higher frequencies (bottom) produce maximum displacement in the basal portion of the cochlea (nearer to the stapes). (Adapted from von Bekesy G. Experiments in Hearing. New York: McGraw-Hill, 1960:448.)

traveling wave displacement pattern appears to move from the base to the apex. On the contrary, experiments with models of the inner ear have shown that the source of vibration (oval window) can be anywhere along the cochlea, including the apex, with no effect on the displacement pattern of the basilar membrane (Vignette 3.2). The primary physical feature of the inner ear responsible for the direction in which the

VIGNETTE 3.2 **Discussion of the traveling-wave paradox**

Regardless of where the vibration is introduced into the cochlea, the traveling wave always travels from base to apex. This phenomenon is known as the traveling-wave paradox. The early tests of hearing that were routinely performed decades ago with tuning forks made use of this phenomenon. A tuning fork was struck, and the vibrating tongs were placed next to the outer ear. The tester asked the listener to indicate when the tone produced by the vibrating tuning fork could no longer be heard. Immediately after the listener indicated that the sound was no

(continued)

VIGNETTE 3.2   **Discussion of the traveling-wave paradox (Continued)**

---

longer audible, the base of the tuning fork was pressed against the mastoid process, the bony portion of the skull behind the ear. If the listener could hear the tone again, it was assumed that the hearing sensitivity of the inner ear alone was better than that of the entire peripheral portion of the auditory system as a whole (outer ear, middle ear, and inner ear).

When the base of the tuning fork was placed on the mastoid process, the skull vibrated. The cochlea is embedded firmly within the temporal bone of the skull, such that skull vibrations produce mechanical vibration of the inner ear. Even though the vibration is not introduced at the oval window by the vibrating stapes, the tone produced by the tuning fork placed against the skull is heard as though it were. The traveling wave within the inner ear behaves the same, regardless of where the mechanical vibration is introduced.

For normal listeners, the typical means of stimulating the inner ear is through the outer and middle ears. This is air conduction hearing. Sound can also be introduced by vibrating the skull at the mastoid process, forehead, or some other location. This is called bone conduction hearing. Whether the tone is introduced into the inner ear by bone conduction or air conduction, the traveling wave and the resulting sensation are the same.

Modern-day air conduction and bone conduction tests are described in more detail in Chapter 4. They are of great assistance in determining which portion of the peripheral auditory system is impaired in listeners with hearing loss.

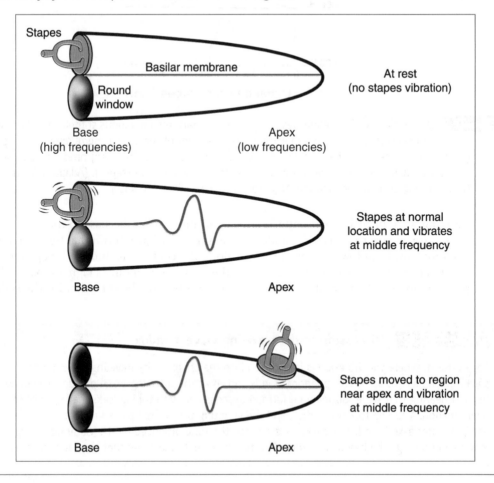

traveling wave progresses is the stiffness gradient of the basilar membrane. The stiffness of the basilar membrane is greatest in the base and decreases from the base to the apex. As we saw in Chapter 2, stiffness offers greatest opposition to displacement for low-frequency vibrations. Thus, the greater stiffness of the basilar membrane in the basal portion of the cochlea opposes displacement when stimulated by low-frequency sound and forces the wave to travel further up the cochlea toward the apex to a region having less stiffness and less opposition to low-frequency vibration.

A more detailed picture of the structures within the scala media is provided in Figure 3.9 The sensory organ of hearing, the organ of Corti, is seen to rest on top of the basilar membrane. The organ of Corti contains several thousand sensory receptor cells called *hair cells*. Each hair cell has several tiny hairs, or cilia, protruding from the top of the cell. As shown in Figure 3.9, there are two types of hair cells in the organ of Corti. The inner hair cells make up a single row of receptors closest to the modiolus, or bony core, of the cochlea. The cilia of these cells are freestanding (i.e., they do not make contact with any other structures). Approximately 90 to 95% of the auditory nerve fibers that carry information to the brain make contact with the inner hair cells. The outer hair cells are much greater in number and are usually organized in three rows. The cilia of the outer hair cells are embedded within a gelatinous structure known as the *tectorial membrane,* draped over the top of the organ of Corti.

The organ of Corti is bordered by two membranes: the basilar membrane below and the tectorial membrane above. The modiolar or medial points of attachment for these two membranes are offset; the tectorial membrane is attached to a structure called the spiral limbus, which is nearer to the modiolus than the comparable point of attachment for the basilar membrane (a bony structure called the spiral lamina). Figure 3.10 illustrates one of the consequences of these staggered points of attachment. When the basilar membrane is displaced upward (toward the scala vestibuli),

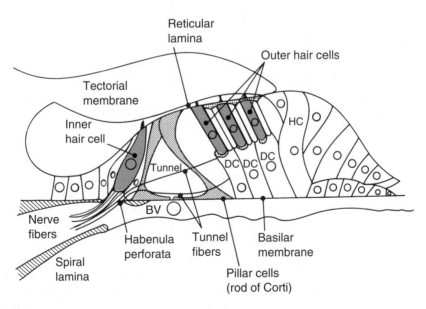

FIGURE 3.9 Detailed cross-section of the organ of Corti. BV, basilar vessel; DC, Deiter cell; HC, Hensen cell. (Adapted from Pickles JO. An Introduction to the Physiology of Hearing. 2nd ed. London: Academic, 1988:29.)

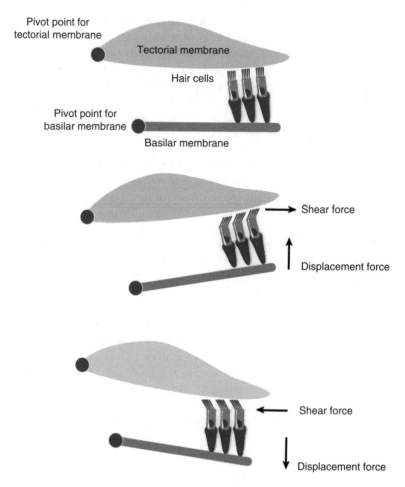

FIGURE 3.10 The mechanism responsible for generation of shearing forces on the cilia of the outer hair cells. Because the pivot points for the tectorial membrane and basilar membrane (*small black circles*) are offset horizontally, vertical displacement of the basilar membrane creates radial shearing forces across the cilia (i.e., a push or pull of the cilia in left to right in the drawings). (Adapted from Zemlin WR. Speech and Hearing Science: Anatomy and Physiology. 2nd ed. Englewood Cliffs, NJ: Prentice-Hall, 1998:484.)

the cilia of the outer hair cells embedded in the tectorial membrane undergo a shearing force in a radial direction (a horizontal direction in the figure). Displacement downward develops a radial shearing force in the opposite direction. This shearing force is believed to be the trigger that initiates a series of electrical and chemical processes within the hair cells. This, in turn, leads to the activation of the auditory nerve fibers that are in contact with the base of the hair cell.

A critical element in the conversion of mechanical movements of the basilar membrane to electrical impulses in the auditory nerve is the transduction function served by the inner and outer hair cells in the organ of Corti. The shearing forces applied to the cilia on the tops of these hair cells in response to acoustic stimulation give rise to electrical potentials known generally as receptor potentials. Receptor potentials are common in sensory cells and are produced only in response to a stimulus, unlike resting potentials, which are present in cells at all times in the living organism. Two types of receptor potentials are found in the cochlea: the cochlear microphonic potential and the summating potential. These potentials are generally referred to as gross electrical potentials in that they are measured with electrodes inserted in the cochlea (and sometimes can be recorded from the ear canal) and represent the collective response of hundreds or even thousands of hair cells. In addition, the cochlear microphonic is an alternating-current (ac) potential that varies in instantaneous amplitude over time (the waveform of the potential mimics that of the stimulating sound, the same way a microphone does). The summating potential is a steady-state direct-current (dc) potential that maintains a constant value in response to sound.

Scientists have been able to record electrical potentials generated by individual hair cells. Again, both resting potentials and receptor potentials have been recorded from individual hair cells. Receptor potentials of single hair cells, referred to as the ac and dc receptor potentials, are somewhat analogous to the grossly recorded cochlear microphonic and summating potentials, respectively. The exact role of the hair cells, their receptor potentials, and the interaction between the two types of hair cells (inner and outer) is unclear. It is clear, however, that damage to the hair cells and the elimination of the receptor potentials produced by the cells greatly diminishes the cochlea's ability to perform a frequency analysis on incoming sounds and reduces the sensory response for sounds of low and moderate intensity.

Some research conducted since the mid 1980s has indicated that the receptor potentials generated by the hair cell trigger mechanical changes in the length of the bodies of the hair cells. When the cilia on the top of the hair cell are sheared in one direction, the receptor potential produced makes the cell body of the hair cell contract. Deflection of the cilia in the opposite direction changes the receptor potential, which causes the body of the hair cell to elongate or stretch. This expansion and contraction of the hair cells along the length of their cell bodies have been likened to similar events in muscle fibers. Although, actin, a protein found in muscle fibers that is critical to the fiber's ability to expand and contract, has also been found in hair cells, it is a different protein, prestin, that supports the contractile properties of the hair cells. The net effect of these mechanical changes in the length of the hair cell is to amplify, or boost, the displacement of the basilar membrane and to create a more vigorous electrical response to the stimulus. The ultimate effect of this elaborate micromechanical system is a much more precise analysis of frequency and a stronger mechanical and electrical response to sounds of low and moderate intensity. Researchers frequently refer to this facilitatory effect of the hair cell movement as the cochlear amplifier because of its enhancement of low- and moderate-intensity sounds (Vignette 3.3).

To understand how changes in the length of the hair cell bodies in response to sound can enhance the basilar membrane's response, consider the following analogy. Imagine that you are bouncing up and down on a large trampoline. You adjust your bounce so that the trampoline is vibrated in an up-and-down motion with a vertical displacement of 1 foot in each direction. A partner is now positioned beneath the trampoline and is wearing a special helmet, the top of which is attached to the underside of the trampoline's surface at the location corresponding to your point of contact with the trampoline. When your partner squats, the trampoline is pulled down, and when he or she stands, it is returned to a horizontal position. By synchronizing your partner's active vertical movements (using the muscles in his or her legs to alternately squat and stand) with the "passive" vertical displacement of the trampoline produced by your

VIGNETTE 3.3 The cochlear amplifier

The ability of the outer hair cells to contract and elongate in response to sound stimulation results in the amplification of the mechanical response of the inner ear (the basilar membrane) at low sound intensities. This has been determined through research involving a variety of techniques and approaches over the years. Some of these techniques involved either temporarily or permanently disabling the outer hair cells while leaving the rest of the inner ear intact. When this is done, the amplitude of vibration measured for the basilar membrane is less at low intensities but unchanged at high intensities. This also affects the frequency-resolving, or filtering, power of the inner ear at low intensities. Both of these effects, on low-intensity displacement and low-intensity tuning or filtering, are illustrated in the nearby figure. These well-established physiologic effects have considerable significance for audiologists, since as noted in subsequent chapters, many cases of sensorineural hearing loss involve primarily the loss of outer hair cells. As a consequence, based on research findings like those illustrated here, one would expect such individuals to have trouble hearing soft sounds but not loud sounds and in performing frequency analysis of low-intensity sounds.

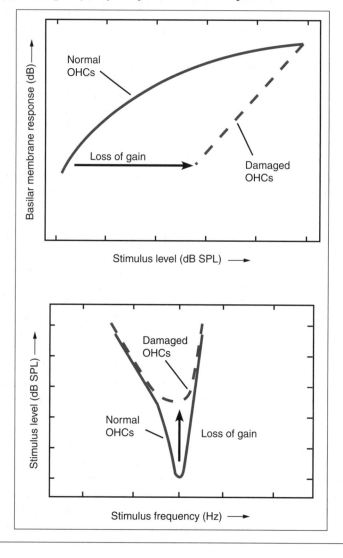

bouncing, the height of your jump (and the displacement of the trampoline) can be increased or amplified considerably. The trampoline surface is like the basilar membrane, and your partner represents the contracting and expanding hair cell body sandwiched between the basilar membrane and the tectorial membrane. The electrical potentials that perfectly mimic the displacement pattern of the basilar membrane (and the waveform of the sound) keep the two partners synchronized to enhance the vertical displacement. Otherwise, without synchronization, your partner could be pushing upward while you were moving downward on the trampoline and effectively cancel the vertical displacement. Working together, however, the combined efforts of you and your partner produce more activity than you could accomplish by yourself.

If such an active cochlear amplifier exists, one would expect to be able to measure vibrations coming out of the inner ear when the hair cells have been pushing and pulling on the basilar membrane. Further, if they vibrate the basilar membrane, the oval window and stapes footplate should also vibrate, which should vibrate the rest of the middle ear ossicles and the eardrum, which in turn should produce a measurable sound in the ear canal. In fact, such sounds, known as otoacoustic emissions (*oto*, of the ear, and *acoustic*, sound), have been the focus of an incredible amount of research since their discovery in 1978. They have been measured by placing a tiny microphone deep inside the ear canal.

There are two broad classes of otoacoustic emissions, or OAEs: spontaneous and evoked. Evoked emissions require a stimulus of some sort to produce them, whereas spontaneous emissions simply occur, as the name implies, spontaneously (without a stimulus). Using the trampoline analogy, spontaneous emissions can be thought of as being produced by your partner's continued up-and-down movement, even when you are no longer on the trampoline. Spontaneous OAEs occur in at least 50% of the normal-hearing young adult population, are more prevalent in females, and are not of much clinical value at present. Evoked OAEs, however, have been demonstrated to be sensitive to damage to the hair cells in the cochlea and have become a key clinical tool for the detection and diagnosis of hearing loss (Vignette 3.4).

There are basically three types of evoked OAEs: (*a*) transient-evoked OAE (TEOAE), (*b*) distortion-product OAE (DPOAE), and (*c*) stimulus-frequency OAE (SFOAE). The SFOAEs are the most difficult to measure and have been studied the least. They are produced by presenting the ear with a pure tone and then examining the sound recorded in the ear canal. The frequency of the emission sound, however, is the same as that of the stimulus tone, and its level is much lower than that of the stimulus. This makes it difficult to measure and study.

TEOAEs were the first OAEs measured in humans. They are recorded by stimulating the ear with a brief click while recording the sound level in the ear canal with a tiny microphone. A click is a brief sound that has energy spread over a wide range of frequencies. Thus, a wide range of the basilar membrane can be stimulated in an instant. Because of the nature of the traveling wave mechanism in the cochlea, the basilar membrane initially responds to a click with maximum displacement in the high-frequency basal region. The peak displacement of the basilar membrane then travels toward the apex, where maximum displacement occurs in response to low-frequency sounds. Thus, even though the click stimulus instantly presents the ear with sounds of low, mid, and high frequency, it takes longer for the low-frequency sounds to travel to the apex and stimulate the basilar membrane. Assuming that it takes 3 ms for the peak displacement to travel from the basal to the apical portion of the basilar membrane, the low frequencies would maximally stimulate the basilar membrane at the appropriate place about 3 ms after the high frequencies present in the click.

VIGNETTE 3.4   Use of OAEs as a screening tool for babies

The development of tools to measure OAEs clinically has led to many exciting applications. For the first time in the history of clinical audiology, a tool to measure the integrity of the sensory receptors in the generally inaccessible inner ear was available.

One of the clinical applications explored and refined during the 1990s was the use of OAEs as a screening tool for hearing loss in infants. Some of the advantages associated with the use of OAEs for this application included the ability to record these responses without requiring the active participation of the infant, the ability to assess each ear separately, and the capability of evaluating a fairly broad range of frequencies. In addition, normal OAE responses would be possible only with normal outer, middle, and inner ears. The focus in OAE-based screening is clearly on the auditory periphery. Problems localized to any of these sections of the auditory periphery, moreover, are most amenable to intervention, either medical (for outer and middle ears) or audiologic (in the form of hearing aids or other prosthetic devices for those with inner ear problems; see Chapter 7).

In recent years many states have adopted legislation to require that all infants be screened for hearing loss at birth (referred to as universal screening; see Chapter 6). Screening tools based on OAEs are among the most commonly used devices in universal newborn screening programs.

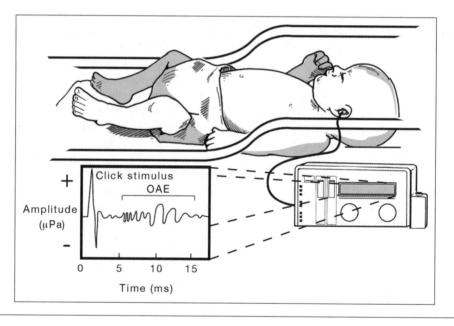

Further, the vibrations producing the emissions travel back out of the cochlea at the same rate, so that low-frequency sounds would come back out of the cochlea and be measurable by a microphone in the ear canal about 6 ms after the high frequencies appeared.

Figure 3.11 illustrates a representative TEOAE from a normal-hearing young adult. The plot is essentially the acoustic waveform that is recorded in the ear canal by the tiny microphone. The first, large, abrupt portion of the waveform is the click stimulus

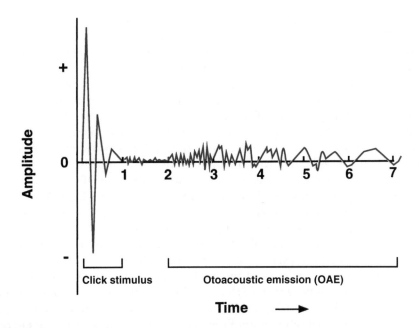

FIGURE 3.11 A TEOAE. The plot is a waveform showing as a function of time the sound levels recorded by a tiny microphone in the ear canal. The large initial portion of the waveform is a recording of the click stimulus presented in the ear canal by the earphone. The lower-level and later-appearing portion of the waveform is the echo coming back out into the ear canal from the inner ear.

presented by the earphone. After a brief period of silence, another waveform emerges: a low-level echo! In fact, TEOAEs have frequently been referred to as cochlear echoes. Careful scrutiny of the echo reveals that the first portion has shorter periods or higher frequencies than the later parts of the echo. This is entirely consistent with the scenario described earlier based on the delays introduced by the traveling wave along the basilar membrane.

TEOAEs are observed only in response to clicks of low and moderate sound level. Animal research has demonstrated that TEOAEs are sensitive to damage, even reversible injury, to the hair cells. If the measurements described in Figure 3.11 were repeated on an individual with hair cell damage in the high-frequency basal portion of the cochlea, the early parts of the echo would be missing and only the later-emerging low-frequency emissions originating from the healthy apical region would be observed.

DPOAEs are also being used for clinical applications. Although DPOAEs can be generated in a variety of ways, the most commonly employed method makes use of two stimulus tones simultaneously introduced into the ear canal. The frequencies of these two pure tones are denoted f_1 and f_2, with f_2 being higher in frequency than f_1. Distortion is a characteristic of many systems, including mechanical systems, and can be measured in a variety of ways. One manifestation of distortion in a system is the emergence of tones in the response or output of the system that were not part of the sound stimulus presented to the system. These additional tones are referred to as distortion products. When two tones are presented to the auditory system, the most prominent distortion product that emerges is one that has a frequency corresponding to $2f_1 - f_2$.

For reasons beyond the scope of this book, this distortion product is often referred to as the cubic difference tone, or CDT. The CDT is lower in frequency than the two input tones. For example, for f_1 = 1000 Hz and f_2 = 1200 Hz, the frequency of the CDT is 800 Hz ([2 × 1000 Hz] − 1200 Hz). Although other distortion products have been explored for measurement of DPOAEs, the CDT has been the most thoroughly studied and is the one receiving the most emphasis clinically. Hereafter, unless noted otherwise, the term DPOAE implies measurement of the CDT distortion product.

Because the DPOAE occurs at a frequency close to but separate from the input frequencies, it is possible to use sounds of longer duration to evoke the emission. The distortion product is separated from the input frequencies by a fast frequency analysis of the sound recorded in the ear canal. Unlike the TEOAE, the DPOAE can be measured over a wide range of sound levels from moderately low to very high. Although there is considerable uncertainty as to whether the same distortion processes are involved over this entire range of sound levels, it appears that the DPOAEs evoked by low-intensity stimuli are just as sensitive to hair cell damage in the cochlea as TEOAEs. They continue to be explored for a variety of clinical applications.

The two primary functions of the auditory portion of the inner ear can be summarized as follows. First, the inner ear performs a frequency analysis on incoming sounds so that different frequencies stimulate different regions of the inner ear. Second, mechanical vibration is amplified and converted into electrical energy by the hair cells. The hair cells are frequently referred to as mechanoelectrical transducers. That is, they convert mechanical energy (vibration) into electrical energy (receptor potentials).

Auditory Nerve

The action potentials generated by auditory nerve fibers are called all-or-none potentials because they do not vary in amplitude when activated. If the nerve fibers fire, they always fire to the same degree, reaching 100% amplitude. The action potentials, moreover, are very short-lived events, typically requiring less than 1 to 2 ms to rise in amplitude to maximum potential and return to resting state. For this reason, they are frequently referred to as spikes. They can be recorded by inserting a tiny microelectrode into a nerve fiber. When this is done, spikes can be observed even without the presentation of an acoustic stimulus, because the nerve fiber has spontaneous activity that consists of random firings of the nerve fiber. The lowest sound intensity that gives rise to a criterion percentage increase (e.g., 20% increase) in the rate at which the fiber is firing is called the threshold for that particular stimulus frequency. As stimulus intensity rises above threshold, the amplitude of the spikes does not change. They always fire at maximum response. The rate at which the nerve fiber responds, however, does increase with stimulus level. This is illustrated in Figure 3.12, in which an input-output function for a single auditory nerve fiber is displayed. The discharge rate, or *spike rate*, increases steadily with input level above the spontaneous rate until a maximum discharge rate is reached approximately 30 to 40 dB above threshold. Consequently, a single nerve fiber can code intensity via the discharge rate over only a limited range of intensities. Again, an increase in intensity is encoded by an increase in the firing rate (more spikes per second), not by an increase in the amplitude of the response.

Solid line c in Figure 3.13 depicts the frequency threshold curve (FTC) of a single auditory nerve fiber. Combinations of stimulus intensity and frequency lying within the *striped area* bordered by the FTC will cause the nerve fiber to increase its firing rate above the spontaneous rate. Combinations of frequency and intensity lying outside

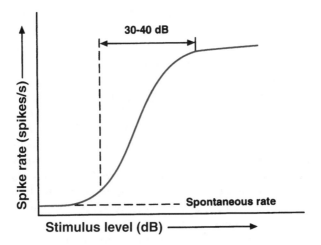

FIGURE 3.12 An input-output function for a single auditory nerve fiber. As stimulus intensity increases, the firing rate of the nerve fiber increases but only over a narrow range of 30 to 40 dB.

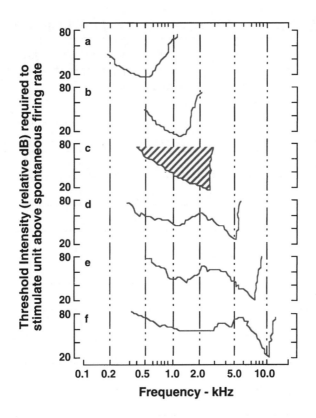

FIGURE 3.13 FTCs for six auditory nerve fibers (*a–f*). The FTC illustrates the intensity required at each frequency to produce a barely measurable response in the nerve fiber. The frequency requiring the lowest intensity for a response is known as the best frequency or characteristic frequency. The best frequency for each of the six nerve fibers increases from top (*a*) to the bottom (*f*). The area within each curve, illustrated in *c* by the striped region, represents the response area of the nerve fiber. Any combination of frequency and intensity represented in that area will yield a response from the nerve fiber.

this region fail to activate the nerve fiber. The *striped region*, therefore, is frequently referred to as the nerve fiber's response area (Vignette 3.5).

The FTC for the nerve fiber in Figure 3.13, area *c*, indicates that the nerve fiber responds best to a frequency of about 2000 Hz; i.e., 2000 Hz is the frequency requiring the least amount of stimulus intensity to evoke a response from the nerve fiber. This frequency is often referred to as the best frequency or characteristic frequency of the nerve fiber. Some nerve fibers have a low characteristic frequency, and some have a high characteristic frequency. This is illustrated in the other areas of Figure 3.13. Fibers with high characteristic frequencies come from hair cells in the base of the cochlea, whereas those with low characteristic frequencies supply the apex. As the nerve fibers exit through the bony core of the cochlea, or modiolus, on their way to the brainstem, they maintain an orderly arrangement. The bundle of nerve fibers composing the cochlear branch of the auditory nerve is organized so that fibers with high characteristic frequencies are located around the perimeter, whereas fibers with low characteristic frequencies make up the core of the cochlear nerve. Thus, the auditory nerve is organized, as is the basilar membrane, so that each characteristic

---

VIGNETTE 3.5   Illustration of response area and FTC of nerve fiber

The FTC of an auditory nerve fiber maps out the response area of the fiber. Combinations of stimulus frequency and intensity falling within the response area produce a response from the nerve fiber, whereas those lying outside this area fail to do so.

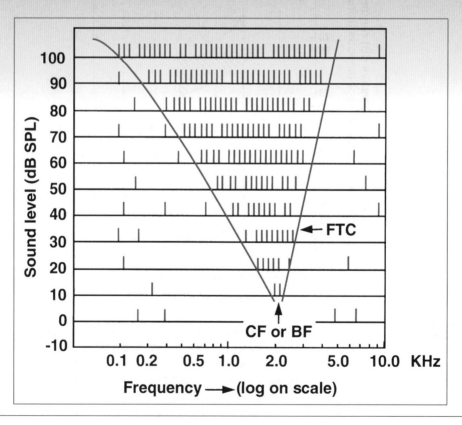

VIGNETTE 3.5   Illustration of response area and FTC of nerve fiber *(Continued)*

The figure illustrates how this area can be mapped out. A series of response histories from an auditory nerve are displayed. The vertical location of these response tracings from the nerve fiber correspond to the level of the sound presented to the ear, as noted along the y-axis. The lowest tracing shows the spikes or action potentials (short vertical lines) recorded from this nerve fiber for a sound that had a level of 0 dB SPL as it increased gradually in frequency from 100 Hz (left-hand portion) to 10,000 Hz (right-hand portion). Only a few spikes occurred during the several seconds required to progress from a sound of 100 Hz to one of 10,000 Hz. This tracing essentially describes the spontaneous activity of the nerve fiber: the sound was not intense enough to produce a response in the nerve fiber.

Next, the sound stimulus is increased to 10 dB SPL (second tracing from bottom) and again gradually increased in frequency from 100 to 10,000 Hz. Now there is an increase in rate of firing (more vertical lines) near the frequency of 2000 Hz. Thus, this particular nerve fiber appears to respond best (i.e., at the lowest sound intensity) at a frequency of 2000 Hz. This frequency corresponds to this nerve fiber's best, or characteristic, frequency (BF or CF).

As the pure tone increases by another 10 dB to a level of 20 dB SPL, the nerve fiber reveals a broader range of frequencies to which it responds at a rate greater than its spontaneous firing rate. This range now extends from approximately 1500 to 2200 Hz. As the level of the tone continues to increase in 10-dB steps and sweeps the frequency from 100 to 10,000 Hz, the frequency range over which the nerve fiber responds continues to broaden. A line connecting the border between spontaneous activity and increased firing rate at each level to those at adjacent levels defines the response area. This border is essentially the FTC for the nerve fiber. The FTC is sometimes referred to as the tuning curve of the nerve fiber because it indicates the frequency to which the nerve fiber is tuned (in this case, 2000 Hz). The FTC indicates the response area of the fiber and its best frequency. With a best frequency of 2000 Hz, this auditory nerve fiber originated from somewhere in the middle of the cochlea between the high-frequency basal portion and the low-frequency apex.

---

frequency corresponds to a place within the nerve bundle. This mapping of the frequency of the sound wave to place of maximum activity within an anatomic structure is referred to as *tonotopic organization*. It is a fundamental anatomic property of the auditory system from the cochlea through the auditory cortex.

Temporal or time domain information is also coded by fibers of the auditory nerve. Consider, for example, the discharge pattern that occurs within a nerve fiber when that stimulus is a sinusoid that lies within the response area of the nerve fiber. The pattern of spikes that occurs under such conditions is illustrated in Figure 3.14. When the single nerve fiber discharges, it always does so at essentially the same location on the stimulus waveform. In Figure 3.14, this happens to be the positive peak of the waveform. Notice also that it may not fire during every cycle of the stimulus waveform. Nonetheless, if one were to record the interval between successive spikes and examine the number of times each interval occurred, a histogram of the results would look like that shown in Figure 3.14. This histogram, known simply as an interval histogram, indicates that the most frequent interspike interval corresponds to the period of the waveform. All other peaks in the histogram occur at integer multiples of the period. Thus, the nerve fiber is able to encode the period of the waveform. This holds true for nerve fibers with characteristic frequencies less than approximately 5000 Hz. As discussed in Chapter 2, if we know the period of a sinusoidal waveform, we know

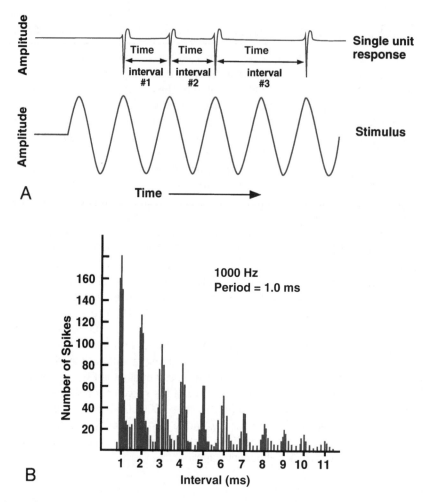

FIGURE 3.14 **A.** The synchronization of nerve fiber firings to the stimulus waveform. The nerve fiber always fires at the same point of the waveform, although it may not fire every cycle. The intervals between successive firings of the nerve fiber can be measured and stored for later analysis. **B.** A histogram of the interspike intervals measured in **A.** An interval of 1 ms was the most frequently occurring interval, having occurred approximately 180 times. This corresponds to the period of the waveform in **A.**

its frequency ($f = 1/T$). Hence, the nerve fibers responding in the manner depicted in Figure 3.14 could code the frequency of the acoustic stimulus according to the timing of discharges. For frequencies up to 5000 Hz, the neural firing is synchronized to the sound stimulus, as in Figure 3.14A. By combining synchronized firings for several nerve fibers, it is possible to encode the period of sounds up to 5000 Hz in frequency.

The electrical activity of the auditory nerve can also be recorded from more remote locations. In this case, however, the action potentials are not being measured from single nerve fibers. Recorded electrical activity under these circumstances represents the composite response from a large number of nerve fibers. For this reason, this composite electrical response is referred to frequently as the whole-nerve action potential. The whole-nerve action potential can be recorded in human subjects from the ear canal or from the medial wall of the middle ear cavity by placing a needle electrode through the eardrum (with local anesthesia applied, of course!). Because the whole-nerve action potential represents the summed activity of several nerve fibers, the more fibers can be made to fire simultaneously, the greater the amplitude of the response. For this reason, brief abrupt acoustic signals, such as clicks or short-duration pure tones, are used as stimuli. Recall, however, that the traveling wave begins in the base and travels toward the apex. It takes roughly 2 to 4 ms for the wave to travel the full length of the cochlea from the base to apex. Even for abrupt stimuli, such as clicks, the nerve fibers are not triggered simultaneously throughout the cochlea. Fibers associated with the basal high-frequency region respond synchronously to the stimulus presentation. Fibers originating farther up the cochlea will fire later (up to 2 to 4 ms later). Those firing in synchrony will provide the largest contribution to the whole-nerve action potential. Consequently, the whole-nerve action potential does not represent the activity of the entire nerve but reflects primarily the response of the synchronous high-frequency fibers associated with the base of the cochlea.

The input-output function for the whole-nerve action potential differs considerably from that described previously for single nerve fibers. For the whole-nerve action potential, the response is measured in terms of its amplitude or latency, not its spike rate. The input-output function of the whole-nerve action potential shows a steady increase in amplitude with increase in stimulus level. This is illustrated in Figure 3.15. Also shown is a plot of the latency of the response as a function of stimulus intensity. Latency refers to the interval between stimulus onset and the onset of the neural response. As stimulus intensity increases, the latency of the response decreases. Thus, as response amplitude increases with intensity, response latency decreases. The plot of response latency as a function of stimulus intensity is called a latency intensity function. The latency intensity function is of primary importance in clinical electrophysiologic assessment of auditory function.

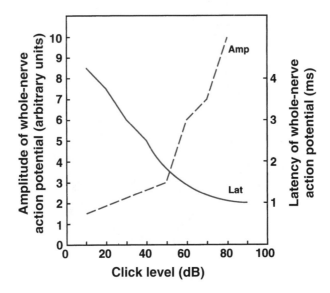

FIGURE 3.15 Amplitude intensity (left ordinate) and latency intensity (right ordinate) functions for the whole-nerve action potential. As intensity increases, the amplitude (Amp) of the action potential increases and the latency (Lat) of the response decreases.

AUDITORY CENTRAL NERVOUS SYSTEM

Once the action potentials have been generated in the cochlear branch of the auditory nerve, the electrical activity progresses up toward the cortex. This network of nerve fibers is frequently referred to as the auditory central nervous system (auditory CNS). The nerve fibers that carry information in the form of action potentials up the auditory CNS toward the cortex form part of the ascending or afferent pathways. Nerve impulses can also be sent toward the periphery from the cortex or brainstem centers. The fibers carrying such information compose the descending or efferent pathways.

Figure 3.16 is a simplified schematic diagram of the ascending auditory CNS. All nerve fibers from the cochlea terminate at the cochlear nucleus on the same side. From here, however, several possible paths are available. Most nerve fibers cross over, or decussate, at some point along the auditory CNS, so that the activity of the right ear is represented most strongly on the left side of the cortex and vice versa. The crossover, however, is not complete. From the superior olives through the cortex, activity from both ears is represented on each side. All ascending fibers terminate in the medial geniculate body before ascending to the cortex. Thus, all ascending fibers within the brainstem portion of the auditory CNS synapse at the cochlear nucleus and at the medial geniculate body, taking one of several paths between these two points, with many paths having additional intervening nerve fibers. Vignette 3.6 describes measurement of the auditory brainstem response and its correlation with anatomic structure.

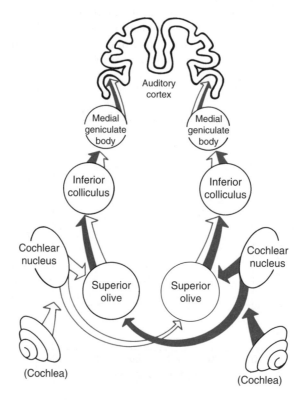

FIGURE 3.16 The ascending pathways of the auditory central nervous system. *Red arrows*, input from the right ear; *white arrows*, input from the left ear. (Adapted from Yost WA, Nielsen DW. Fundamentals of Hearing: An Introduction, 2nd ed. New York: Holt, Rinehart, & Winston, 1985:98.)

VIGNETTE 3.6   Auditory brainstem response measurements

It was mentioned earlier that the whole-nerve action potential represented the summed response of many single nerve fibers firing synchronously in response to an abrupt acoustic signal. It was also mentioned that this potential could be recorded remotely from the ear canal. The left-hand portion of the drawing that accompanies this vignette shows a patient with electrodes pasted to the skin of the forehead, the top of the head (vertex), and the area behind the pinna (the mastoid prominence). The tracing in the right-hand portion of this illustration shows the electrical activity recorded from the patient. The acoustic stimulus is a brief click that produces synchronized responses from nerve fibers in the cochlea and the brainstem portion of the auditory CNS. The tracing represents the average of 2000 stimuli presented at a moderate intensity at a rate of 11 clicks per second. Approximately 3 minutes is required to present all 2000 stimuli and to obtain the average response shown here. The time scale for the x-axis of the tracing spans from 0 to 10 ms. This represents a 10-ms interval beginning with the onset of the click stimulus. The tracing shows several distinct bumps or waves, with the first appearing at approximately 1.5 ms after stimulus onset. This first wave, labeled *I*, is believed to be a remote recording of the whole-nerve action potential from the closest portion of the auditory nerve.

Approximately 1 ms later, 2.5 ms after stimulus onset, wave *II* is observed. This wave is believed to be the response of the more distant portion of the auditory nerve. Another millisecond later the electrical activity has traveled to the next center in the brainstem, the cochlear nucleus, and produces the response recorded as wave *III*. Wave *IV* represents the activity of the superior olivary complex. Wave *V* represents the response of the lateral lemniscus, a structure lying between the superior olives and the inferior colliculus. Waves *VI* and *VII* (the two unlabeled bumps after wave *V*) represent the response of the latter brainstem structure.

The response shown in the right-hand tracing is known as an auditory brainstem response (ABR). It has proved very useful in a wide variety of clinical applications, from assessment of the functional integrity of the peripheral and brainstem portions of the ascending auditory CNS to assessment of hearing in infants or difficult-to-test patients. Additional related information may be found in the advanced material section at the end of this chapter.

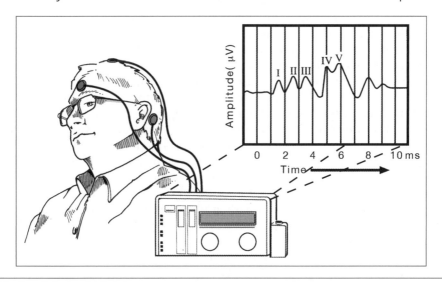

We have already reviewed the simple coding of information available in the responses of the auditory nerve fibers. The mapping of frequency to place within the cochlea, for example, was preserved in the responses of the nerve fibers in that fibers having high characteristic frequencies originated from the high-frequency base of the cochlea. The period of the waveform could also be coded for stimulus frequencies less than 5000 Hz. In addition, the intensity of the stimulus was coded over a limited range (30 to 40 dB) by the discharge rate of the fiber. At the level of the cochlear nucleus, it is already apparent that the ascending auditory pathway begins processing information by converting this fairly simple code into more complex codes. The coding of timing information, for example, is much more complex in the cochlear nucleus. In addition, some nerve fibers within the cochlear nucleus have a much broader range of intensities (up to 100 dB) over which the discharge rate increases steadily with sound intensity. As one probes nerve fibers at various centers within the auditory CNS, a tremendous diversity of responses is evident.

Despite this increasing anatomic and physiologic complexity, one thing that appears to be preserved throughout the auditory CNS is tonotopic organization. At each brainstem center and within the auditory portions of the cortex, there is an orderly mapping of frequency to place. This can be demonstrated by measuring the characteristic frequency of nerve fibers encountered at various locations within a given brainstem center or within the cortex.

Another principle underlying the auditory CNS is redundancy. That is, information represented in the neural code from one ear has multiple representations at various locations within the auditory system. Every auditory nerve fiber, for example, splits into two fibers before entering the cochlear nucleus, with each branch supplying a different region of the cochlear nucleus. In addition, from the superior olives through the auditory areas of the cortex, information from both ears is represented at each location in the auditory CNS.

Our knowledge of the ascending pathway of the auditory CNS is far from complete. We know even less about the descending pathways. This is a result, in part, of the small number of efferent nerve fibers involved in this pathway. There are approximately 2 descending efferent fibers for every 100 ascending afferent nerve fibers. Essentially, the same brainstem centers are involved in the descending pathway as were involved in the ascending path, although an entirely separate set of nerve fibers is used. The last fiber in this descending pathway runs from the superior olivary complex to enter the cochlea on the same side or the cochlea on the opposite side. These fibers are referred to as either the crossed or the uncrossed olivocochlear bundles. Most (60–80%) of these fibers cross over from the superior olivary complex on one side to the cochlea on the other side and innervate the outer hair cells. The remaining fibers make up the uncrossed bundle and appear to innervate the inner hair cells.

Not all descending fibers terminate at the cochlear nerve fibers. Descending fibers may modify incoming neurally coded sensory information at any of the centers along the auditory CNS. In addition, they may either facilitate or inhibit responses along the ascending auditory pathway. In other words, electrical stimulation of some descending fibers increases the discharges recorded from fibers at lower centers, whereas stimulation of other descending fibers results in decreased activity at lower centers. Thus, the descending efferent system regulates, modifies, and shapes the incoming sensory information.

Reflexive contractions of the middle ear muscles caused by the presentation of a sound stimulus may also be considered a regulating mechanism for the incoming sensory information. The reflex pathway is illustrated schematically in Figure 3.17.

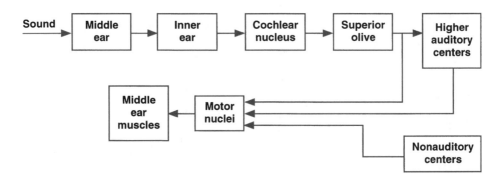

FIGURE 3.17   The reflex arc for the middle ear muscle reflex.

Incoming sensory information enters through the peripheral auditory system and ascends to the superior olive. If the sound is sufficiently intense, descending information is routed to motor nuclei that control the contraction of the middle ear muscles. This explains why the reflexive contraction of middle ear muscles caused by sound stimuli is a consensual phenomenon, as mentioned previously. Information from the cochlear nucleus goes to both superior olives, so that sound stimulation on one side yields middle ear muscle contraction on both sides.

CLINICAL AUDITORY ELECTROPHYSIOLOGY

In our discussion of auditory electrophysiology earlier in this chapter, we focused primarily on peripheral electrophysiology, mainly the cochlear receptor potentials and the action potentials from the auditory nerve. Much of the information reviewed was for receptor potentials from individual hair cells or action potentials from individual nerve fibers.

Although this is the most fundamental form of electrophysiologic information, clinical electrophysiology never makes use of electrical potentials from individual cells. Rather, clinical auditory electrophysiology involves the recording of gross electrical potentials representing the activity of hundreds or thousands of individual hair cells or nerve fibers. These tiny electrical potentials are usually recorded from remote locations on the surface of the head and require amplification and computer averaging of at least several hundred stimulus presentations to be visible.

To give you some perspective on the size and temporal sequence of many of the more common electric potentials used in audiology, consider the hypothetical electrical waveform in Figure 3.18. We have assumed that a special recording electrode has been placed in each ear canal and that a third electrode has been applied to the top of the scalp (vertex). The stimulus is a 2-ms burst of a 2000-Hz pure tone, as shown in the top waveform. This stimulus is presented 1000 times at 11 tone bursts per second, and the electrical potentials recorded have been averaged to produce the electrical waveform in the lower portion of the figure. The first electrical potentials to be recorded are the gross cochlear microphonic (*CM*), which looks like a miniature version of the sound stimulus, and the summating potential (*SP*), which appears as a vertical shifting of the CM away from the zero line. Next is the whole-nerve action potential (WNAP), which also corresponds to waves I and II of the auditory brainstem

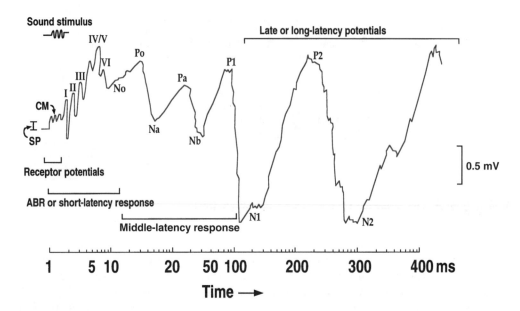

FIGURE 3.18 Hypothetical clinical electrophysiologic response recorded from the scalp of a human, showing the electrical responses from early responses of the auditory nerve through later responses from the higher centers of the auditory system (bottom portion) in response to a brief (2-ms) 2000-Hz pure tone (top portion). CM, cochlear microphonic; SP, summating potential.

response (ABR). The ABR consists of a series of five to seven bumps or waves in the electrical waveform that appear in the first 10 ms after the stimulus has been presented. Next we have a larger and later electrical response known as the middle latency response (MLR), followed by a still larger and later potential referred to as the late evoked potential. The MLR is believed to originate from the upper portions of the auditory brainstem, and the late potential comes from the auditory cortex. Thus, the hypothetical electrical waveform shows the progression of electrical activity from the cochlea to the auditory cortex. This waveform is hypothetical in that the recording procedures and stimulus characteristics that are ideal for one type of electrical potential are often not the same ones used to record one of the other potentials. Nonetheless, it suffices to introduce the various electrical potentials that can be recorded easily from surface electrodes by the audiologist.

Of the electrical potentials available to the audiologist, the one that has received the most investigation and most frequent use clinically is the ABR. The ABR is of value because it is very robust and can be recorded reliably and easily, yet it is sensitive to dysfunction occurring from the auditory periphery to the upper brainstem portions of the auditory central nervous system. Thus, it is useful in assisting with detection of neurologic problems along a large portion of the auditory CNS; also, it can be used to estimate the hearing loss in a patient. Although a normal ABR waveform does not indicate normal auditory function (i.e., a problem could lie further up the auditory pathway), an abnormal or absent ABR waveform in response to acoustic stimulation does indicate significant hearing loss or neurologic dysfunction in approximately 95% of such cases. ABR has been used to screen the hearing of newborns and to estimate hearing thresholds in patients who are difficult to test. It is an extremely valuable clinical tool for the audiologist. Vignette 3.7 illustrates how the combined use of OAEs and the ABR led to the discovery of an intriguing disorder referred to as auditory neuropathy.

Audiologists are keenly interested in applying emerging science and technology to obtain a better understanding of challenging cases encountered in the clinic. Although ABR has been used as a clinical tool since the 1970s, widespread clinical application of OAEs emerged only in the mid 1990s. In many diagnostic evaluations, both the ABR and OAEs were obtained from the same patients. After doing so with hundreds or thousands of cases, some clinicians began to notice a surprising pattern in some of these patients.

A robust ABR could not be measured or wave latencies were prolonged considerably, despite the presence of perfectly normal OAEs! The presence of normal OAEs, as noted previously, is an indication that the entire auditory periphery, from the outer ear to the outer hair cells within the inner ear, is normal. Yet the ABR suggested that pathology was present in the auditory system at or below the brainstem. Most often, the abnormalities in ABR waveforms appeared first in the early waves of the response. Subsequent radiologic or surgical investigation of many of these individuals failed to detect the presence of significant brainstem or auditory nerve pathology, such as tumors. This pattern of results in the OAE and ABR measures is called auditory neuropathy and is believed to indicate a dysfunction of the inner hair cells or the first-order afferent fibers of the auditory nerve. It has been suggested that another common feature of such cases is difficulty understanding speech, especially in noisy conditions, which is greater than one would expect given the measured hearing loss. Although auditory neuropathy is believed to be a fairly rare clinical disorder, further research is being conducted to further validate its existence and to establish its prevalence. The case of auditory neuropathy, however, is just a relatively recent example of how audiologists attempt to capitalize on emerging hearing science to solve sometimes puzzling clinical problems, whether of a diagnostic or rehabilitative nature.

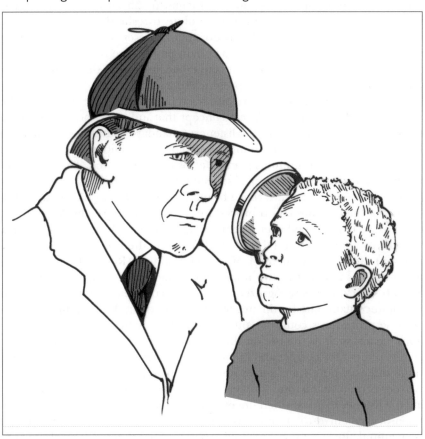

THE PERCEPTION OF SOUND

The basic structure and some key aspects of the physiologic function of the auditory system have been reviewed; the remainder of this chapter reviews some fundamental aspects of the perception of sound by humans. We have examined the acoustics involved in the generation and propagation of a sound wave and have reviewed its conversion into a complex neural code. This code of incoming sensory information can influence the behavior of a human subject, whether the sound is the loud whistle of an oncoming train or the cry of a hungry infant. The study of behavioral responses to acoustic stimulation is referred to as psychoacoustics.

Psychoacoustics

Psychoacoustics is the study of the relationship between the sound stimulus and the behavioral response it produces in the subject. We have already discussed how the important parameters of the acoustic stimulus can be measured. Much of psychoacoustics concerns itself with the more challenging task of appropriately measuring the listener's response. Two primary means have evolved through which the psychoacoustician measures responses from the listener. The first, known generally as the discrimination procedure, is used to assess the smallest difference that would allow a listener to discriminate between two stimulus conditions. The end result is an estimate of a threshold of a certain type. A tone of specified amplitude, frequency, and starting phase, for example, can be discriminated from the absence of such a signal. In this particular case, one is measuring the absolute threshold for hearing. That is, the absolute threshold is a statistical concept that represents the lowest sound pressure level at which the tone can be heard a certain percentage of the time. This threshold is often referred to as a detection threshold because one is determining the stimulus parameters required to detect the presence of a signal.

Discrimination procedures have also been used to measure difference thresholds. A difference threshold is a statistical concept that indicates the smallest change in a stimulus that can be detected by the listener. A standard sound that is fixed in intensity, frequency, starting phase, and duration is employed. A comparison stimulus that differs typically in one of these stimulus parameters is then presented. The difference threshold indicates how much the comparison stimulus must differ from the standard signal to permit detection of the difference by the listener a certain percentage of the time.

Many of the discrimination procedures used to measure absolute and difference thresholds were developed over a century ago. Three such procedures, referred to as the classic psychophysical methods, are (*a*) the method of limits, (*b*) the method of adjustment, and (*c*) the method of constant stimuli. Research conducted in more recent years has resulted in two important developments regarding the use of these procedures. First, it was recognized that thresholds measured with these procedures were not uncontaminated estimates of sensory function. Rather, thresholds measured with these procedures could be altered considerably by biasing the subject through various means, such as the use of different sets of instructions or different schedules of reinforcement for correct and incorrect responses. The threshold for the detection of a low-intensity pure tone, for example, can be changed by instructing the listener to be very certain that a tone was heard before responding accordingly or by encouraging the listener to guess when uncertain. The magnitude of sensation evoked within the sensory system during stimulus presentation should remain unchanged under these manipulations. Yet the threshold was noticeably affected. Threshold as measured with any of these traditional psychophysical procedures is affected by factors other than the magnitude of sensation evoked by the signal. For the audiologist, however, the traditional psychophysical procedures have proven to be valid and reliable tools with which to measure various aspects of hearing in clinical settings as long as care is used in instructing the listeners and administering the procedures.

The second recent development that led to a modification of the classic psychophysical procedures was the creation of adaptive test procedures. The current procedure advocated for the measurement of absolute threshold of hearing (discussed in Chapter 4) uses an adaptive modification of the method of limits. Adaptive procedures increase the efficiency of the paradigm without sacrificing the accuracy or reliability of the procedure.

In addition to discrimination procedures, a second class of techniques has been developed to quantify a subject's responses to acoustic signals. These procedures, known generally as scaling techniques, attempt to measure sensation directly. In the study of hearing, they are used most frequently to measure the sensation of loudness, though they have also been used to quantify other sensations, such as pitch. The results from one of these procedures, magnitude estimation, are shown in Figure 3.19. In the magnitude estimation technique, subjects simply assign numbers to the perceived loudness of a series of stimuli. In the case shown in Figure 3.19, the stimuli differed only in intensity. The average results fall along a straight line when plotted on log-log coordinates. Both the x-axis and the y-axis in Figure 3.19 are logarithmic. Recall that the decibel scale, the x-axis in this figure, involved the logarithm of a pressure ratio: sound pressure level in decibels = $20 \log (p_1/p_2)$. Comparable results have been obtained for other sensations, such as brightness, vibration on the fingertip, and electric shock. In all cases, a straight line fits the average data very well when plotted on log-log coordinates. From these extensive data, a law was developed to relate the perceived magnitude of sensation (S) to the physical intensity of the stimulus (I) in the following manner: $S = kI^x$, where k is an arbitrary constant and x is an exponent that varies with the sensation under investigation. This law is known as Stevens' power law in honor of the scientist S. S. Stevens, who discovered and developed it.

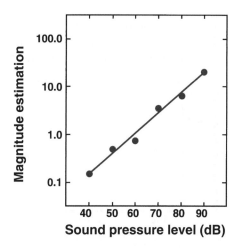

FIGURE 3.19 Hypothetical results from a magnitude estimation experiment in which the perceived loudness was measured for various sound levels. The results fall along a straight line when both axes are logarithmic (recall use of logarithms in the calculation of decibels).

A convenient feature of a power function plotted on log-log coordinates is that the slope of the line fit to the data is the exponent, *x*.

Finally, a procedure that has been used extensively in psychoacoustics to measure auditory sensations via the subject's response is the matching procedure. The matching procedure is a cross between discrimination procedures and scaling procedures. The technique is similar to that of the method of adjustment (one of the classic psychophysical methods), but its goal is to quantify a subjective attribute of sound, such as loudness or pitch. The matching procedures enable the experimenter to determine a set of stimulus parameters that all yield the same subjective sensation. A pure tone fixed at 1000 Hz and 70 dB SPL, for example, may be presented to one ear of a listener and a second pure tone of 8000 Hz presented to the other ear in an alternating fashion. The subject controls the intensity of the 8000-Hz tone until it is judged to be equal in loudness to the 1000-Hz, 70-dB SPL reference tone. Data in the literature indicate that the 8000-Hz tone would have to be set to 80 to 85 dB SPL to achieve a loudness match in the case presented above.

Hearing Threshold

Let us now examine how these procedures have been applied to the study of the perception of sound. The results obtained from the measurement of hearing thresholds at various frequencies are depicted in Figure 3.20. The sound pressure level that is just detectable varies with frequency, especially below 500 Hz and above 8000 Hz. The slope of the function in the low frequencies is a result of the attenuation of lower frequencies by the middle ear. The frequency contour of the hearing threshold has a minimum in the 2000- to 4000-Hz range. This is attributable, in large part, to the amplification of signals in this frequency range by the outer ear, as discussed earlier in this chapter. The range of audibility of the normal-hearing human ear is described frequently as 20 to 20,000 Hz. Acoustic signals at frequencies above or below this range typically cannot be heard by the normal human ear.

Masking

The phenomenon of masking has also been studied in detail. Masking refers to the ability of one acoustic signal to obscure the presence of another acoustic signal so that it cannot be detected. A whisper might be audible, for example, in a quiet environment.

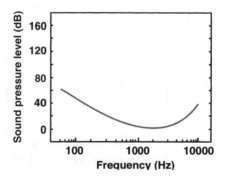

FIGURE 3.20 Average normal threshold SPL plotted as a function of frequency for binaural (two-ear) listening in a free field. (Adapted from Sivian LJ, White SD. Minimum audible pressure and minimum audible field. J Acoust Soc Am 4:288–321, 1933.)

In a noisy industrial environment, however, such a weak acoustic signal would be masked by the more intense factory noise.

The masking of pure tone signals by noise has been studied extensively. To consider the results, however, we must first examine some important acoustic characteristics of the masking noise. Briefly, two measures of intensity can be used to describe the level of a noise. These two measures are the total power (TP) and the noise power per unit (1-Hz) bandwidth, or spectral density (N_o). The TP in decibels SPL is the quantity measured by most measuring devices, such as sound level meters. The N_o of the noise is not measured directly with a sound level meter. Rather, it is calculated from the following equation: $10 \log_{10} N_o = 10 \log_{10} TP + 10 \log_{10} BW$, where BW is the bandwidth of the noise in hertz. The quantity $10 \log10 N_o$ is the spectrum level in units of decibels SPL per hertz and represents the average noise power in a 1-Hz band. For broadband noises, the spectrum level determines the masking produced at various frequencies.

Figure 3.21 illustrates data obtained from one of the early studies of masking produced by broadband noise. These data have been replicated several times since. The lowest curve in this figure depicts the threshold in a quiet environment; all other curves represent masked thresholds obtained for various levels of the noise masker. These levels are expressed as the spectrum level of the masker. The lowest noise levels are not effective maskers at low frequencies. That is, hearing thresholds measured for low-frequency pure tones in the presence of a broadband noise having $N_o = 0$ dB SPL/Hz are the same as thresholds in quiet. At all frequencies, however, once the noise begins to produce some masking, a 10-dB increase in noise intensity produces a 10-dB increase in masked threshold for the pure tone. Once the noise level that just begins to produce masking has been determined, the desired amount of masking can be produced simply by increasing the noise level by a corresponding amount.

How might the masking produced by a noise be affected by decreasing the bandwidth of the noise? Figure 3.22 illustrates data obtained several decades ago from a now-classic masking experiment. The results of this experiment, referred to frequently

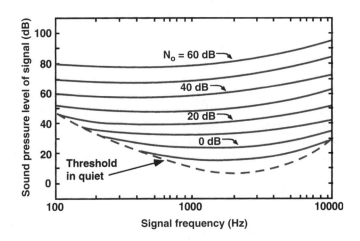

FIGURE 3.21 Threshold in quiet and masked threshold for various noise spectrum levels (N_o). Threshold was measured at several frequencies in the presence of a broadband noise. (Adapted from Hawkins JE Jr, Stevens SS. The masking of pure tones and of speech by white noise. J Acoust Soc Am 22:6–13, 1950.)

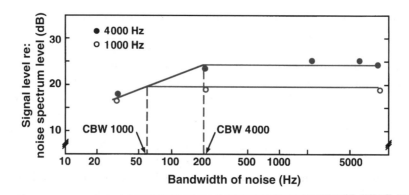

FIGURE **3.22** Results from a band-narrowing experiment. Data for two frequencies, 1000 and 4000 Hz, are shown. The critical bandwidths at each frequency are illustrated by dashed vertical lines. For bandwidths greater than the critical bandwidth (CBW), masking remained unchanged. (Data from Fletcher H. Auditory patterns. Rev Mod Physics 12:47–65, 1940.)

as the band-narrowing experiment, have been replicated several times since. Masked threshold in decibels SPL is plotted as a function of the bandwidth of the masker in hertz. Results for two different pure-tone frequencies are shown. The *open circles* represent data for a 1000-Hz pure tone, and the *solid circles* depict data for a 4000-Hz pure tone. When the band of masking noise was narrowed, the tone was kept in the center of the noise, and the spectrum level of the noise was held constant. For both frequencies, the masked threshold remains the same as the bandwidth decreases to a level called the critical bandwidth. Continued decreases in bandwidth beyond the critical bandwidth reduce the masking produced by the noise, as reflected in the decrease in masked threshold.

The critical bandwidth, first derived from the band-narrowing masking experiment, has proved to apply to a wide variety of psychoacoustic phenomena. For the audiologist, however, one of the most important implications drawn from the band-narrowing experiment is that noise having a bandwidth just exceeding the critical bandwidth is as effective a masker for a pure tone centered in the noise as a broad-band noise of the same spectrum level. As Chapter 4 shows, the audiologist frequently must introduce masking into a patient's ear. A broadband masking noise can be uncomfortably loud to a patient. The loudness can be reduced by decreasing its bandwidth while maintaining the same spectrum level. A masking noise having a bandwidth only slightly greater than the critical bandwidth will be just as effective as broadband noise in terms of its masking but much less loud. The narrow band of noise is more appropriate for use as a masking sound when measuring hearing threshold for pure tones in patients because of its reduced loudness but equal masking capability.

Loudness

Loudness is another psychoacoustic phenomenon that has been studied extensively. The effects of signal bandwidth on loudness, alluded to in the discussion of masking, have been investigated in detail. Basically, as the bandwidth of the stimulus increases beyond the critical bandwidth, an increasing number of adjacent critical bands are stimulated, resulting in an increase in loudness. Thus, broadband signals are louder than narrow-band signals at the same spectrum level.

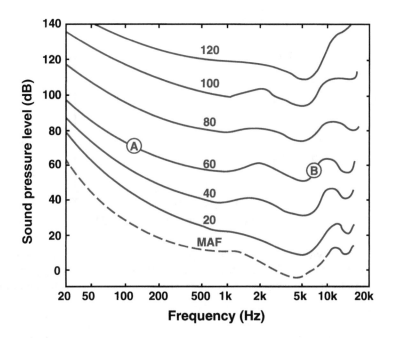

FIGURE 3.23 Equal-loudness contours. Each curve displays the combinations of frequency and intensity judged to be equal in loudness to a 1000-Hz tone having SPL as indicated above each contour. Point A indicates that a 125-Hz tone at 75 dB SPL is as loud as a 1000-Hz tone at 60 dB. (Frequency scale is logarithmic.) MAF, minimum audible field, or the threshold contour for free-field testing. (Adapted from Fletcher H, Munson WN. Loudness, its definition, measurement, and calculation. J Acoust Soc Am 5:82–108, 1933.)

For pure tones, loudness also varies with frequency. This has been established using the matching procedure described previously. Figure 3.23 depicts so-called equal-loudness contours that have been derived with this technique. A given contour displays the SPL at various frequencies necessary to match the loudness of a 1000-Hz pure tone at the level indicated by the contour. For example, on the curve labeled *20*, the function coincides with a sound pressure level of 20 dB SPL at 1000 Hz, whereas on the curve labeled *60*, the function corresponds to 60 dB SPL at 1000 Hz. The contour labeled *60* indicates combinations of frequencies and intensities that were matched in loudness to a 60-dB SPL, 1000-Hz pure tone. All combinations of stimulus intensity and frequency lying along that contour are said to have a loudness level of 60 phons (pronounced *phones*, as in *telephones*). Thus, a 125-Hz pure tone at 70 dB SPL (point labeled *A* in Fig. 3.23) and an 8000-Hz tone at 58 dB SPL (point labeled *B*) are equivalent in loudness to a 60-dB SPL, 1000-Hz pure tone. All three of those stimuli have a loudness level of 60 phons.

In Figure 3.23 stimulus intensity must be increased by 110 dB to go from a loudness level of 10 phons (threshold) to 120 phons at 1000 Hz. At 100 Hz, only an 80-dB increase is required to span that same change in loudness. From this we can conclude that loudness increases more rapidly at low frequencies than at intermediate frequencies. It took only an 80-dB increase in sound level to go from a sound that was just audible (10 phons) to one that was uncomfortably loud (120 phons) at 100 Hz, whereas an increase of 110 dB was needed to cover this same range of loudness at 1000 Hz.

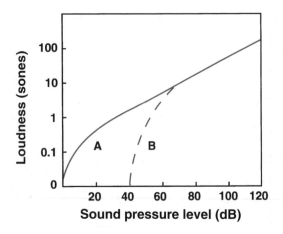

FIGURE 3.24   The growth of loudness with intensity in quiet **(A)** and in the presence of a background noise that produced 40 dB of masking **(B)**. (Loudness scale is logarithmic.) Functions comparable to **B** are also obtained in listeners who have sensorineural hearing loss.

Another scale of loudness is the sone scale, derived by first defining the loudness of a 1000-Hz, 40-dB SPL pure tone as 1 sone. Next, the listener is asked to set the intensity of a second comparison stimulus so that it produces a loudness sensation either one-half or twice that of the 1-sone standard stimulus. These intensities define the sound levels associated with 0.5 and 2 sones, respectively. This procedure is repeated, with the sound having a loudness of either 0.5 or 2 sones serving as the new standard signal. Figure 3.24 illustrates the relationship between the increase of loudness in sones and the increase in sound intensity. Consistent with Stevens' law, described previously, we find that the loudness-growth function is a straight line, with the exception of intensities near threshold, when plotted on log-log coordinates. The slope of this line is 0.6, indicating that Stevens' law for loudness is: $L = k P^{0.6}$, where L is loudness, k is a constant, and P is sound pressure. Over the linear range of the function in Figure 3.24, a 10-dB increase in sound pressure level yields a doubling of loudness. At 1000 Hz, an increase in sound pressure level from 40 to 50 dB SPL or from 80 to 90 dB SPL corresponds to a doubling of loudness.

The *dashed line* in Figure 3.24 illustrates a loudness growth function obtained at 1000 Hz in the presence of a broadband masking noise. The intersection of the x-axis by the *dashed line* at 40 dB SPL indicates that the threshold has been elevated 40 dB (from 0 to 40 dB SPL) because of the masking noise. As intensity increases slightly above threshold, comparison of the two functions indicates that the loudness of a 50-dB SPL tone is greater in the quiet condition (2 sones) than in the masked condition (0.2 sones). At higher intensities, however, the two functions merge, so that an 80-dB SPL tone has a loudness of 16 sones in both cases. Thus, in the masked condition, loudness grows very rapidly to catch up with the loudness perceived in the unmasked condition. This rapid growth of loudness is also a characteristic of ears that have sensorineural hearing loss, which affects the hair cells in the cochlea. The rapid growth of loudness in ears with sensorineural hearing loss is known as loudness recruitment. Its presence helps signify that the hearing loss is caused by pathology within the cochlea. Unfortunately, loudness recruitment presents the audiologist with considerable difficulties in attempting to fit affected patients with amplification devices, such as hearing aids. Low-level sounds must be amplified a specified amount to make them audible to the listener with hearing loss. If high-level sounds are amplified by the same amount, however, they are uncomfortably loud, just as they would be in a normal ear.

Loudness is clearly one of the more salient perceptual features of a sound, and it has considerable clinical importance. Pitch is another very salient perceptual feature of sound, but it has less clinical relevance. Some basic aspects of pitch perception in normal listeners have been summarized in Vignette 3.8 as illustrated through the case of the missing fundamental.

VIGNETTE 3.8   Pitch perception and the case of the missing fundamental

The pitch of a sound is often one of its most salient perceptual characteristics. Musicians and hearing scientists have been interested in how humans perceive pitch for centuries, but probably the greatest progress in our understanding of pitch perception occurred during the 20th century.

In the late 19th century, probably the most widely accepted theory of pitch perception was based on a "place principle" akin to tonotopic organization, described in the discussion of basic auditory structure and function. Although many details of early place principle theories of pitch perception were incorrect, the basic premise that certain portions of the auditory system, especially the inner ear, were tuned to specific frequencies was correct. Basically, low-frequency pure tones produced a low pitch sensation and high-frequency pure tones produced a high pitch sensation because each frequency stimulated a different region or place within the inner ear.

In the late 19th and early 20th centuries, however, several researchers in the Netherlands produced a low-frequency pitch using sounds that were composed of only higher frequencies. An example of the amplitude spectrum for one such sound is shown in the figure. This sound is composed of pure tones at frequencies of 800, 1000, 1200, and 1400 Hz. Yet the pitch of this sound was judged to be 200 Hz by listeners. A frequency of 200 Hz would correspond to the fundamental frequency of these sounds, with 800 Hz being the fourth harmonic of 200 Hz (i.e., 800 Hz = 4 × 200 Hz), 1000 Hz being the fifth harmonic, 1200 Hz being the sixth harmonic, and 1400 Hz being the seventh harmonic of 200 Hz. For this reason, the pitch of such a series of pure tones is often referred to as the missing fundamental.

Now, the place theorists simply argued that the equipment or the ear (the middle ear was believed to be the culprit at the time) generated a distortion product that corresponded to the 200-Hz frequency, and the listener's pitch perception was dominated by this low-frequency distortion tone. Therefore, the fundamental frequency (200 Hz) wasn't really missing after all. In this way, the results were entirely consistent with the place theory. The complex of four pure tones from 800 to 1400 Hz generated a distortion product at 200 Hz, and this 200-Hz distortion product stimulated the place associated with a 200-Hz pure tone yielding a corresponding pitch.

To counter this argument, the Dutch researchers conducted the following experiment. A low-frequency noise was introduced with enough acoustical energy below 400 Hz to mask low-frequency tones of moderate intensity (as demonstrated with a pure tone at 200 Hz, for example). The four pure tones from 800 to 1400 Hz were played in this background of low-frequency noise, and a pitch of 200 Hz was again perceived. Basically, the low-frequency masking noise rendered the low-frequency region of the inner ear unusable, and yet a low-frequency pitch was still perceived when the four tones from 800 to 1400 Hz were presented. Clearly, the place theory could not account for these findings.

(continued)

VIGNETTE 3.8 **Pitch perception and the case of the missing fundamental** *(Continued)*

Recognizing the limitations of the place theory as a single explanation for the perception of pitch, hearing scientists began to focus on possible timing, or periodicity, cues in the four-tone complex. Today, although several details of pitch perception remain unexplained, most findings can be described by a duplex theory. This theory relies on exclusive use of place cues above approximately 5000 Hz (synchronization of nerve fiber firing breaks down at frequencies above approximately 5000 Hz, making periodicity cues unavailable). It also rests on exclusive use of timing cues for very low frequencies, below approximately 50 Hz, and a combination of periodicity and place cues for frequencies from 50 to 5000 Hz.

Incidentally, there is a standardized scale of pitch sensation, the mel scale (no, not named after a famous scientist named Mel but derived from *melody*). A pure tone of 1000 Hz at 40 dB SPL is said to have a pitch of 1000 mels (as well as a loudness of 1 sone and a loudness level of 40 phons). A sound with a pitch judged to be twice as high as this standard would have a pitch of 2000 mels, whereas one with half the pitch of the standard sound would be assigned a pitch value of 500 mels. Often, however, pitch is measured by matching the frequency of a pure tone to the perceived pitch of the sound under evaluation.

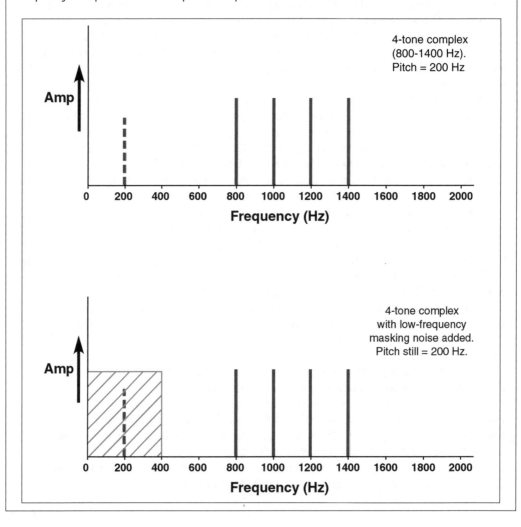

Binaural Hearing

The final section of this chapter deals with the manner in which the information encoded by one ear interacts with that encoded by the other ear. The processing of sound by two ears is referred to as binaural hearing.

The localization of sound in space is largely a binaural phenomenon. A sound originating on the right side of a listener will arrive first at the right ear because it is closer to the sound source. A short time later, the sound will reach the more distant left ear. This produces an interaural (between-ear) difference in the time of arrival of the sound at the two ears. The ear being stimulated first will signal the direction from which the sound arose. As might be expected, the magnitude of this interaural time difference will increase as the location of the sound source changes from straight ahead (called 0° azimuth) to straight out to the side (90° or 270° azimuth). As shown in Figure 3.25A when the sound originates directly in front of the listener, the length

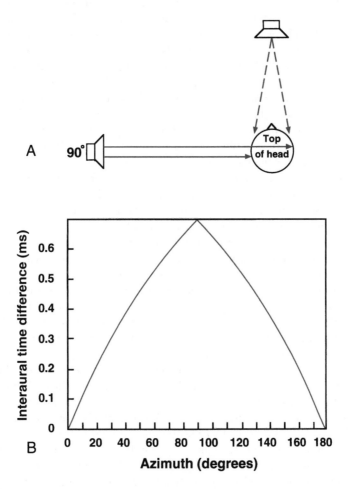

FIGURE 3.25   **A.** Path lengths from sound source to the left and right ears for 0° azimuth (*dashed lines*) and 90° azimuth (*solid lines*). **B.** The interaural time differences as a function of azimuth for the spherical head assumed in **A**. At 0° and 180°, the sound arrives at the left and right ears simultaneously, resulting in no interaural time difference. The maximum interaural time difference occurs at 90°.

of the path to both ears is the same, and there is no interaural difference in time of arrival of the sound. At the extreme right or left, however, the difference between the length of the path to the near ear and the length of the path to the far ear is greatest (and corresponds to the width of the head). This then will produce the maximum interaural time difference. Figure 3.25B illustrates the dependence of the interaural time difference on the azimuth of the sound source.

For frequencies below approximately 1500 Hz, the interaural time difference could also be encoded meaningfully into an interaural phase difference. Figure 3.25B shows that a 60° azimuth results in an interaural time difference of approximately 0.5 ms. This occurs for all frequencies. For a pure tone that completes one cycle in 1 ms (frequency = 1000 Hz), this means that the signal to the far ear would be starting 0.5 cycle after the signal to the near ear. The two signals therefore would have a 180° phase difference between the two ears. A pure tone of 500 Hz having a 2-ms period and originating from 60° azimuth, however, would only be delayed one-fourth of the period (0.5 ms/2.0 ms), corresponding to a 90° interaural phase difference. Thus, although interaural time differences are the same for all frequencies, the interaural phase differences resulting from these time differences vary with frequency.

Interaural intensity differences are also produced when a sound originates from a location in space. These differences result from a sound shadow being cast by the head. Recall from Chapter 2 and Vignette 2.5 that when the wavelength of the sound is small relative to the dimensions of the object, a sound shadow is produced. The magnitude of the sound shadow created by the head increases with frequency above 500 Hz. It produces interaural intensity differences of 20 dB at 6000 Hz for 90° or 270° azimuth. The intensity of a 6000-Hz pure tone at the near ear is 20 dB greater than that measured at the far ear when the sound originates straight to the side of the listener (90° or 270° azimuth). At 500 Hz, the maximum interaural intensity difference is less than 4 dB. The interaural intensity difference decreases to 0 dB at all frequencies for 0° azimuth (sound source straight ahead).

Thus, there are two primary acoustic cues for the localization of sound in space (specifically, the horizontal plane): interaural time differences and interaural intensity differences. The duplex theory of sound localization in the horizontal plane (left to right) maintains that both cues may be used over a wide range of frequencies by the listener in identifying the location of a sound source but that interaural time differences predominate at low frequencies and interaural intensity differences predominate at high frequencies. In contemporary theories of sound localization, several additional monaural and binaural cues are included, but interaural time and intensity differences are considered the strongest cues.

Masking has also been explored in considerable detail in the binaural system. Experiments conducted in the late 1940s and the 1950s indicated that certain combinations of binaural signals and maskers could make the signal more detectable than others. Consider the following example. A noise masker and a pure-tone signal are presented equally and identically to both ears. The signal threshold, that is, the sound level of the signal required to make it barely heard in the presence of the noise, is determined. Then the pure-tone signal is removed from one ear and the signal becomes *easier* to detect! This release from masking, named the masking level difference (MLD), corresponds to the change in threshold between two test conditions. The initial or reference threshold is usually determined for identical maskers and signals delivered to both ears. This is referred to as a diotic condition. Diotic stimulus presentations are those that deliver identical stimuli to both ears. Sometimes the reference threshold involves a masker and signal delivered to only one ear. This is called a monotic or monaural condition. After establishing the masked threshold in one of these reference conditions, the signal threshold is measured again under any one of several dichotic conditions. A dichotic test condition is one in which different stimuli are presented to the two ears. In the example in which the signal was removed from one ear, the removal of the signal made that condition a dichotic one. That is, one ear received the masker and the pure-tone signal, while the other received only the masker. In general, a signal is more readily detected under dichotic masking conditions than under diotic or monaural masking conditions. For a given dichotic condition, the MLD is greatest at low frequencies (100 to 500 Hz), increases with the intensity of the masker, and is typically 12 to 15 dB under optimal stimulus conditions.

SUMMARY

In this chapter, we review the structure and function of the auditory system. The anatomy and physiology of the auditory system are discussed in the first portion. The amplification and impedance-matching functions of the outer and middle ear are reviewed. The importance of both a temporal or timing code and a place code (tonotopic organization) within the auditory system is emphasized. Perceptual phenomena, such as loudness and masking, are also reviewed, with an emphasis on those features of clinical relevance.

References and Suggested Readings

Durrant JD, Lovrinic JH. Bases of Hearing Science. 3rd ed. Baltimore: Williams & Wilkins, 1995.

Geisler CD. From Sound to Synapse. New York: Oxford University, 1998.

Gelfand SA. Hearing: An Introduction to Psychological and Physiological Acoustics. 4th ed. New York: Marcel Dekker, 2004.

Hall JW. Handbook of Auditory Evoked Responses. Needham, MA: Allyn & Bacon, 1992.

Kidd J. Psychoacoustics. In Katz J, ed. Handbook of Clinical Audiology. 5th ed. Philadelphia: Lippincott Williams & Wilkins, 2002.

Möller AR. Auditory Physiology. New York: Academic, 1983.

Moore BCJ. An Introduction to the Psychology of Hearing. 5th ed. London: Academic, 2003.

Pickles JO. An Introduction to the Physiology of Hearing. 2nd ed. London: Academic, 1988.

Probst R, Lonsbury-Martin BL, Martin G. A review of otoacoustic emissions. J Acoust Soc Am 89:2027–2067, 1991.

Shaw EAG. The external ear. In Keidel WD, Neff WD, eds. Handbook of Sensory Physiology, vol 1. New York: Springer-Verlag, 1974:455–490.

von Bekesy G. Experiments in Hearing. New York: McGraw-Hill, 1960.

Wever EG, Lawrence M. Physiological Acoustics. Princeton, NJ: Princeton University, 1954.

Yost WA. Fundamentals of Hearing: An Introduction. 5th ed. New York: Academic, 2006.

Zemlin WR. Speech and Hearing Science: Anatomy and Physiology. 2nd ed. Englewood Cliffs, NJ: Prentice-Hall, 1988.

Zwicker E, Fastl H. Psychoacoustics. 3rd ed. Berlin: Springer-Verlag, 2007.

PART 2

Assessment of Auditory Function

Audiologic Measurement

Following completion of this chapter, the reader should be able to:

- Understand the procedures for measuring pure-tone threshold by air conduction and by bone conduction.
- Understand the procedures for measuring hearing sensitivity for speech (speech recognition threshold) and speech recognition.
- Identify situations requiring the use of contralateral masking and understand the concept of masking.
- Recognize the special modifications of these basic measurements needed for application to pediatric populations.
- Understand acoustic immittance measurements.
- Appreciate the way in which each test result represents just one aspect of the complete basic audiologic test battery.
- Appreciate and understand the basic concepts associated with the measurement of auditory brainstem responses and otoacoustic emissions.

The nature of auditory impairment depends on such factors as the severity of the hearing loss, the age at onset, the cause of the loss, and the location of the lesion in the auditory system. The hearing evaluation plays an important role in determining some of these factors. Audiometric measurement can (*a*) determine the degree of hearing loss, (*b*) estimate the location of the lesion, (*c*) help establish the cause of the problem, (*d*) estimate the extent of the disability produced by the hearing loss, and (*e*) help to determine the client's needs and the appropriate means of filling those needs. This chapter focuses on the tests used most commonly in the evaluation of auditory function. This battery of tests includes pure-tone audiometry, speech audiometry, and acoustic immittance measures.

CASE HISTORY

Before the audiologic evaluation begins, the audiologist obtains a history from the client. For adults, this history may be supplied by completing a printed form before the evaluation. The form contains pertinent identifying information for the client, such as home address, patient identification number, and referral source. Questions regarding the nature of past and present hearing problems, other medical problems, and prior use of amplification are also usually included. The written responses are followed up during an interview between the audiologist and the client before any testing.

For children, the case history form is usually more comprehensive than the adult version. In addition to questions such as the ones mentioned for adults, detailed questions about the mother's pregnancy and the child's birth are included. The development of gross and fine motor skills and of speech and language are also probed. The medical history of the child is reviewed in detail, with special emphasis on childhood diseases capable of producing a hearing loss (e.g., measles, mumps) (see Chapter 5).

PURE-TONE AUDIOMETRY

Pure-tone audiometry is the basis of a hearing evaluation. With pure-tone audiometry, hearing thresholds are measured for pure tones at various test frequencies. Hearing threshold is typically defined as the lowest (softest) sound level needed for a person to detect a signal approximately 50% of the time. Threshold information at each frequency is plotted on a graph known as an audiogram. Before examining the audiogram, however, we describe the equipment used to measure hearing.

Audiometer

An audiometer is the primary instrument used to measure hearing threshold. Audiometers vary from the simple, inexpensive screening devices used in schools and public health programs to the more elaborate and expensive diagnostic audiometers found in hospitals and clinics. Certain basic components are common to all audiometers. Figure 4.1 shows one of these basic units. A frequency selector dial permits selection of different pure-tone frequencies. Ordinarily, these frequencies are available at octave intervals ranging from 125 to 8000 Hz. An interrupter switch or presentation button allows presentation of the tone to the listener. A hearing-level dial controls the intensity of the signal. Most audiometers can deliver signals spanning a 100-dB range in 5-dB steps. An output selector determines whether the pure tone will be presented to the earphones for air conduction testing (for either the right or the left ear) or whether the tone is to be sent to a bone vibrator for bone conduction testing. Many audiometers also have a masking-level dial, which controls the intensity of any masking noise presented to the nontest ear. The more elaborate diagnostic audiometers not only can generate masking noise and pure-tone signals but also provide a means for measuring understanding of speech signals.

Audiogram

The audiogram is a graph used to record the hearing thresholds and other test results. Figure 4.2 shows an audiogram and the associated symbol system recommended by the American Speech-Language-Hearing Association (ASHA). The audiogram is shown

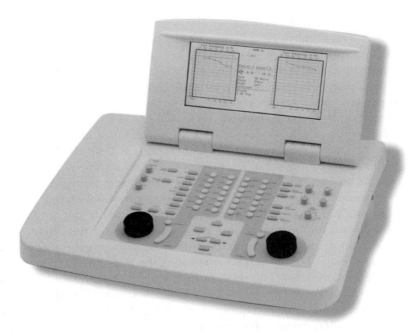

FIGURE 4.1 An example of the control panel of a pure-tone audiometer.

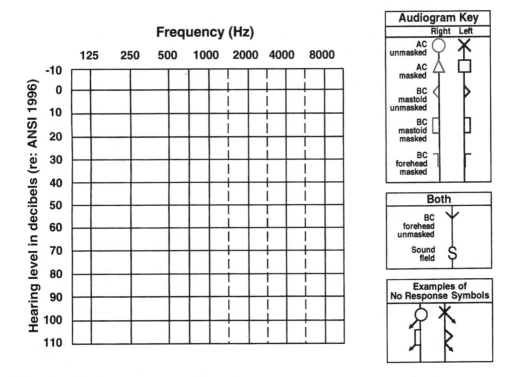

FIGURE 4.2 (Left) Audiogram used for plotting pure-tone air and bone conduction thresholds. (Right) The audiogram key displays the symbols commonly used in audiograms. AC, air conduction; BC, bone conduction.

with the signal frequencies (in hertz) on the x-axis and the hearing level (in decibels) on the y-axis. The graph is designed in such a manner that one octave on the frequency scale is equal in size to 20 dB on the hearing level scale.

The horizontal line at 0 dB hearing level (HL) represents normal hearing sensitivity for the average young adult. However, as described in Chapter 3, the human ear does not perceive sound equally well at all frequencies. Recall that the ear is most sensitive to sound in the intermediate region from 1000 to 4000 Hz and is less sensitive at both the higher and lower frequencies. In normal ears more sound pressure is needed to elicit a threshold response at 250 Hz than at 2000 Hz. The audiometer is calibrated to correct for these differences in threshold sensitivity at various frequencies. Consequently, when the hearing level dial is set at zero for a given frequency, the signal is automatically presented at the normal threshold sound pressure level required for the average young adult to hear that particular frequency (Vignette 4.1).

Results plotted on the audiogram can be used to classify the extent of a hearing disability. This information plays a valuable role in determining the needs of a hearing-impaired individual. Classification schemes using the pure-tone audiogram are based on the fact that there is a strong relationship between the threshold for frequencies known to be important for hearing speech (500, 1000, and 2000 Hz) and the lowest level at which speech can be recognized accurately 50% of the time. The latter measure is generally called the speech recognition threshold, or SRT. Given the pure-tone thresholds at 500, 1000, and 2000 Hz, one can estimate the hearing loss for speech and the potential handicapping effects of the impairment. This is done by simply calculating the average (mean) loss of hearing for these three frequencies. This average is the three-frequency pure-tone average. Figure 4.3 shows a typical classification system based on the pure-tone average. This scheme, adapted from several other systems, reflects the different classifications of hearing loss and the likely effects of the hearing loss on an individual's ability to hear speech. The hearing loss classes, ranging from mild to profound, are based on the pure-tone average at 500, 1000, and 2000 Hz. The classification of normal limits extends to 25 dB HL, and hearing levels within this range have typically been thought to produce essentially no problems with even faint speech. Some evidence indicates, however, that losses from 15 to 25 dB HL can have negative effects educationally on children. Children with hearing loss in this range should be considered for relatively unobtrusive ways to amplify the teacher's speech in the classroom that will also provide benefit to children with normal hearing in the same classroom (see Chapter 7 for more details).

Measurement of Hearing

In pure-tone audiometry, thresholds are obtained by both air conduction and bone conduction. In air conduction measurement, the different pure-tone stimuli are transmitted through earphones. The signal travels through the ear canal, across the middle ear cavity via the three ossicles to the cochlea, and on to the auditory central nervous system, as reviewed in Chapter 3. Air conduction thresholds reflect the integrity of the total peripheral auditory mechanism. When a person exhibits a hearing loss by air conduction, it is not possible to determine the location of the pathology along the auditory pathway. The hearing loss could be the result of (a) a problem in the outer or middle ear, (b) a difficulty at the level of the cochlea, (c) damage along the neural pathways to the brain, or (d) some combination of these. When air conduction measurements are combined with bone conduction measurements, however, it is possible to differentiate outer and middle ear problems (conductive hearing loss) from inner ear problems (sensorineural hearing loss).

VIGNETTE 4.1 **The relation between decibels SPL and decibels HL**

The accompanying figure depicts the relation between the dB HL scale and the dB SPL scale of sound intensity. The circles in the upper panel are the data for hearing thresholds of normal-hearing young adults. The triangles in the upper panel are hearing thresholds obtained from an individual with a high-frequency hearing loss. Increasing hearing loss is indicated by higher SPLs at threshold. At 4000 Hz, for example, the average threshold for normal-hearing young adults is 10 dB SPL; the patient's threshold is 80 dB SPL, indicating a hearing loss of 70 dB. These same data have been plotted on the dB HL scale in the lower panel. The normal-hearing threshold has been set to 0 dB HL on this scale at all frequencies. Increasing intensity is shown in a downward direction on the audiogram. The threshold for the subject with hearing loss at 4000 Hz is 70 dB HL. This threshold value itself directly indicates the magnitude of hearing loss relative to normal hearing. There is no need to subtract the normal-hearing threshold value from the value observed in the impaired ear, as was the case for the dB SPL scale.

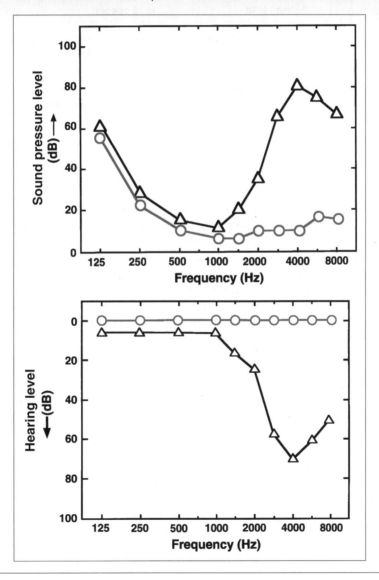

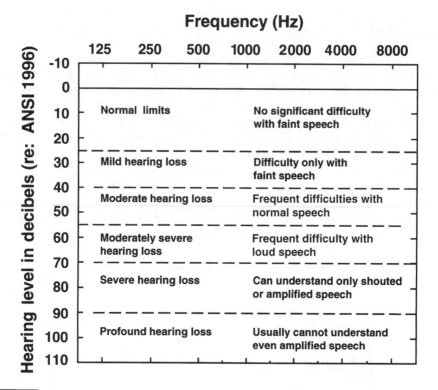

FIGURE 4.3 Classification of hearing loss in relation to disability for speech recognition.

In bone conduction measurement, signals are transmitted via a bone vibrator that is usually placed on the mastoid prominence of the skull (a bony prominence behind the pinna, slightly above the level of the concha). The forehead is another common position for placement of the bone vibrator. A signal transduced through the vibrator causes the skull to vibrate. The pure tone directly stimulates the cochlea, which is embedded in the skull, effectively bypassing the outer ear and middle ear systems. If an individual exhibits a reduction in hearing sensitivity when tested by air conduction yet shows normal sensitivity by bone conduction, the impairment is probably a result of an obstruction or blockage of the outer or middle ear. This condition is a conductive hearing loss. Figure 4.4 gives an audiometric example of a young child with a conductive hearing loss caused by middle ear disease. The bone conduction thresholds (right-ear thresholds; left-ear thresholds) appear close to 0 dB HL for all test frequencies. Such a finding implies that the inner ear responds to sound at normal threshold levels. The air conduction thresholds (O-O, right ear; X-X, left ear), however, are much greater than 0 dB HL. Greater sound intensity is needed for this child to hear the air-conducted pure-tone signals than is required by the average normal hearer. Because the bone conduction thresholds suggest that the inner ear is normal, the loss displayed by air conduction must result from a conductive lesion affecting the outer or middle ear.

The difference between the air conduction threshold and the bone conduction threshold at a given frequency is called the air-bone gap. In Figure 4.4, at 250 Hz there is a 30-dB air-bone gap in the right ear and a 40-dB gap in the left ear. Conductive hearing loss is especially prevalent among preschool-aged and young school-aged

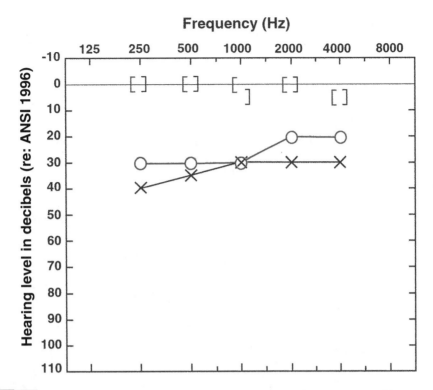

FIGURE 4.4 Pure-tone audiogram demonstrating the relation between air and bone conduction thresholds typifying mild conductive hearing loss.

children who have repeated episodes of otitis media (middle ear infection). Other pathologic conditions known to produce conductive hearing loss include congenital atresia (absence of ear canals), blockage or occlusion of the ear canal (possibly by cerumen, or earwax), perforation or scarring of the tympanic membrane, ossicular chain disruption, and otosclerosis. These pathologies are described in detail in Chapter 5.

Hearing thresholds better than a hearing level of 25 dB HL are considered normal. Air-bone gaps of 10 dB or more, however, indicate a significant conductive hearing loss and may require medical referral, even if the air conduction thresholds are less than 25 dB at all frequencies.

A sensorineural hearing loss is suggested when the air conduction thresholds and bone conduction thresholds are approximately the same (65 dB) at all test frequencies. Sensorineural hearing impairment may be either congenital or acquired. Some of the congenital causes include heredity, complications of maternal viral and bacterial infections, and birth trauma. Factors producing acquired sensorineural hearing loss include noise, aging, inflammatory diseases (e.g., measles or mumps), and ototoxic drugs (e.g., aminoglycoside antibiotics). Many of these disorders are also described in Chapter 5. Figure 4.5 gives three examples of sensorineural hearing loss. Figure 4.5A shows the audiogram of an adult with a hearing loss resulting from the use of ototoxic antibiotics. This audiogram displays a moderate bilateral sensorineural impairment with a greater hearing loss in the high-frequency region. Figure 4.5B shows the audiogram of a child whose hearing loss resulted from maternal rubella (German measles). It can be seen that the magnitude of this hearing loss falls in the profound category

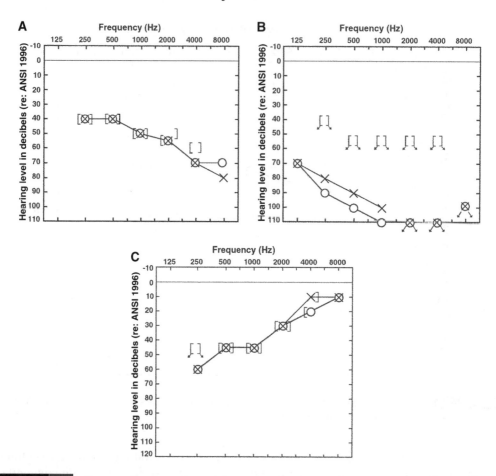

FIGURE 4.5 Three pure-tone air and bone conduction audiograms. **A.** Moderate bilateral sensorineural hearing loss. **B.** Profound bilateral sensorineural hearing loss. **C.** Low-frequency bilateral sensorineural hearing loss.

in the region of the critical frequencies for hearing speech (500 to 2000 Hz). In fact, the loss is so severe that bone conduction responses could not be obtained at the maximum output of the audiometer at all test frequencies. This is indicated by the downward-pointing arrows attached to the audiometric symbols. Air conduction thresholds also could not be obtained at frequencies above 1000 Hz because the hearing loss was so great.

Most sensorineural hearing losses are characterized by audiometric configurations that are flat, trough-shaped, or slightly to steeply sloping in the high frequencies. The latter is probably the most common configuration associated with acquired sensorineural hearing loss. Occasionally, however, patients display a sensorineural hearing loss that is greatest at low and intermediate frequencies, with normal or nearly normal hearing at the high frequencies. Figure 4.5C shows a typical low-frequency hearing loss. Low-tone hearing loss most commonly results from either some type of hereditary deafness or Ménière disease. (See Chapter 5.) Young children whose audiograms display low-frequency hearing loss are difficult to identify and are sometimes the unfortunate victims of misdiagnosis. Because of their nearly normal hearing sensitivity in the high frequencies, these children may respond to whispered speech and broadband stimuli at low intensity levels. In addition, unlike children with a high-frequency hearing loss, their articulation of speech is usually good. These manifestations are not typical of sensorineural hearing loss in children, which makes them particularly prone to misdiagnosis.

When both air conduction thresholds and bone conduction thresholds are reduced in sensitivity but bone conduction yields better results than air conduction, the term *mixed hearing loss* is used, meaning the patient's hearing loss is partially conductive and partially sensorineural. Figure 4.6 shows an audiogram depicting mixed hearing loss. Even though hearing loss is evident for both bone and air conduction thresholds, bone conduction sensitivity is consistently better across all test frequencies. This suggests that there has been some damage to the hair cells or nerve endings in the inner ear, causing a reduction in bone conduction thresholds, which is added to the reduction in air conduction thresholds resulting from malfunction of the outer ear or middle ear.

Vignette 4.2 provides a little more detail about the mechanisms underlying air conduction and bone conduction hearing tests. It also further explains the interpretation of thresholds from air conduction and bone conduction testing to pinpoint the location of the pathology in the auditory periphery.

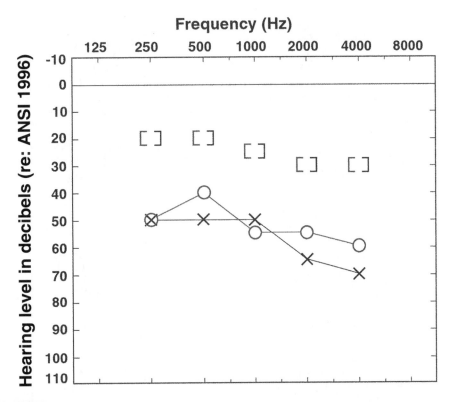

FIGURE 4.6 Pure-tone audiogram demonstrating the relation between air and bone conduction thresholds indicating a mixed (conductive and sensorineural) type of hearing loss.

VIGNETTE 4.2 Mechanisms underlying air conduction and bone conduction thresholds

This series of panels is designed to explain the nature of hearing thresholds obtained by air conduction and by bone conduction. Panel A schematically shows the sound wave and resulting mechanical energy traveling from the outer ear, through the middle ear, and stimulating the cochlea in the inner ear. Panel B illustrates the mechanical vibration of the bony skull with a bone oscillator and a mechanical pathway directly stimulating the cochlea. The bone conduction pathway for the most part can be viewed as bypassing the outer and middle ears to stimulate the inner ears directly (recall that both cochleae are stimulated through skull vibration). The symbol in the next two panels, C and E, represents the location of

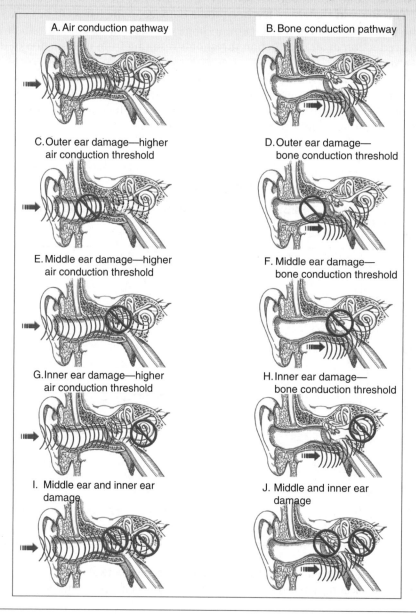

A. Air conduction pathway

B. Bone conduction pathway

C. Outer ear damage—higher air conduction threshold

D. Outer ear damage— bone conduction threshold

E. Middle ear damage—higher air conduction threshold

F. Middle ear damage— bone conduction threshold

G. Inner ear damage—higher air conduction threshold

H. Inner ear damage— bone conduction threshold

I. Middle ear and inner ear damage

J. Middle and inner ear damage

VIGNETTE 4.2 **Mechanisms underlying air conduction and bone conduction thresholds (Continued)**

---

pathology in the outer ear (C) and middle ear (E). Clearly, the pathology in these two areas would impair the transmission of mechanical energy through the normal air conduction pathway. To get through the blockage posed by the pathology in the outer or middle ear, the sound intensity for air conduction stimulation would have to be increased. In other words, a hearing loss would be measured for air conduction stimuli.

What about bone conduction stimulation in the case of outer or middle ear pathology? This situation is illustrated schematically in panels D and F. The mechanical bone conduction pathway is not affected by outer ear or middle ear pathologies, and bone conduction hearing is essentially normal. Consequently, air conduction thresholds reveal elevated hearing thresholds and bone conduction thresholds do not, which results in an air-bone gap.

Now consider the case of inner ear pathology as shown in panels G and H. The inner ear pathology occurs at the end of both the air conduction and bone conduction pathways. As a result, hearing thresholds for air and bone conduction stimulation are impaired by the same amount. In other words, both thresholds show the same amount of hearing loss and so there will be no air-bone gap.

Finally, the bottom two panels, I and J, depict the situation for a mixed hearing loss with pathology in both the middle ear and inner ear. The air conduction pathway (I) is obstructed by both pathologies, whereas the bone conduction pathway (J) is obstructed only by the inner ear pathology. As a result, bone conduction thresholds will be higher than normal, but air conduction thresholds, having to surmount both the middle ear and inner ear pathology will be even higher. In other words, an air-bone gap will exist, and the bone conduction thresholds will indicate the presence of sensorineural (inner ear) hearing loss.

Procedures for Obtaining Threshold

The hearing examination is generally conducted in a sound-treated room where noise levels are kept at a minimum and do not interfere with or influence the hearing test results. Pure-tone audiometry begins with air conduction measurements at octave intervals ranging from 125 or 250 Hz to 8000 Hz; these are followed by bone conduction measurements at octave intervals ranging from 250 to 4000 Hz. (Air conduction measurements at 125 Hz are optional. Some audiometers do not include this frequency.) The initial step in measuring threshold is to instruct the patient as to the listening and responding procedures. The listener is instructed to respond to the pure-tone signals no matter how soft they might be, to respond as soon as the tone is heard, and to stop responding when the sound becomes inaudible. The most common form of response is merely raising or lowering the forefinger. Earphones should be placed carefully and snugly on the patient's head so that the signal source is directed toward the opening of the ear canal.

Because 1000 Hz is considered the frequency most easily heard under headphones, and the threshold at this frequency is the most reliable, it is used as the initial test frequency and is administered first to the better ear. The right ear is tested first if the patient indicates that hearing sensitivity is the same in both ears. The most common procedure for establishing threshold is known as the ascending technique. Figure 4.7 shows this threshold procedure. An interrupted signal is presented at a hearing level of approximately 30 dB. If the listener is unable to perceive the tone at this level, the signal

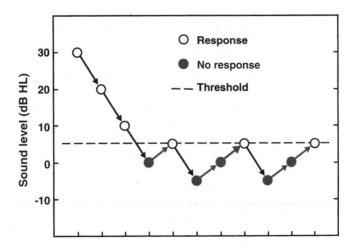

FIGURE 4.7 Alternating descending and ascending sound level presentations commonly used in obtaining pure-tone thresholds. The x-axis simply shows the temporal sequence of tone presentations from beginning (left) to end (right).

is increased by 20 dB and presented again. This procedure is continued until the listener indicates that a signal has been perceived. For the case shown in Figure 4.7, the initial presentation level of 30 dB HL produced a response in the listener. After each positive response, the intensity dial setting is decreased in 10-dB steps until there is no response on the part of the listener. Once the patient fails to respond to the signal, the actual ascending technique begins. After a failure to obtain a response, the signal is increased in 5-dB increments until a response is obtained. Every time a positive response is obtained, the signal is decreased by 10 dB. As soon as the listener's response changes to no response, an ascending series of 5-dB steps is begun again. This process is continued until the listener responds positively at least 50% of the time to an intensity level in an ascending series. This level is recorded as the threshold. In practice, if the listener responds at the same ascending level for two of two, two of three, two of four, or three of five presentations, this level is considered the threshold. Once this procedure has been completed at 1000 Hz, the examiner goes on to the higher test frequencies (2000, 4000, and 8000 Hz) and then returns to 1000 Hz for a reliability check. The lower frequencies, 500 and 250 Hz, are presented last. After testing all of the frequencies in one ear, the examiner switches the signal to the opposite ear and repeats the procedures.

Essentially the same procedures are used for obtaining the bone conduction thresholds, except that only frequencies from 250 through 4000 Hz are used. A bone vibrator is attached by a tension band to the mastoid prominence of the test ear or to the forehead so that the signal is transmitted via the bone pathways of the skull, bypassing the outer and middle ear. Once pure-tone thresholds have been established using the same procedures as those described for air conduction, the bone vibrator, if placed on the mastoid prominence, may be removed and placed on the opposite mastoid prominence for completion of the bone conduction threshold measurements, depending on the agreement observed between the air conduction and bone conduction measurements and the need for masking (Fig. 4.7). If the bone vibrator is placed on the forehead, both inner ears can be evaluated from this location and there is no need to move the bone vibrator.

Factors That Can Influence Threshold

To ensure accurate threshold measurement, it is important to take every precaution to eliminate extraneous variables that can influence the threshold test. The following factors are known to be significant.

Proper Maintenance and Calibration of the Audiometer

Like all electronic equipment, the audiometer is subject to malfunction, especially with extensive use. It is critical that the audiometer be handled carefully to ensure reliable results and that it be checked electroacoustically and biologically (listening checks) on a periodic basis. Such services can usually be obtained at a university hearing clinic or at the manufacturer's distributorship.

Test Environment

Threshold measurement may also be affected if ambient noise levels are high at the time of the test. The evaluation should be conducted in a sound-treated environment designed specifically for hearing threshold measurement. If such facilities are not available, every precaution should be taken to perform the evaluation in the quietest room possible.

Earphone Placement

Inadequate positioning of the earphones can produce threshold errors as great as 10 to 15 dB. The audiologist should be sure that the tension band holding the earphones offers a snug yet comfortable fit and that the phones are placed carefully over the ear canal openings. The problems of earphone placement may be especially difficult with hyperactive children, very young children (under 2 years of age), or elderly adults. A popular alternative to conventional earphones is described in Vignette 4.3.

Placement of the Bone Vibrator

In testing for bone conduction, the vibrator is usually positioned on the prominence of the mastoid bone. Thresholds can vary, however, depending on the placement. To ensure the most accurate placement, it is advisable to introduce a comfortably loud pure tone at 1000 Hz and vary the position of the vibrator on the mastoid while asking the subject to report where the signal is loudest. With younger children, such a practice may not be feasible, and special care must be taken to position the vibrator on a prominent portion of the mastoid bone.

The tension of the headband should also be checked on a periodic basis. After extensive use, the headbands for bone vibrators begin to lose tension and reduce the force that holds the vibrator against the mastoid process. Bone conduction thresholds are known to vary depending on the force applied to the vibrator. Again, because most tension bands were designed for adult-sized heads, special care must be taken when positioning the bone vibrator on the head of a child.

Procedures for Young Children

The procedures for pure-tone audiometry previously described are those recommended for older children and adults. Considerable modification of these techniques is required for testing the hearing of younger children. This section focuses on behavioral procedures used with infants and children aged approximately 5 months to 5 years.

> ### VIGNETTE 4.3   Insert earphones: an alternative to conventional headphones
>
> The drawing that accompanies this vignette illustrates insert earphones, a popular alternative to conventional headphones for testing hearing. As shown in the drawing, a tube 292 mm long is used to conduct the sound from a pocket-sized electronic device to a soft foam cylindrical ear insert that can be compressed temporarily by rolling it between the fingers. While it is compressed, it is inserted deep into the ear canal and held in place for about 1 minute. This allows the foam material to expand and fit snugly in the ear canal. The pocket-sized electronic device is connected to the audiometer just like typical headphones.
>
> Insert earphones have become increasingly popular among audiologists for several reasons. When they are calibrated appropriately, the thresholds measured with them are the same as those measured with conventional headphones. The insert earphones also reduce environmental noise more than conventional headphones. This enables them to be used in somewhat noisier test areas without the ambient noise affecting test results. The insert phones are also more comfortable to wear and fit children as well as they do adults. Finally, masking (discussed later in this chapter) is needed less frequently for testing by air conduction. They also have some advantages when used to deliver sounds used in clinical electrophysiology, such as the measurement of gross cochlear receptor potentials and the ABR.
>
>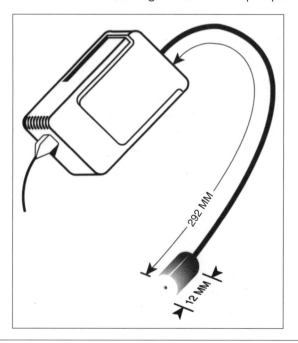

Young infants exhibit developmental changes in behavioral responses to sounds, especially during the first year of life. Figure 4.8 illustrates the developmental changes that occur among infants in response to speech noise as a function of age. Clearly, such normative data are critical to appropriate interpretation of threshold estimations. It is also noteworthy that infants exhibit different types of behavioral responses at different age levels.

Table 4.1 shows an index of the expected auditory responses to various sounds for normal-hearing infants. The responses during the early months are typically arousal or startle oriented, whereas more sophisticated sound localization responses, such as head turns or eye movements in the direction of the loudspeaker producing the sound,

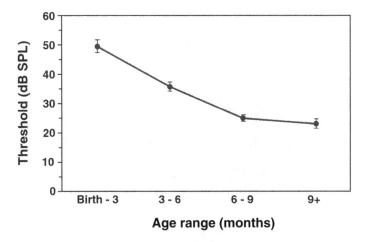

FIGURE 4.8 Developmental changes of infants' response to speech noise as a function of age. (Adapted from Tharpe AM, Ashmead DH. A longitudinal investigation of infant auditory sensitivity. Am J Audiol 10:104–112, 2001.)

occur with the older infants. Although one can make behavioral observations of younger infants' responses to sound, these responses are highly variable and not reliable for auditory assessment. As noted in the advanced material from Chapter 3, however, clinical electrophysiologic measures, such as the auditory brainstem response, can also be used to provide indirect estimates of hearing threshold in many difficult-to-test populations, including infants and young children. These methods are considered indirect estimators of hearing threshold. This is because unlike the behavioral procedures described next, an electrophysiologic response measured with electrodes does not always reflect perception of the sound or the sensation of hearing. Behavioral methods are generally required to verify the perception of sound by the listener.

TABLE 4.1 Expected Auditory Responses to Sound by Normal-Hearing Infants[a]

Age	Stimulus & Expected Detection Level (dB SPL)	Typical Responses at Suprathreshold Levels
Neonate	Broadband, high frequency, 45–55	Slow head turn toward off-center sound[b]; response disappearing after a few weeks
1–3 mo	Speech-shaped noise, 45–55	Eyes widening, quieting, arousal from sleep
3–6 mo	Speech-shaped noise, 35–40	Eyes widening, quieting, arousal from sleep; return of head orientation toward sounds
6–9 mo	Speech-shaped noise, 25–30	Localization on horizontal plane
9–12 mo	Speech-shaped noise, 20–25	More precise localization on horizontal plane

[a]Adapted from Tharpe AM, Ashmead DH. A longitudinal investigation of infant auditory sensitivity. Am J Audiol 10:104–112, 2001.

[b]Clifton RA. Development of spatial hearing. In: Werner LA, Rubel EW, eds. Developmental Psychoacoustics. Washington: American Psychological Association, 1992.

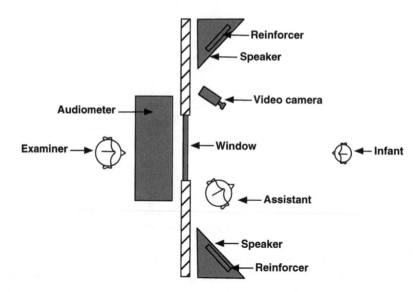

FIGURE 4.9 Typical sound-field test arrangement for infants and young children. The infant is typically in the mother's lap or seated in a high chair.

Testing the Younger Infant, 5 Months to 2 Years Old

A child aged 5 months to 2 years is considerably easier to evaluate than a newborn because the child's increased maturity results in more sophisticated and reliable responses. By approximately 5 to 7 months of age, reliable head-turn responses to sound are elicited easily, and the infant is able to determine the location of the sound source in the horizontal plane. The audiologist's assessment of hearing in this age category is generally centered on behavioral observation of this head turn response conducted in a sound-field setting or under earphones. Figure 4.9 shows a typical test arrangement for sound-field audiometry. The infant is placed in a high chair or on the mother's lap between two loudspeakers flanking the child at a 45° or 90° angle. Controlled auditory signals are presented and behavioral responses (head turns) are observed. The signal is decreased systematically in 10- to 20-dB steps for each positive response and increased 10 dB for each negative response. Threshold is usually defined as the lowest presentation level at which an infant responds 50% of the time. Some type of visual reinforcement is used to maintain the response and to reward the infant for responding appropriately.

The nature of the signal varies. Some clinicians favor the use of various noisemakers, such as a squeeze toy, bell, rattle, or spoon in a cup. Although these signals are considered favorable in that they maintain a certain amount of interest on the part of the child and appear to be effective for eliciting arousal responses in young infants, they have uncontrolled frequency characteristics. Most noisemakers contain energy at several frequencies. This makes it difficult to define the way in which the hearing loss varies with frequency and in many cases to determine whether a hearing loss is present. If, for example, the infant has normal or near-normal hearing for low frequencies, the use of noisemakers that have energy at low and high frequencies will always produce a normal response in this infant even though a severe or profound high-frequency hearing loss might be present. Most clinicians favor the use of electronically generated signals, such as narrowband and complex noise, warble tones (tones that change slightly in frequency over time), and speech. More recently, some clinicians have begun to use digitally generated speech noise as the preferred stimulus for threshold measurement. With these types of test signals, the relevant stimulus parameters, such as intensity and frequency, can be carefully controlled and specified. Clinical experience suggests that a combination of warble tones (frequency modulated sounds), narrowband noise, and filtered speech is valuable in the hearing assessment of young infants.

The use of a visual reinforcer in the measurement of hearing for very young infants is extremely important. Delivery of a visual stimulus after the appropriate head-turn response serves to enhance the response behavior by delaying habituation and leads to a more accurate threshold measurement. This technique is sometimes called the conditioned orientation reflex or visual reinforcement audiometry (VRA). Visual reinforcers range from a simple blinking light to a more complex animated toy animal.

The scoring of a child's responses is also an important variable in the assessment of very young children. Although one person is capable of conducting this type of assessment, it is usually helpful to have two people involved. The clinician controlling the audiometer is involved with the appropriate presentation of the auditory signals and looks for the head-turn response. It is desirable to have an assistant in the examination room with the child to help keep the child content and facing forward.

There are limitations to the use of sound-field audiometry with young infants. The most obvious limitations are (a) the inability to obtain thresholds from each ear separately, (b) the inability to obtain bone conduction thresholds, and (c) failure to obtain responses from young children who have severe or profound hearing losses. The latter drawback results simply from the output limitations of typical audiometers when the sound is presented over loudspeakers. For these reasons, clinicians are encouraged to conduct VRA using earphones. Lightweight insert earphones are readily accepted by most infants, and infants will typically turn their head or move their eyes in the direction corresponding to the ear that has been stimulated.

Testing Children 2 to 5 Years Old

A child of 2 to 5 years of age has matured sufficiently to permit the use of more structured procedures in the hearing evaluation. The techniques used most frequently are conditioned-play audiometry, tangible reinforcement operant conditioning audiometry (TROCA) or visual reinforcement operant conditioning audiometry (VROCA), and conventional (hand-raising) audiometry.

Conditioned-play audiometry is the best-accepted procedure for measuring the hearing thresholds of children in this age group. The child participates in some form of play activity (e.g., placing a ring on a cone, putting blocks in a box, or placing pegs in a hole) each time the signal is heard. The play activity serves as both the visible response for the clinician and the reinforcement for the child. Usually, social reinforcement also accompanies an appropriate response. The child is prevented from playing the game if an inappropriate response is made. The evaluation consists of a conditioning period in which the child is trained to perform the play activity in response to the delivery of a sound stimulus that is clearly audible. This is followed by a threshold-seeking period. The technique may be employed in a sound-field condition or with earphone and bone conduction measurements. The application of play audiometry is limited to youngsters above age 2 years and to children who do not have multiple handicaps.

TROCA is a highly structured test procedure that was introduced originally as a means of assessing the hearing sensitivity of developmentally delayed children. Although TROCA test procedures vary somewhat from clinic to clinic, the principle is that a tangible material, such as candy or trinkets (reinforcer), is automatically dispensed if the child depresses a button when a tone is perceived. If an inappropriate response is made, the child does not receive the reinforcement. TROCA incorporates specialized instrumentation that electromechanically controls the stimulus presentation, monitors the responses, and dispenses the tangible reinforcers. Like conditioned-play audiometry, this technique may be employed either in a sound field or with earphone and bone conduction measurements. The use of TROCA has been extended from the developmentally delayed population to young children, particularly those classified as difficult to test, such as distractible and hyperactive children. It is also considered useful when frequent retesting is required, because reconditioning is seldom needed once the child is trained. The TROCA approach is not considered very successful with children below the age of 2 years.

VROCA differs from TROCA only in that a visual reinforcement is used in place of a tangible reinforcer. Those who desire more detail on the audiometric procedures used with children should consult one of the relevant readings suggested at the end of this chapter.

Masking

When hearing is assessed under earphones or with a bone vibrator, sometimes the ear that the clinician desires to test is *not* the one that is stimulated. Sometimes the non-test ear is stimulated by the sound. This situation occurs because the two ears are not completely isolated from one another. Air-conducted sound delivered to the test ear through conventional earphones mounted in typical ear cushions is decreased or attenuated approximately 40 dB before stimulating the other ear via skull vibration. The value of 40 dB for interaural (between-ear) attenuation is actually a minimum value. The amount of interaural attenuation for air conduction varies with the frequency of the test signal but is always more than 40 dB. The minimum interaural attenuation value for bone conduction is 0 dB. Thus, the bone oscillator placed on the mastoid process behind the left ear vibrates the entire skull, such that the effective stimulation of the right ear is essentially equivalent to that of the left ear. It is impossible, therefore, when testing by bone conduction, to discern whether the right ear or the left ear is responding without some way of eliminating the participation of the nontest ear (Vignette 4.4).

Masking enables the clinician to eliminate the nontest ear from participation in the measurement of hearing thresholds for the test ear. Essentially, the audiologist introduces into the nontest ear an amount of masking noise that is sufficient to make any sound crossing the skull from the test ear inaudible.

There are two simple rules for deciding whether to mask the nontest ear; one applies to air conduction testing and the other to bone conduction measurements. Regarding air conduction thresholds, masking is required at a given frequency if the air conduction threshold of the test ear exceeds the bone conduction threshold of the nontest ear by more than 35 dB. Recall that the bone conduction threshold may be equivalent to or better than the air conduction threshold but never poorer. Thus, if one observes a 50-dB difference between the air conduction thresholds of the two ears at a particular frequency, the difference will be at least that great when the air conduction threshold of the test ear is compared with that of the nontest ear. Consequently, one need not always determine the bone conduction threshold of the nontest ear before deciding whether to mask for air conduction. The following example will clarify this.

VIGNETTE 4.4   Understanding the need for masking

In the drawing that accompanies this vignette, two gremlins named Lefty and Righty sit in adjacent rooms. The two rooms are separated by a wall that decreases sound intensity by 40 dB. The gremlins' job is to listen for pure tones. When they hear a sound, they are to signal by pushing a button to light a neon sign containing the words "I heard that!" Righty hears a 10-dB SPL sound coming from the loudspeaker in his room and presses the button. By using softer and louder intensities, we determine the sound intensity that Righty responds to 50% of the time and call this his threshold. Righty has a threshold of 10 dB SPL. This is the typical, or normal, threshold for most gremlins.

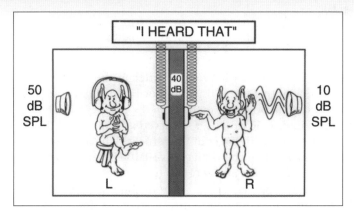

Next we measure Lefty's hearing threshold. Unbeknownst to us, Lefty has decided to wear earmuffs. (You have to be careful with gremlins.) The earmuffs reduce the sound reaching his ears by 60 dB. As we try to measure Lefty's threshold, we gradually increase the intensity of the sound coming from the loudspeaker in the left room. Finally we get a response. Approximately 50% of the time, we see the neon light flash above the rooms when the presentation level of the sound is 50 dB SPL. We conclude that Lefty's threshold is 50 dB SPL.

Is our conclusion correct? Probably not. We said that the earmuffs decrease the sound reaching Lefty's ears by 60 dB and that the typical threshold for gremlins is 10 dB SPL. If the sound level from the speaker in the left room is 50 dB SPL and the earmuffs decrease it by 60 dB, the sound level reaching Lefty's ears is ‾10 dB SPL. This is well below threshold for gremlins. Yet we clearly saw the neon light flash 50% of the time when the left speaker presented a sound level of 50 dB SPL. By now you have probably reasoned that it was Righty, not Lefty, responding to the sound from the left speaker. The wall decreases sound by 40 dB. A 50-dB SPL sound from the left speaker is 10 dB SPL in the right room. Righty's threshold is 10 dB SPL, and he responds accordingly by pushing the button and lighting the neon sign. Whenever the sound level presented to one room is 40 dB or more above the threshold of the gremlin in the other room, we can't be sure which gremlin is turning on the neon light.

If we used the loudspeaker in Righty's room to present a noise loud enough to make Righty's threshold higher than 10 dB SPL, we could then proceed to increase the sound from the left speaker above levels of 50 dB SPL. By introducing enough masking noise into Righty's room, we could eventually measure Lefty's real threshold of 70 dB SPL (10 dB SPL normal threshold plus 60 dB from earmuffs).

(continued)

VIGNETTE 4.4   **Understanding the need for masking *(Continued)***

The gremlins in the drawing are like our inner ears, and the loudspeakers are like the headphones. The wall of 40 dB is the separation between the ears provided by the skull, known as the interaural (between-ear) attenuation. Masking noise is often needed to determine which ear is really responding to sound. This is true especially when testing by bone conduction, because there is no interaural attenuation between the two inner ears when the skull is vibrated. Essentially, the 40-dB wall has been removed for bone conduction testing, and the gremlin with the better hearing always responds. The hearing of the better inner ear is always measured via unmasked bone conduction testing regardless of where the bone vibrator is placed on the skull.

The patient indicates that hearing is better in the right ear, and air conduction testing is initiated with that ear. A threshold of 10 dB HL is observed at 1000 Hz. After completion of testing at other frequencies in the right ear, the left ear is tested. An air conduction threshold of 50 dB HL is observed at 1000 Hz. Is this an accurate indication of the hearing loss at 1000 Hz in the left ear? The audiologist can't be sure. The air conduction threshold for the right ear is 10 dB HL and indicates that the bone conduction threshold for that ear at 1000 Hz is not greater than this value. Thus, there is at least a 40-dB difference between the air conduction threshold of the test ear at 1000 Hz (50 dB HL) and the bone conduction threshold of the nontest ear (≤10 dB HL). If the skull attenuates the air-conducted sound delivered to the test ear by only 40 dB, a signal level of approximately 10 dB HL reaches the nontest ear. The level of the crossed-over signal approximates the bone conduction threshold of the nontest ear and may therefore be detected by that ear. Now assume that a masking noise is introduced into the nontest ear to raise that ear's threshold to 30 dB HL. If the air conduction threshold of the test ear remains at 50 to 55 dB HL, it is safe to conclude that the observed threshold provides an accurate indication of the hearing loss in that ear. Why? Because if the listener was actually using the nontest ear to hear the sound presented to the test ear, making the hearing threshold 20 dB worse in the nontest ear (from 10 to 30 dB HL) would also shift the threshold in the test ear by 20 dB (from 50 to 70 dB HL).

For testing hearing by bone conduction, masking is needed whenever the difference between the air conduction threshold of the test ear and the bone conduction threshold of the test ear at the same frequency (the air-bone gap) is 10 dB or more. Because the interaural attenuation for bone conduction testing is 0 dB, the bone conduction threshold is always determined by the ear having the better bone conduction hearing. Consider the following example. Air conduction thresholds obtained from both ears reveal a hearing loss of 30 dB across all frequencies in the left ear, whereas thresholds of 0 dB HL are obtained at all frequencies in the right ear. Bone conduction testing of each ear indicates thresholds of 0 dB HL at all frequencies. Is the 30-dB air-bone gap observed in the left ear a real indication of a conductive hearing loss in that ear? Without the use of masking in the measurement of the bone conduction thresholds of the left ear, the clinician can't answer that question confidently.

We know that the bone conduction thresholds of the nontest (right) ear will be less than or equal to the air conduction threshold of that ear (0 dB HL). Thus, when we observe this same bone conduction threshold when testing the test (left) ear, either of two explanations is possible. First, the bone conduction threshold could be providing a valid indication of the bone conduction hearing in that ear. This means that a conductive hearing loss is present in that ear. Second, the bone conduction threshold of the test ear could actually be poorer than 0 dB HL but could simply be reflecting the response of the better ear (the nontest ear with a threshold of 0 dB HL). Masking of the nontest ear allows selection of one of these two explanations for the observed bone conduction threshold of the test ear. If the bone conduction threshold of the test ear remains unchanged when sufficient masking noise is introduced into the nontest ear, it is safe to conclude that it provides an accurate indication of bone conduction hearing in that ear.

As we have seen, the need to mask the nontest ear and the rules for when to mask are relatively straightforward. A variety of procedures have been developed to determine how much masking is sufficient. A detailed description of all of these procedures is beyond the scope of this text, but one particular approach, the plateau method, is used as follows.

This method is very simple and quite popular. Once the audiologist has determined that masking is needed for either air or bone conduction measurements, a low-intensity noise is delivered to the nontest ear. The noise might be a narrowband noise with frequency content similar to that of the test tone, or it might be a broadband noise. Once introduced into the nontest ear, the noise is increased in 5-dB steps. If threshold for the tone in the test ear never changes while the noise level in the nontest ear increases to high intensities, this is the true threshold of the test ear.

Frequently, however, this is not the case. At some point, the noise level in the nontest ear reaches a point at which the tone in the test ear is inaudible. At this point, threshold for the tone in the test ear is measured again while the noise remains in the nontest ear. The noise level is increased 5 dB again, and the threshold is reestablished. Frequently during this portion of the plateau method, the level of the noise and tone are alternately increased by 5 dB several times. This is because both the tone and the noise are heard in the nontest ear. The tone is heard in that ear because it crosses over through the skull from the test ear, while the noise is introduced directly into the nontest ear.

Eventually, the noise level will rise by 5 dB several times with no change in threshold for the pure tone. At this point, the noise has eliminated the participation of the nontest ear in the detection of the tone, and the tone is producing sensation in the test ear. Increasing the noise level under these circumstances causes no shift in hearing threshold for the pure tone because the noise is in the nontest ear and the tone is being heard in the test ear. The range of noise levels that fail to shift the threshold for the tone is the plateau. The level of the tone during the plateau is the true threshold of the test ear at that frequency. Figure 4.10 illustrates the gradual increase in masking noise level up to the plateau, which occurs at a hearing level corresponding to the true hearing threshold of the test ear. Generally, the plateau should be 20 to 30 dB in width before termination of the masking procedure.

If the noise level in the nontest ear is increased beyond the plateau, the threshold of the pure tone will eventually begin to increase again (Fig. 4.10). This overmasking occurs when the noise in the nontest ear crosses over through the skull to the test ear and begins to mask the pure tone. During overmasking, the tone and noise will again be alternately increased in 5-dB steps, depending on the intensity of the noise during the plateau and the output limits of the audiometer. Minimum masking occurs at the noise level that first produces the plateau, and maximum masking occurs at the noise level at the end of the plateau, just before overmasking.

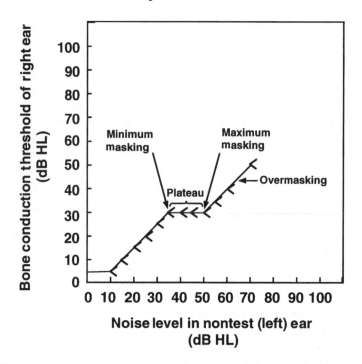

FIGURE 4.10 Plateau method of clinical masking. Masked bone conduction threshold in the right ear (y-axis) is plotted as a function of the masking noise level delivered by a headphone to the nontest (left) ear (x-axis). The unmasked air conduction threshold in the test ear was 30 dB HL, whereas both bone conduction thresholds and the air conduction threshold in the left ear were all 10 dB HL. Thus, there is a 20-dB air-bone gap in the right ear, according to the unmasked thresholds. However, the masked bone conduction threshold of the right ear increases to 30 dB HL at the plateau, indicating that the 30-dB hearing loss in the right ear is sensorineural and not conductive. (The air-bone gap has diminished to 0 dB under masking.)

Additional details about masking methods are beyond the scope of this text. The reader is referred to Hood (1960), Studebaker (1964), and Martin (1974) for additional details about the plateau method and alternative procedures.

SPEECH AUDIOMETRY

Although pure-tone thresholds reveal much about the function of the auditory system, they do not provide a precise measure of a person's ability to understand speech. Speech audiometry, a technique designed to assess a person's ability to hear and understand speech, has become a basic tool in the overall assessment of hearing handicap. This section reviews some of the applications of speech audiometry in the basic hearing evaluation.

Before proceeding to a more detailed description of speech audiometry, a brief note regarding the actual sequence of basic audiologic testing procedures is in order. Although it makes more sense conceptually in a textbook to discuss pure-tone audiometry by air and bone conduction before proceeding to speech audiometry, it would be inappropriate to assume that this is the most common sequence for testing. As noted later, speech audiometry is typically assessed by air conduction only. As a result, from a procedural standpoint, it is often most efficient for the audiologist to complete all air conduction testing first, then remove the earphones and proceed to bone conduction testing. Thus, it is very common for the audiologist to proceed from the case history to air conduction pure-tone audiometry, then to speech audiometry, and then to bone conduction pure-tone audiometry

Speech Audiometer

Speech audiometry generally requires a two-room test suite—a control room, which contains the audiometric equipment and the audiologist, and an evaluation room, where the patient is seated (Fig. 4.11). Most diagnostic audiometers include the appropriate circuitry for both pure-tone measurement and speech audiometric evaluation. The speech circuitry portion of a diagnostic audiometer consists of a calibrated amplifying system having a variety of options for input and output of speech signals. Most commonly, the speech audiometer accommodates inputs for a microphone, tape recorder, and compact disc (CD) player. It is possible to conduct speech testing using live speech (microphone) or recorded materials. The output of the speech signal may be directed to earphones, a bone vibrator, or a loudspeaker in the test room. Speech audiometric testing via air conduction can be conducted in one ear (monaurally), in both ears (binaurally), or in a sound-field environment. Bone conduction testing is also possible. Many diagnostic audiometers employ a dual-channel system that enables the examiner to use two inputs at the same time and to direct these signals to any of the available outputs.

To ensure valid and reliable measurements, just as with pure-tone audiometry, the circuitry of the speech audiometer must be calibrated on a regular basis. The acoustic output of the speech audiometer is calibrated in decibels relative to normal hearing

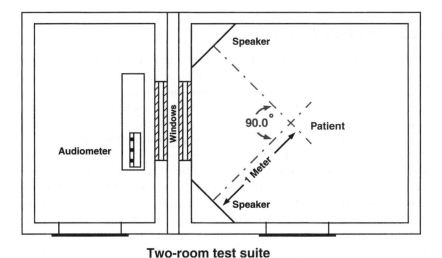

Two-room test suite

FIGURE 4.11 Typical two-room test setup for speech audiometry. Two enclosed rooms are needed, including one for the examiner, because speech is often presented using live voice and a microphone. The enclosed room for the audiologist helps to minimize pickup of unwanted environmental sounds by the microphone during such testing.

threshold (dB HL). According to our most recent standards for speech audiometers, 0 dB HL is equivalent to 20 dB SPL when measured through earphones. There is a difference of approximately 7.5 dB between earphone and sound-field threshold measurements for speech signals. Consequently, 0 dB HL in the sound field corresponds to an output from a loudspeaker of approximately 12 dB SPL. This calculated difference in audiometric zero for earphones and loudspeakers allow us to obtain equivalent speech thresholds in decibels HL under these two listening conditions.

Assessment of Speech Recognition Threshold

SRT is the intensity at which an individual can identify simple speech materials approximately 50% of the time. It is included in the basic hearing evaluation for two specific reasons. First, it serves as an excellent check on the validity of pure-tone thresholds. There is a strong correlation between the average of the pure-tone thresholds obtained at the frequencies known to be important for speech (i.e., 500, 1000, and 2000 Hz) and the SRT. Large discrepancies between the SRT and this pure-tone average (PTA) may suggest functional, or nonorganic, hearing loss. A second important reason for including the SRT in the hearing evaluation is that it provides a basis for selecting the sound level at which a patient's speech recognition abilities should be tested. Finally, besides its use in the basic hearing evaluation, the SRT is useful in the determination of functional gain in the hearing aid evaluation process (see Chapter 7).

Speech Threshold Materials

The most popular test materials used by audiologists to measure SRT are spondaic words. Spondaic words are two-syllable words spoken with equal stress on each syllable (e.g., baseball, cowboy). A carrier phrase, such as "say the word," may precede each stimulus item. The spondaic words used most widely by audiologists are taken from the Central Institute for the Deaf (CID) Auditory Test W-1.

Speech Threshold Procedures

Several procedures have been advocated for determining the SRT using spondaic words. The procedure recommended by the Committee on Audiometric Guidelines of the ASHA uses most of the 36 spondaic words from the CID W-1 word list. The testing begins with presentation of all of the spondaic words to the client at a comfortable level. This familiarizes the patient with the words to be used in the measurement of threshold.

The actual test procedure is a descending threshold technique that consists of a preliminary phase and a test phase. In the preliminary phase, the first spondaic word is presented at 30 to 40 dB above the estimated threshold (pure-tone average) or at 50 dB HL if an estimate cannot be obtained. If the client fails to respond at this level or responds incorrectly, the starting level is increased 20 dB. This is continued until a correct response is obtained. A correct response is followed by a 10-dB decrease in level until the response changes to an incorrect one. At this level, a second spondee is presented. The level is decreased in 10-dB steps until two consecutive words have been missed at the same level. The level is then increased 10 dB above the level at which two consecutive spondees were missed. This is the starting level for the test phase.

During the test phase, two spondaic words are presented at the starting level and at each successive 2-dB decrement in level. If five of the first six spondees are repeated correctly, this process continues until five of the last six spondees are responded to incorrectly. If five of the first six stimuli were not repeated correctly, then the starting level is increased 4 to 10 dB, and the descending series of stimulus presentations is initiated.

The descending procedure recommended by the ASHA begins with speech levels above threshold and descends toward threshold. At the first few presentation levels, approximately 80% (five of six) of the items are correct. At the ending level, approximately 20% (one of six) of the spondees are repeated correctly. A formula is used to then calculate the SRT. The SRT represents the lowest hearing level at which an individual can recognize 50% of the speech material.

Assessment of Suprathreshold Speech Recognition

Although the speech threshold provides an index of the degree of hearing loss for speech, it does not offer any information regarding a person's ability to make distinctions among the various acoustic cues in spoken language at conversational intensity levels. Unlike the situation with the SRT, attempts to calculate a person's ability to understand speech presented at comfortably loud levels based on data from the pure-tone audiogram have not been successful. Consequently, various suprathreshold speech recognition tests have been developed to estimate a person's ability to understand conversational speech. Three of the more common types of speech recognition tests are phonetically balanced word lists, multiple-choice tests, and sentence tests.

Phonetically Balanced Word Lists

The most popular phonetically balanced (PB) word lists are listed in Table 4.2. These word lists are called phonetically balanced because the phonetic composition of all lists are equivalent and representative of everyday English speech. All of the PB word lists use an open-set response format. The listener is not presented with a closed set of alternatives for each test item, one of which is the monosyllabic word spoken by the examiner. Rather, the set of possible responses to a test item is open, that is, limited only by the listener's vocabulary.

For comparative purposes, representative performance intensity functions for many of these lists appear in Figure 4.12. As evidenced by Figure 4.12, a performance intensity function describes performance (for either a group or an individual) in percentage-correct recognition of the test items as a function of the intensity of the speech signal. The intensity of the speech signal is usually specified in decibels above SRT (i.e., decibels sensation level with reference to SRT, abbreviated dB SL). Because two different recordings of one set of items, the CID W-22 lists, are widely used, both of their performance intensity functions are illustrated in Figure 4.12. This figure readily demonstrates that tests do differ. The most difficult test among these monosyllabic materials is the Psychoacoustic Laboratory (PAL) PB-50s. On the most linear portion of the curve (20–80% correct), identification performance for this test increases most slowly, at 3.8% per decibel. Note the differences between the functions of the two recorded versions of the CID W-22s (labeled 3 and 5 in Fig. 4.12). Results for the most recent recording (5) are displaced to higher sensation levels than are the results for the original version (3). Such differences illustrate clearly that two different recordings of the same material can yield significantly different performance functions. It is the recorded words that comprise the test and not simply the printed list of words.

TABLE 4.2 A Summary of the Features of Several Common Speech Recognition Tests for Adults

Response Format	Test	No. of Items (Alt.)[a]	No. of Lists[b]	Source
Open	PAL PB-50	50	20	Egan (1948)
	CID W-22	50	4	Hirsh, Davis, Silverman, et al. (1952)
	Northwestern University Auditory Test 6 (Nu-6)	50	4	Tillman and Carhart (1966)
Closed	MRHT	50 (6)	6	House, Williams, Hecker, Kryter (1965)
	CCT	100 (4)	2	Owens, Schubert (1977)
	CUNY NST	67–102 (7–9)	1[c]	Levitt and Resnick (1978)

[a]Alt, number of alternatives in the multiple-choice, closed response-set tests.
[b]Lists refer to sets of unique words.
[c]Although the same nonsense syllables are used, 14 randomizations of these materials are available, 7 with a female talker and 7 with a male talker.
PAL, psychoacoustic laboratory.

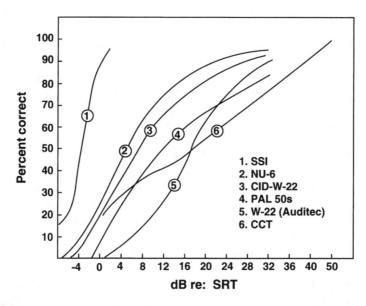

FIGURE 4.12 Performance intensity functions of different suprathreshold speech recognition tests. Functions 3 and 5 represent two different recordings of the W-22 material.

VEST	REST
NEST	TEST
BEST	WEST

FIGURE 4.13 A test ensemble used in the Modified Rhyme Hearing Test.

Multiple-Choice Tests

Some clinicians, unsatisfied with the conventional open-set PB words, directed their attention to alternative formats for word recognition testing. The closed-set format inherent in multiple-choice tests was one of the most popular alternatives developed. The closed-set tests provide several advantages over open-set word recognition tests. The closed-set format eliminates the need to familiarize a subject with the test vocabulary and reduces the potential for a practice effect. Other advantages of the closed-set format include elimination of examiner bias, ease of administration, and simplified scoring techniques.

Table 4.2 lists the features of several popular multiple-choice tests. The most widely recognized, the Modified Rhyme Hearing Test (MRHT), was introduced as a recorded clinical test of speech recognition in 1968. A sample test ensemble is shown in Figure 4.13. In this and other multiple-choice tests, the choices available to the listener usually differ from one another by only one speech sound.

Another development in multiple-choice tests occurred with the introduction of the California Consonant Test (CCT), a consonant identification test developed for and standardized on a population with hearing loss. The CCT is composed of two different scramblings of 100 test items, each of which is arranged within an ensemble of four consonant-vowel-consonant monosyllabic words. For each item, the words are assembled so that either the initial two phonemes are the same, with the final phoneme varying, or conversely, the final two phonemes are the same, with the initial phoneme varying. Of the 100 test items, 36 have consonants in the initial position, whereas 64 consonants are found in the final position. Figure 4.14 shows four test ensembles.

Figure 4.12 shows the performance intensity function for the CCT (labeled 6). The function for the CCT is distinct from the functions for the other test materials. The slope of the function is only 1.6% per decibel. In addition, maximum intelligibility is not reached until signal intensity reaches 50 dB SL (with reference to SRT).

BACK	_____	GAVE	_____
BAT	_____	GAME	_____
BATCH	_____	GAZE	_____
BATH	_____	GAGE	_____
THIN	_____	LEASE	_____
TIN	_____	LEASH	_____
SIN	_____	LEAF	_____
SHIN	_____	LEAP	_____

FIGURE 4.14 Four test ensembles used in the California Consonant Test (CCT).

Another development in speech audiometry is the emergence of closed-set nonsense syllable tests. One such test, the City University of New York (CUNY) Nonsense Syllable Test (NST), is composed of consonant-vowel and vowel-consonant syllables categorized into 11 subtests of 7 to 9 syllables each. The syllables in these subtests differ in (a) consonant voicing (voiced or voiceless), (b) syllable position of the consonant (initial or final position), and (c) vowel context (/a, u, i/). With this test, it is possible to obtain a somewhat detailed picture of the type of errors made by the listener and not just an indication of the total number of errors. More detailed knowledge of the types of perceptual errors made by the patient should lead to more effective remediation of their speech understanding difficulties.

Sentence Tests

In an attempt to approximate everyday speech more closely, several speech identification tests have been developed using sentences as the basic test item. An advantage of sentence materials over other types of tests is that sentences approximate the spectral and contextual characteristics of everyday conversational speech while controlling for sentence length and semantic content. This increases the test's face validity.

The first sentence test designed to clinically assess speech recognition ability was developed and recorded at the CID. At present, however, there are no commercial recordings of these materials. Consequently, the clinical application of the CID sentences is somewhat limited.

One popular sentence test is the Synthetic Sentence Identification (SSI) test. The sentences used in this test were constructed such that each successive group of three words in the sentence was itself meaningful but the entire sentence was not. The following is an example of a test item from the SSI: "Forward march said the boy had a."

Figure 4.12 shows a sample performance intensity function for the SSI. Clearly, this test is much easier than other materials represented in this figure. In an effort to increase the difficulty of this test, a competing speech message was mixed with the sentences. For clinical evaluation purposes, it was recommended that the SSI be administered at a message-to-competition ratio of 0 dB; in other words, the speech and the competition are delivered at the same intensity level. This amount of competition yielded performance scores in normal listeners that were comparable with scores obtained with phonetically balanced materials in a quiet environment.

Another sentence identification test, the Speech Perception in Noise (SPIN) test, has also been developed and evaluated clinically. The eight available lists of the revised SPIN test are each composed of 50 sentences, each 5 to 8 words in length. The last word of each sentence is the test item; 25 of the sentences contain test items that are classified as having high predictability, which means that the word is readily predictable given the context of the sentence. Conversely, 25 sentences have test items with low predictability. An example of a sentence containing a high-predictability test item is "The boat sailed across the bay," whereas an example of a sentence with low predictability using the same test word is "John was talking about the bay." The test's developers also provide a recording of a background of babble-type competition composed of 12 voices reading simultaneously.

Finally, an increasingly popular speech recognition test especially for use in the evaluation of hearing aids makes use of sentences connected in brief, meaningful passages. This is the Connected Speech Test (CST). For this test, a passage consisting of a series of sentences on a central topic is presented, and the listener is told of the passage's topic before testing. Each passage contains a total of 25 keywords. The recorded materials are paused after each sentence and the listener is asked to repeat the sentence. The number of keywords correct is tallied for each passage and a percent correct score, typically based on at least two passages (50 keywords), is calculated. Given the high context of these materials, the test is most frequently administered in a background of competing speech.

Speech Materials for the Pediatric Population

This section reviews some speech materials commonly used to assess the word recognition skills of children. The major modification required in the evaluation of children is to ensure that the speech material is within the receptive vocabulary of the child being tested. The required response, moreover, must be appropriate for the age tested. It would not be appropriate, for example, to ask for written responses from a 4-year-old child on a word recognition task. Common speech recognition tests used for children are listed in Table 4.3.

Some of the more popular tests for use with the pediatric population are (*a*) the Phonetically Balanced Kindergarten test (PBK-50s), (*b*) the Bamford-Koval-Bench Sentence test (BKB), (*c*) the Word Intelligibility by Picture Identification (WIPI) test, (*d*) the Children's Perception of Speech (NU Chips), and (*e*) the Pediatric Speech Intelligibility Test (PSI).

The open-response PBK-50s seems to be most suitable for children aged 6 to 9 years. For many younger children, the open-response design of the PBK-50s and BKBs provides a complicated task, which causes difficulty in administration and scoring. For example, a child with a speech problem is difficult to evaluate because oral responses may not indicate what the child actually perceived. In addition, children sometimes lose interest in the task because of its tedium. Many children's lists have a closed-set response format to minimize some of these problems.

One of the most widely used multiple-choice tests for children with hearing loss is the WIPI test. This test consists of four 25-word lists of monosyllabic words within the vocabulary of preschool-aged children. For a given test item, the child is presented

TABLE 4.3 Features of Common Speech Recognition Tests for Children

Response Format	Test	Materials	No. of Items	No. of Lists	Age Range (y)	Reference
Open	PBK	Monosyllables	50	4	6–9	Haskins (1949)
	BKB	Sentences	21 11	16 16	8–15	Bench, Koval, and Bamford (1979)
Closed	WIPI	Monosyllables	50	4	3–6	Ross and Lerman (1970)
	NU Chips	Monosyllables	50	4	≥3	Katz and Elliott (1978)
	PSI	Monosyllables Sentences	20 10	1 2	3–10	Jerger, Lewis, Hawkins and Jerger (1980)

with a page containing six pictures, one of which is a picture of the test item. The appropriate response of the child is to select the picture corresponding to the word perceived. The WIPI test is most appropriate for children aged 3.5 to 6 years. Other popular tests for children that incorporate a closed-set format include the NU Chips, a word picture identification test, and the PSI, a picture identification task for mono-syllables and sentences (Table 4.3).

Clinical Decisions in the Assessment of Speech Recognition

The speech recognition score can be influenced (sometimes to a large extent) by several variables, most of which are related to the procedures used in test administration. Because of their important implications for the audiologist, several of these variables are considered next.

Mode of Test Presentation

The audiologist must think about the details of test presentation. Speech recognition scores can be affected dramatically by speaker differences, methods used in recording the test materials, and characteristics of the test equipment. The protocol for presenting the test materials seems to entail three issues of special concern to the clinician: (*a*) whether to use recorded materials or a monitored live-voice presentation, (*b*) whether to use a carrier phrase, and (*c*) how to determine the appropriate intensity level for administering the test materials.

Generally, recorded materials offer greater test reliability than monitored live-voice presentations. The score on retest is more similar to results obtained just before retest when recorded materials are used. With many clinical populations, however, greater flexibility is needed than is offered by a tape-recorded test. This is frequently the case, for example, when testing young children. Under these circumstances, monitored live-voice presentation is preferred.

A common practice in the assessment of speech recognition is to preface each test item with a carrier phrase such as "Say the word," "You will say," or "Write the word." Carrier phrases are used for two purposes. First, they prepare the listener for the upcoming stimulus item, and second, they help the clinician monitor the intensity of the speech signal during monitored live-voice presentation.

Another important consideration for the audiologist is determining the intensity level that is most appropriate for administering a speech recognition test. The objective is usually to estimate the listener's maximum ability to understand speech, often called the PB-max, when phonetically balanced monosyllabic materials are used. The only true means of obtaining the best speech recognition score is to obtain a complete performance intensity function. To do so, several lists should be presented at successively higher intensity levels. Such a procedure, however, is clinically impractical because of the time required. Instead, clinicians attempt to estimate maximum speech recognition ability from just one intensity level, usually 40 dB above the SRT. The intensity needed to yield a maximum recognition score will vary with the test material used. Figure 4.12 shows the variation in scores that may occur as a function of material. For example, for the CCT an intensity of 50 dB SL is required to achieve a maximum score, whereas with the original recordings of the W-22 materials, only 25 dB SL is needed to reach a best score.

Ideally, it is recommended that the clinician administer the speech recognition test at two or three successively higher intensity levels if time permits. Understandably, however, such a practice is simply not always practical in the clinical milieu. Sometimes the clinician has to select one intensity level for estimating the PB-max.

Mode of Response

In scoring the responses to a speech recognition test, the most common practice is for the clinician to judge whether the listener's oral response was correct or in error. However, if the patient is able and if time permits, a written response should be used in an effort to minimize any biases of the clinician. The patient's written responses are easiest to implement for multiple-choice tests.

Listening Conditions

There are limitations associated with the assessment of speech recognition ability in a quiet environment. First, many tests fail to differentiate among listeners with hearing loss when administered in a quiet test condition. The tests simply do not appear difficult enough to identify the problems of many listeners with hearing loss. A second disadvantage with performing speech audiometry in quiet is that such a testing condition does not reflect the typical environment encountered in everyday listening situations.

In an attempt to increase the difficulty of the identification task and simulate a more realistic listening environment, audiologists have turned to the use of various background noises and competing messages in the assessment of speech recognition. In 1968, Carhart emphasized the need for clinicians to assess speech recognition ability under conditions that more closely approximated typical listening situations. Carhart's impressions on this subject can best be summarized by this statement: ". . . once we have developed good methods for measuring a patient's capacity to understand speech under adverse listening conditions we will possess the audiologic tools for dealing much more insightfully with his everyday listening problems" (Carhart, 1968). Unfortunately, to date there are no standardized procedures for assessing recognition under adverse listening conditions, even though there is an abundance of literature in this area.

Several types of background noises or competition have been used in speech recognition tests, including white noise, filtered and shaped noise, modulated white noise, cafeteria noise, and spoken messages from one to several talkers. All such background signals are known to degrade the perception of the speech signal to various degrees. Unfortunately, the addition of background noise also increases the variability of test results and reduces the reliability of the data. Nonetheless, by measuring recognition under adverse listening conditions, the clinician is able to assess more adequately the communication handicap imposed by the patient's hearing loss.

Masking

In speech audiometry, just as in pure-tone measurements, crossover from the test ear to the nontest ear can occur. Consequently, when the level of the speech signal presented to the test ear exceeds the bone conduction threshold of the nontest ear by more than 35 dB, masking may be necessary.

ACOUSTIC IMMITTANCE MEASUREMENT

Impedance, as mentioned in Chapter 2, is defined as opposition to the flow of energy through a system. When an acoustic wave strikes the eardrum of the normal ear, a portion of the signal is transmitted through the middle ear to the cochlea, while the remaining part of the wave is reflected out the external canal. The reflected energy forms a sound wave traveling outward with an amplitude and phase that depend on the opposition encountered at the tympanic membrane. The energy of the reflected wave is greatest when the middle ear system is stiff or immobile, as in such pathologic conditions as otitis media with effusion and otosclerosis. On the other hand, an ear with ossicular-chain interruption will reflect considerably less sound into the canal because of the reduced stiffness. A greater portion of the acoustic wave will be transmitted to the middle ear under these circumstances. The reflected sound wave, therefore, carries information about the status of the middle ear system.

The reciprocal of impedance is admittance. An ear with high impedance has low admittance and vice versa. Admittance describes the relative ease with which energy flows through a system. Some devices measure quantities related to acoustic impedance of the middle ear, whereas others measure quantities related to acoustic admittance. In an effort to provide a common vocabulary for results obtained with either device, professionals have decided to use the term *immittance.* Immittance itself is not a physical quantity but simply a term that can be used to refer to either impedance data or admittance data.

The measurement of acoustic immittance at the tympanic membrane is an important component of the basic hearing evaluation. This sensitive and objective diagnostic tool has been used to identify the presence of fluid in the middle ear, to evaluate eustachian tube and facial nerve function, to predict audiometric findings, to determine the nature of hearing loss, and to assist in diagnosing the site of auditory lesion. This technique is considered particularly useful in the assessment of difficult-to-test persons, including very young children.

Figure 4.15 shows how this concept may be applied to actual practice. A pliable probe tip is inserted carefully into the ear canal, and an airtight seal is obtained so that varying amounts of air pressure can be applied to the ear cavity by pumping air into

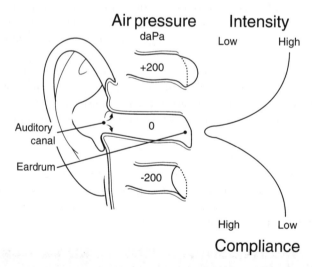

FIGURE 4.15 Concepts of immittance applied in practice. The *middle column* shows three air pressures (+200, 0, and −200 daPa) developed in the ear canal, and the *dotted line* in the drawings at the top and bottom of this column represent the resting position of the eardrum (at 0 daPa). The *right column* shows both the sound intensity of the probe tone recorded in the ear canal as the air pressure is changed from +200 daPa (*top*) to −200 daPa (*bottom*) and the corresponding changes in the compliance of the middle ear.

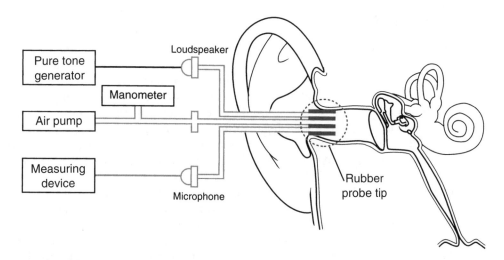

FIGURE 4.16   Components of an immittance instrument.

the ear canal or suctioning it out. A positive amount of air pressure (usually $+200$ daPa)[1] is then introduced into the airtight ear canal, forcing the tympanic membrane inward. The eardrum is now stiffer than usual because of the positive pressure in the ear canal. A low-frequency pure tone is introduced, and a tiny microphone measures the level of the sound reflected from the stiffened eardrum. A low-frequency tone is used because this is the frequency region most affected by changes in stiffness (see Chapter 2). With the intensity of the probe tone in the ear canal constant, the pressure is reduced slowly, causing the tympanic membrane to become more compliant (less stiff). As the tympanic membrane becomes increasingly compliant, more of the acoustic signal will pass through the middle ear, and the level of reflected sound in the ear canal will decrease. When the air pressure in the ear canal equals the air pressure in the middle ear, the tympanic membrane will move with the greatest ease. As the pressure is reduced further, the tympanic membrane is pulled outward, and the eardrum again becomes less mobile. As before, when the eardrum becomes less compliant, more low-frequency energy is reflected off the tympanic membrane, and the sound level within the ear canal increases.

Figure 4.16 illustrates the basic components of most immittance instruments. The probe tip is sealed in the ear canal, providing a closed cavity. The probe contains three small ports that are connected to (*a*) a sound source that generates a low-frequency (usually 220- or 660-Hz) pure tone, (*b*) a microphone to measure the reflected sound wave, and (*c*) an air pump and manometer for varying the air pressure within the ear canal.

Immittance Test Battery

Three basic measurements—tympanometry, static acoustic immittance, and threshold of the acoustic reflex—commonly make up the basic acoustic immittance test battery.

---

[1]daPa is a measure of air pressure in units of dekaPascals. 1 daPa = 10 Pa = 1.02 mm H_2O. *Millimeters of water* refers to the amount of pressure to push a column of water in a special tube to a given height in millimeters. For measurements of immittance, air pressure is generally expressed relative to ambient air pressure. That is, ambient air pressure is represented as 0 daPa, and a pressure of 100 daPa above ambient pressure is represented as 1 100 daPa.

Tympanometry

Acoustic immittance at the tympanic membrane of a normal ear changes systematically as air pressure in the external canal varies above and below ambient air pressure (Fig. 4.15). The normal relationship between air pressure changes and changes in immittance is frequently altered in the presence of middle ear disease. Tympanometry is measurement of the mobility of the middle ear when air pressure in the external canal varies from +200 to −400 daPa. Results from tympanometry are plotted on a graph, with air pressure along the x-axis and immittance, or compliance, along the y-axis.[2] Figure 4.17 shows patterns of tympanograms commonly seen in normal and pathologic ears.

Various estimates have been made of the air pressure in the ear canal that results in the least amount of reflected sound energy from normal middle ears. This air pressure is routinely called the peak pressure point. A normal tympanogram for an adult (Fig. 4.17a) has a peak pressure point between −100 and +40 daPa, which suggests that the middle ear functions optimally at or near ambient pressure (0 daPa). Tympanograms that peak at a point below the accepted range of normal pressures (Fig. 4.17b) suggest malfunction of the middle ear pressure-equalizing system. This malfunction might be a result of eustachian tube malfunction, early or resolving serous otitis media, or acute otitis media. (These and other disorders are described in detail in Chapter 5.) Ears that contain fluid behind the eardrum are characterized by a flat tympanogram at a high impedance or low admittance value without a peak pressure point (Fig. 4.17c). This implies an excessively stiff system that does not allow for an increase in sound transmission through the middle ear under any pressure state.

The amplitude (height) of the tympanogram also provides information about the compliance, or elasticity, of the system. A stiff middle ear (as in, for example, ossicular-chain fixation) is indicated by a shallow amplitude, suggesting high acoustic impedance or low admittance (Fig. 4.17d). Conversely, an ear with abnormally low acoustic impedance or high admittance (as in an interrupted ossicular chain or a hypermobile tympanic membrane) is revealed by a tympanogram with a very high amplitude (Fig. 4.17e).

Most tympanograms are measured using low-frequency probe tones introduced into the ear canal; frequencies of 220 and 660 Hz are most commonly used. In recent years, however, there has been increased interest in the use of multiple probe tone frequencies in which a family of tympanograms is obtained for a wide range of probe frequencies. This has usually been accomplished by sweeping the probe tone frequency from a low to a high value at each of several air pressure values or by sweeping the air pressure from positive to negative (or vice versa) at each of several probe tone frequencies. Use of multiple probe tone frequencies allows measurement and specification of the resonant frequency of the middle ear. Although it has been suggested that changes in the resonant frequency observed with multiple-frequency tympanograms can improve the diagnostic capabilities of tympanometric measurements, the clinical usefulness of this additional information remains to be firmly established. It does seem, however, that multiple-frequency tympanograms may be more useful in detecting the presence of fluid in the middle ears of infants under 4 months of age than those obtained using only a 220-Hz or 660-Hz probe tone.

---

[2]Throughout this text, we have assumed that immittance measurements are made with an impedance meter. With such a device, immittance values are described in arbitrary units, frequently labeled *compliance*. These devices do not actually measure compliance.

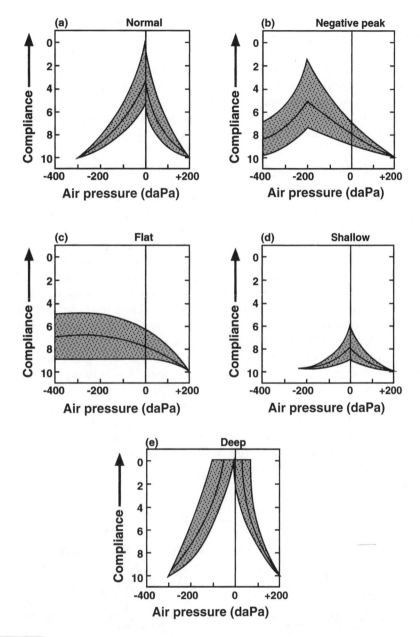

FIGURE 4.17 Tympanometric configurations for normal and pathologic ears. Measured tympanograms falling in the dotted regions are classified according to the label at the top of each tympanogram (e.g., normal, negative peak, flat).

Static Acoustic Immittance

Static acoustic immittance measures the ease of flow of acoustic energy through the middle ear. To obtain this measurement, immittance is first determined under positive pressure (+200 daPa) artificially induced in the canal. Very little sound is admitted through the middle ear under this extreme positive pressure, with much of the acoustic energy reflected into the ear canal. Next, a similar determination is made with the eardrum in its most compliant position, which maximizes transmission through the middle ear cavity. The arithmetic difference between these two immittance values, usually recorded in cubic centimeters of equivalent volume, provides an estimate of immittance at the tympanic membrane. Compliance values less than or equal to 0.25 cm³ of equivalent volume suggest low acoustic immittance (indicative of stiffening pathology), and values of 2.0 cm³ or above generally indicate abnormally high immittance (suggestive of ossicular discontinuity or healed tympanic membrane perforation).

Acoustic Reflex Threshold

The acoustic reflex threshold is defined as the lowest possible intensity needed to elicit a middle ear muscle contraction. Contraction of the middle ear muscles evoked by intense sound results in a temporary increase in middle ear impedance. As noted in Chapter 3, the acoustic reflex is a consensual phenomenon; acoustic stimulation to one ear will elicit a muscle contraction and subsequent impedance change in both ears. Usually the acoustic reflex is monitored in the ear canal contralateral to the ear receiving the sound stimulus. Figure 4.18 shows how it is measured. A headphone is placed on one ear, and the probe assembly is inserted into the contralateral ear. When the signal transduced from the earphone reaches an intensity sufficient to evoke an acoustic reflex, the stiffness of the middle ear is increased in both ears. This results in more sound being reflected from the eardrum, and a subsequent increase in sound pressure is observed on the immittance instrument. In recording the data, it is standard procedure to consider the ear stimulated with the intense sound as the ear under test. Because the ear stimulated is contralateral to the ear in which the reflex is measured, these reflex thresholds are called contralateral reflex thresholds. It is also frequently possible to present the loud reflex-activating stimulus through the probe assembly itself. In this case, the reflex is activated and measured in the same ear. This is called an ipsilateral acoustic reflex.

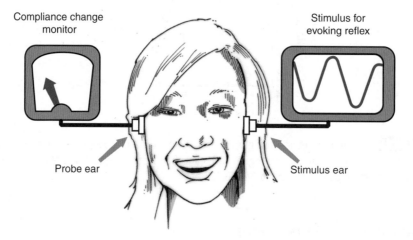

FIGURE 4.18 How an acoustic reflex is obtained for contralateral stimulus presentation. Essentially, for ipsilateral measurements, the functions of the probe tip and the earphone are combined so that the reflex-eliciting stimulus and the immittance change that results from the muscle contraction can be measured in the same ear.

In the normal ear, contraction of middle ear muscles occurs with pure tones ranging from 65 to 95 dB HL. A conductive hearing loss, however, tends either to elevate or to eliminate the reflex response. When acoustic reflex information is used in conjunction with tympanometry and static acoustic immittance measurements, it serves to substantiate the existence of a middle ear disorder. With unilateral conductive hearing loss, failure to elicit the reflex depends on the size of the air-bone gap and on the ear in which the probe tip is inserted. If the stimulus is presented to the good ear and the probe tip is placed on the affected side, an air-bone gap of only 10 dB will usually abolish the reflex response. If, however, the stimulus is presented to the pathologic ear and the probe is in the normal ear, a gap of 25 dB is needed to abolish or significantly elevate the reflex threshold.

Acoustic reflex thresholds can also be useful in differentiating whether a sensorineural hearing loss is caused by a lesion in the inner ear or to one in the auditory nerve. For hearing losses ranging from mild to severe, the acoustic reflex threshold is more likely to be elevated or absent in ears with neural pathology than in those with cochlear damage. The pattern of acoustic reflex thresholds for ipsilateral and contralateral stimulation across both ears, moreover, can aid in diagnosing brainstem lesions affecting the reflex pathways in the auditory brainstem. (See Chapter 3 for a brief overview of these pathways.)

Special Considerations in the Use of Immittance with Young Children

Immittance can be most valuable in the assessment of young children, although it does have some diagnostic limitations. Further, although electroacoustic immittance measures are ordinarily simple and quick to obtain, special consideration and skills are required to obtain these measures successfully from young infants.

Although immittance tests may be administered to neonates and young infants with a reasonable amount of success, tympanometry may have limited value with children younger than 7 months of age. Below this age, there is a poor correlation between tympanometry and the actual condition of the middle ear. In very young infants, a normal tympanogram does not necessarily imply that there is a normal middle ear system. However, a flat tympanogram obtained in an infant strongly suggests a diseased ear. Consequently, it is still worthwhile to administer immittance tests to this population.

Another limitation of immittance measurements is the difficulty of obtaining measurements from a hyperactive child or a child who is crying, yawning, or continually talking. A young child who exhibits excessive body movement or head turning will make it almost impossible to maintain an airtight seal with the probe tip. Vocalization produces middle ear muscle activity that in turn causes continual alterations in the compliance of the tympanic membrane, making immittance measurements impossible. With difficult-to-test and younger children, specialized techniques are needed to keep the child relatively calm and quiet. For young children, it is always recommended that a second person be involved in the evaluation. While the child is sitting on the parent's lap, one person can place the earphone and insert the probe tip and a second person can manipulate the controls of the equipment. With infants below 2 years of age, placing the earphones and headband on the child's head is often distracting. It may be helpful to remove the earphone from the headband, rest the band over the mother's shoulder, and insert the probe tip into the child's ear. It is also helpful to use some distractive techniques that will occupy the child's attention during the test (Vignette 4.5).

VIGNETTE 4.5   Distractive techniques used in evaluating young children with immittance

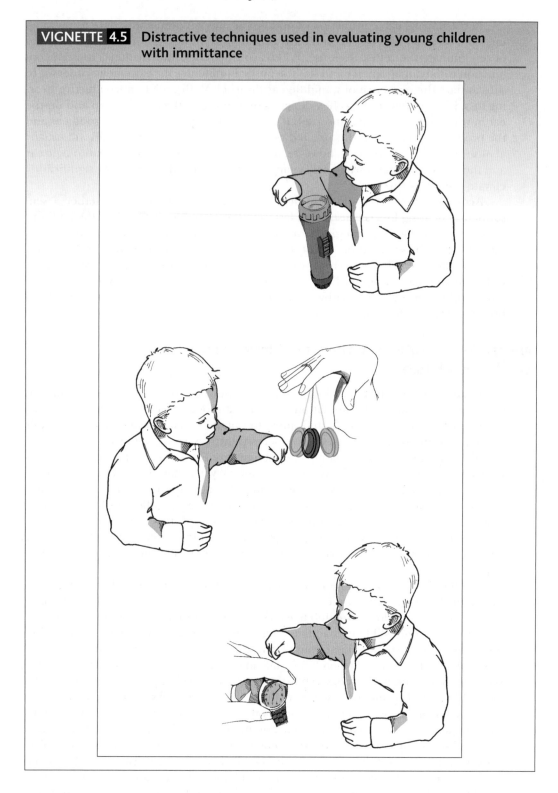

VIGNETTE 4.5 **Distractive techniques used in evaluating young children with immittance** *(Continued)*

DESIRABLE DISTRACTORS

Flashlight Direct the light toward the child or shine it on objects or people well within the child's visual field. Constantly change the rate of movement from slow to fast. If habituation occurs, take the child's hand and repeatedly place it over the light source.

Cotton swab Gently brush the back of the child's hand, arm, or leg in a slow, even motion. Make the distraction visual as well as tactile by making oscillatory or exaggerated movements of the swab.

Pendulum Using a bright and unusually shaped object, make a pendulum with about an 18-inch string. This technique is highly effective if the examiner swings the pendulum about in various motions within various areas of the infant's vision. Swing the pendulum rather slowly in short excursions, permitting easy visual following. Frequently stop or alter the swinging motion to provide novelty to the pendular action.

Mirror To an infant less than 1 year of age who is capable of reacting and attending to faces, a large mirror is sometimes irresistible, at least for a period sufficiently long to place a probe tip and to perform the impedance test battery.

Watch In front of the child, simply remove the wristwatch and manipulate or wind it well out of reach of the child or point to it.

Shoe A simple yet effective technique is to begin lacing and unlacing a child's shoe, either on or off his foot. This should be carefully timed to coincide with the insertion of the test tip into the ear. Move slowly and methodically and do not appear to have any object in mind except to lace and unlace the shoe.

Wad of cotton or tissue A cotton ball balanced on the hand, arm, or knee of the child or on the hand of the assistant can facilitate effective passive attention. It can be squeezed or otherwise manipulated; it can be blown or allowed to fall repeatedly from the hand. A tissue can also be used as a parachute, torn slowly into shapes, rolled into small balls and placed in the child's hand, waved, punctured, and so forth.

Tape A roll of adhesive or paper surgical tape has been found to be one of the most effective distractive devices available in the clinic. Bits of tape can be torn off or stuck on various parts of the child's or examiner's anatomy. The child can be allowed to pull the tape off, objects can be picked up with the adhesive side of the tape, fingers can be bound together, links can be made with small strips, rings can be formed, fingernails covered, and innumerable other meaningless manipulations can be performed. Tape works wonders for the few seconds necessary for obtaining immittance measures.

Miscellaneous devices Tongue blades, cotton swabs, colored yarn, or similar devices are all effective as distractive devices. They are best used in the hands of the examiner. If the child insists, he or she can be allowed to manipulate the device. Care must be taken to permit only passive action so as to reduce movement artifact while the test is proceeding.

LESS DESIRABLE DISTRACTORS AND THOSE TO BE USED WITH CAUTION

Animated toys Introduce animated toys only as required at critical times necessary to complete the test. Avoid movement artifacts by keeping the toy well out of the reach of the child.

Toys that produce sounds Toys or other devices that emit intense sounds should be avoided because they may evoke an acoustic or other reflexive response from the child. Toys that produce softer sounds in no way interfere with the test and can be used effectively, especially if the sound is novel.

(continued)

VIGNETTE 4.5   Distractive techniques used in evaluating young children with immittance *(Continued)*

Food Children, like adults, seem to enjoy sweets, and although swallowing and sucking movements are notorious for producing artifacts in the tympanogram and reflex measures, food can still be used as a distractive technique. Flavored gelatin or soft-drink powder in water, honey, or sweetened lemon juice can be dropped into the child's mouth at intervals during the test. Avoid taking measurements until the reflexive sucking action has subsided. Administering small amounts of liquid at well-spaced intervals can keep the child occupied for many minutes.

Action toys A variety of toys perform repetitive actions, such as a monkey that climbs down a stick pole. Often these are not the best distractive devices, because children 1 year and older often wish to handle or manipulate this type of toy.

Lollipop A lollipop can be used when the child is cradled and partially immobilized in the examiner's or parent's arm. The examiner can stroke the child's lips or tongue with the lollipop. Careful spacing of the lollipop sampling permits completion of the entire immittance test pattern.

Adapted from Northern JL. Acoustic impedance in the pediatric population. In Bess FH, ed. Childhood Deafness: Causation, Assessment and Management. New York: Grune & Stratton, 1977.

BASIC AUDIOLOGIC TEST BATTERY

In the measurement of auditory function, the most meaningful information can be gleaned only when the entire test battery of pure-tone and speech audiometry together with immittance measurements is used. If just one or two of these procedures are used, valuable clinical information will be lost, because each of these clinical tools offers a unique and informative set of data. In particular, the reader should keep in mind the differences between pure-tone measures and electroacoustic immittance measurements. Pure-tone audiometry does not measure the immittance of the middle ear, just as immittance does not measure hearing sensitivity. Although an abnormal audiogram strongly suggests hearing loss, abnormal immittance does not. Abnormal immittance findings in the absence of significant hearing loss, on the other hand, can be sufficient grounds for medical referral. A test battery approach is essential. Vignettes 4.6 to 4.8 show applications of the test battery.

VIGNETTE 4.6   A 6-year-old child with bilateral otitis media

The accompanying charts show a mild to moderate bilateral hearing loss for air conduction; bone conduction thresholds are normal in both ears. Such a discrepancy between air conduction and bone conduction thresholds suggests a conductive loss. The SRTs are compatible with the pure-tone data. Also, when the signal is made comfortably loud, suprathreshold speech recognition is excellent in both ears. Good speech recognition is consistent with a middle ear disorder. Immittance confirms the impression of a conductive loss. The shaded areas on the tympanogram and static immittance forms represent normative data. The tympanograms are flat, the static immittance is well below normal, and acoustic reflexes are absent in both ears. This general

---

VIGNETTE 4.6   A 6-year-old child with bilateral otitis media *(Continued)*

pattern is consistent with a middle ear complication and strongly suggests a fluid-filled middle ear, which requires a medical referral. If, however, there is no evidence of previous middle ear problems and the child has no complaints, a recheck should be recommended in 3 weeks. If the same results are obtained, the child should be referred to the family physician.

Educationally, such a problem can be relatively serious if medical intervention does not result in a speedy return to completely normal hearing. Such children are likely to appear listless and inattentive in the classroom, and their performance soon begins to deteriorate. Both the teacher and the parents should receive an explanation of these probable consequences from the audiologist. In counseling the teacher, emphasis should be placed on establishing favorable classroom seating, supplementing auditory input with visual cues, articulating clearly and forcefully, and frequently reiterating assignments. If the condition does not respond readily to medical treatment, amplification, along with other remedial measures, such as speech reading instruction and training in listening skills, should not be ruled out. Above all, the child will need patient understanding while the hearing level is diminished and sometimes fluctuating from one day to the next.

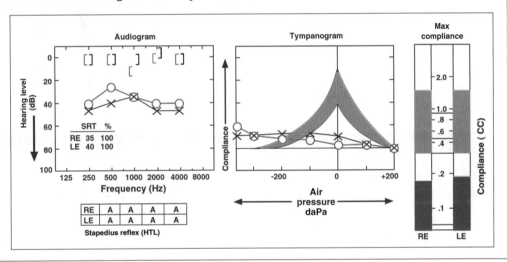

VIGNETTE 4.7   An 8-year-old child with a bilateral severe to profound hearing loss

The pure-tone results in the accompanying figure display a severe to profound sensorineural hearing loss. Bone conduction responses could not be obtained at the maximum output limits of the audiometer. The SRTs using selected spondees were compatible with the pure-tone data. Suprathreshold speech recognition scores could not be tested because of the severity of the loss. Immittance results on both ears show tympanograms and static immittance values to be within the normal range. Acoustic reflexes are absent in both ears, but these usually cannot be elicited with a hearing loss in excess of 85 dB HL.

(continued)

VIGNETTE 4.7   **An 8-year-old child with a bilateral severe to profound hearing loss** *(Continued)*

These audiologic results confirm the irreversibility of the hearing loss, which is so severe that the best possible special education opportunities must be made available. Periodic audiologic evaluations are highly important in the optimal educational management of such children. Frequently they have ear infections that further reduce their already greatly depressed level of sensitivity. At such times, the amplification program that has been recommended for them must be modified temporarily while medical treatment is being obtained.

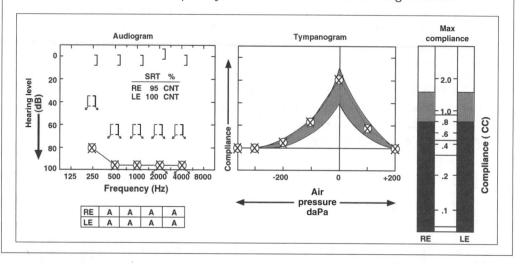

ADDITIONAL ELECTROPHYSIOLOGIC MEASURES

The basic audiologic test battery determines whether a patient has a hearing loss, the affect of any loss on speech understanding, and whether the nature of the hearing loss is conductive, sensorineural, or a combination of the two (mixed).

The immittance battery can also evaluate tympanic membrane and middle ear function regardless of whether a measurable hearing loss is present. Moreover, it can help raise clinical suspicion for potential auditory nerve or brainstem lesions, which may manifest as an absent or elevated acoustic stapedial reflex.

Thus, the basic audiologic test battery is able to determine where in the peripheral portion of the auditory system a particular disease process may be. Additional special testing is sometimes needed to substantiate or augment results from the basic audiologic test battery (i.e., children who are difficult to test) or to determine whether lesions are present beyond the inner ear (cochlea) in the more central portions of the ascending auditory nervous system pathway such as the acoustic nerve, brainstem, or cortex.

A patient with a tumor affecting the cochlear segment of the acoustic nerve, for example, will frequently present with a high-frequency sensorineural hearing loss. It is important, in this case, to differentiate a neural from a sensory etiology underlying the observed sensorineural hearing loss. However, such lesions that arise within the brainstem, beyond the cochlea, often do not produce hearing loss. In this case, additional tests aid in the diagnosis of an auditory disorder that has gone undetected by the basic audiologic test battery.

Other components of the basic hearing test battery may also provide some characteristic signs pointing to an acoustic nerve tumor. In such cases, the high-frequency

---

VIGNETTE 4.8 Adult with a bilateral mild to moderate sensorineural hearing loss

The pure-tone results accompanying this vignette show a bilateral sloping sensorineural hearing loss in an elderly adult. The SRTs are compatible with the pure-tone data, and suprathreshold speech recognition is only fair to good, even when the signal is made comfortably loud. Immittance results show normal tympanograms and static immittance for both ears, with acoustic reflexes present but elevated bilaterally.

Most adults with this battery of results are successful users of individual amplification, highly competent speech readers, or both. It may still be necessary to provide special assistance in the form of training in auditory and visual (speech reading) communication skills.

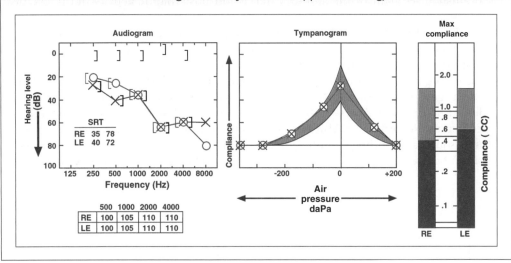

sensorineural hearing loss most often is unilateral (in one ear), with the opposite (contralateral) ear unaffected. In addition, speech recognition scores in the impaired ear can be reduced much more than would be explainable on the basis of the pure-tone hearing loss. Finally, acoustic reflex thresholds for the affected ear are typically elevated above the normal range (100 dB HL or more), or they are absent. The development and refinement of contemporary electrophysiologic measures to complement the basic audiologic test battery have made it possible to corroborate behavioral test data objectively and in many instances to identify retrocochlear lesions. Two electrophysiologic measures used most frequently by the audiologist include auditory brainstem response (ABR) and evoked otoacoustic emissions (OAE). Although detailed descriptions of these procedures are beyond the scope of this book, it is important for the beginning student to develop at least a cursory understanding of these two important measures, which have become essential to the clinical assessment of patients with hearing loss. The reader is encouraged to review the basic concepts of auditory electrophysiology and otoacoustic emissions introduced in Chapter 3 prior to reading the sections that follow next.

The Auditory Brainstem Responses (ABR)

Chapter 3 (see Vignette 3.5) revealed that the peripheral and central auditory nervous system generates a series of electrical signals in response to a transient acoustic stimulus, such as a click. These signals, synchronized electrical impulses from the auditory nerve through the brainstem, can be recorded as a series of waves from electrodes placed on the scalp and earlobes, respectively. The time it takes from the onset of the click to the response defines the classification of the auditory evoked potential. The ABR is divided into what can be called short-latency component waveforms that appear within the first 10 ms following the onset of the transient click stimulus.

For clinical use, the ABR consists of a series of five primary waves labeled with Roman numerals as illustrated in Figure 4.19. Each of the five waves arises from one or more neural generator sites beginning at the auditory nerve and ending in the brainstem. It is generally believed that wave I arises from the cochlear portion of the auditory nerve before it enters the brainstem. Wave II, which can be viewed as the second component of the auditory nerve, is thought to be generated by the brainstem segment of the auditory nerve and postsynaptic activity in the cochlear nucleus.

Beyond wave II, the ABR reflects multiple neural generator sources. Wave III arises mostly from the superior olivary complex with some additional contribution from the cochlear nucleus. Wave IV appears to originate primarily from fibers of the ascending lateral lemniscal pathway just below the inferior colliculus. Finally, wave V, the largest peak in the ABR, is thought to emanate either from the inferior colliculus itself or from fibers of the lateral lemniscus that terminate in the inferior colliculus. Recording an ABR requires a computer instrument that includes (*a*) stimulus sources, including stimulus intensity control, (*b*) preamplifiers, (*c*) a data acquisition board, (*d*) digital amplifiers, (*e*) filters, (*f*) digital signal processor or averager,

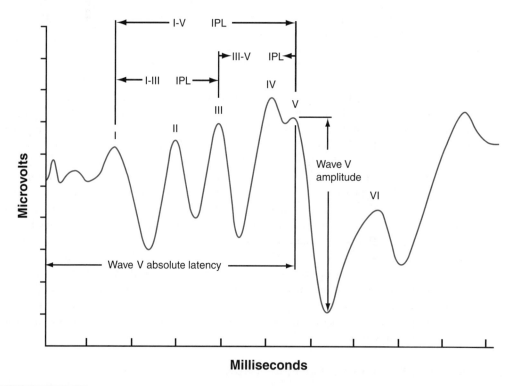

FIGURE 4.19 The ABR waveform from a normal-hearing adult; calculation of absolute and interpeak latencies (IPL) and peak-to-trough amplitude.

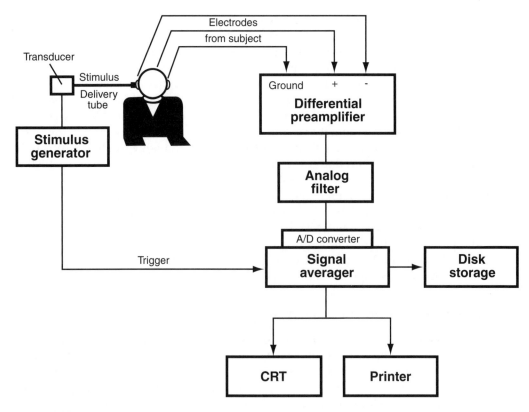

FIGURE 4.20 Basic components for conducting ABR measures.

(*g*) a display screen (CRT) with measurement cursors, and (*h*) data storage. A schematic of the necessary components recording an ABR is shown in Figure 4.20. Very briefly, these components function to generate and present via a transducer (e.g., earphones or bone conduction oscillator) an auditory stimulus that is used to excite a chain of neural events beginning at the auditory nerve and traversing the brainstem pathway. The signal from the neuroauditory way stations described earlier is picked up by the electrodes placed on the scalp similar to an electroencephalogram (EEG). Because the amplitudes of these electrical impulses are so small relative to the background brain electrical activity, they must first be amplified, filtered, and averaged to extract the neural events that are time-locked to the acoustic stimulus from among those that are occurring randomly in the background. The resulting ABR is displayed on a monitor, where the latency in milliseconds and amplitude in microvolts of each wave peak can be determined. These electrophysiologic waveforms and the latency and amplitude values derived from them can be saved for later retrieval on the computer hard drive.

To record the electrical activity, surface electrodes are placed on the scalp with a conductive gel or paste. One of the electrodes is placed on the vertex (center point on the scalp) and additional electrodes are placed on the earlobe or mastoid process of each ear. A fourth electrode, the ground electrode, is usually affixed to the forehead. The electrical activity measured at the vertex is compared to the electrical activity measured at the earlobe or mastoid process of the stimulated ear.

To conduct the ABR test for neurodiagnostic purposes, high-intensity (80–95 dB nHL) clicks are delivered to the ear at a rate ranging from about 9.1 to 21.1 per second. The reference *nHL*, used frequently with ABR measurements, indicates the intensity of the click stimulus relative to the hearing threshold for that same stimulus, transducer, and equipment that has been established by the clinic in a group of normal-hearing young adults. The ABR signals recorded from this rapid sequence of clicks are averaged until there is clear definition of the waveforms. The number of averages necessary varies with the signal-to-noise ratio, that is, the relative size of the response in relation to the background brain electrical activity. In asleep patients, a highly resolved ABR can be seen in only a few hundred averages; however, this number can increase to 1000 or more in a more active patient. Although this seems like a lot of stimuli to present, at 20 clicks per second, only about 50 seconds is necessary to present 1000 stimuli.

The ABR is an invaluable clinical tool that can be used a number of ways, including estimating auditory sensitivity, screening newborns for hearing loss, diagnosing auditory nerve or brainstem lesions, and monitoring the auditory nerve and brainstem pathways intraoperatively, or during surgery. A brief description of each of these clinical applications appears next.

Estimation of Auditory Sensitivity

Perhaps the most common application of ABR is the prediction of hearing sensitivity in young infants, children, or adults who are unable to provide voluntary behavioral responses. In fact, a significant advantage of ABR is that infants and very young children can be evaluated in a natural sleep or with mild sedation. To obtain predictions of hearing loss, wave V of the ABR is used, since it is the most robust wave and resilient to decreasing intensity. Hence, it correlates best with behavioral threshold measurements. Typically, a click or tone burst is presented first at a high intensity and subsequently at lower intensities. As the intensity of the click decreases, most of the ABR waves disappear except wave V, which can be elicited within 10 to 20 dB of the behavioral threshold for a click. As shown in Figure 4.21, as the intensity of the click decreases, there is a corresponding decrease in the amplitude of wave V and an increase in latency (time elapsed between the onset of a stimulus and the response). To estimate the auditory sensitivity, ABR wave forms are recorded at progressively decreasing intensities until wave V is no longer discernible. This level is thought to correspond closely with the behavioral threshold, especially with high-frequency pure-tone thresholds. Once the threshold ABR to clicks has been established, low-frequency tone bursts may be used to predict the possible degree of hearing loss in the lower-frequency range of the audiogram.

Newborn Hearing Screening

Another important application of ABR is newborn hearing tests. As set forth in Chapter 6, the overall purpose for hearing screening is to distinguish within the population at large those who exhibit a significant hearing loss from those who do not. Today, many states mandate universal newborn screening for hearing loss. Because the ABR is considered an excellent indicator of auditory sensitivity, the test has become a popular tool for newborn screening. Several automated ABR systems have been developed. One of the first is the ALGO, which uses a low-level click stimulus at 35 dB HL to elicit the ABR. A computer-based detection algorithm (hence, ALGO) is used to decide whether a response is present by comparing incoming data to a template of a normal

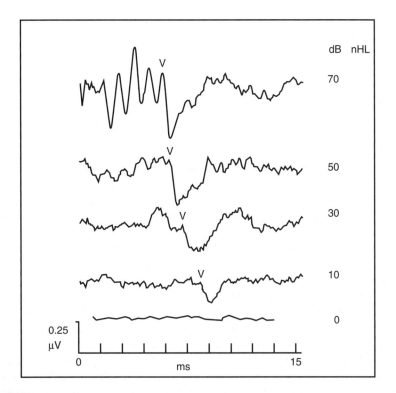

FIGURE 4.21 Estimation of auditory sensitivity using the ABR. ABR intensity series is obtained from a normal-hearing subject at click levels ranging from 70 to 0 dB nHL. Note the wave V latency increases (shifts out in time) as the intensity level is decreased.

wave form stored in memory. The result of such a comparison yields either a pass or refer outcome, depending upon whether the response is detected. Additional automated ABRs have been developed by other manufacturers, and all of these systems are commonly used to screen the hearing of newborns in intensive care units and well-baby nurseries. Automated systems are advantageous in that little technical expertise is needed to administer the test. That is, the screening device can be used by nonprofessionals such as technicians or volunteers, which increases the cost effectiveness of the screening process. Large-scale clinical trials have confirmed the accuracy, simplicity, cost effectiveness, and clinical viability of automated ABR systems.

Neurodiagnosis

The clinical use of auditory evoked potentials in neurodiagnosis has changed over time. Progressive advances in magnetic resonance imaging (MRI) have limited the frequency of evoked-response studies in clinical practice. Yet MRI largely remains an anatomic imaging test, while the ABR explains the functional integrity of the auditory nerve and brainstem pathway. In other words, the MRI gives more accurate information about structural problems, while the ABR provides information about auditory physiology. While the two may be complementary, most clinical questions regarding presence of tumor or other structural lesion are answered better by MRI than ABR.

Regardless, the ABR can be useful as a test to assist in screening for an acoustic tumor or other lesions of the brainstem such as meningiomas, demyelinating (damage to the myelin sheath covering the nerve) diseases (i.e., multiple sclerosis), brainstem stroke, or closed head trauma.

The diagnostic interpretation of the ABR is based on the latencies and amplitudes of the component waves shown previously in Figure 4.19. The absolute (individual peak) and interpeak (difference between peak components) latencies of waves I, III, and V are calculated and charted against a data set of previously established normative values within a range of 2.5 to 3.0 standard deviations. If the interpeak latency (IPL) of waves I to III, III to V, or I to V exceeds the outer limits of this normative range, it suggests a conduction block secondary to a neural lesion. The interpeak latencies of the suspect ear can also be compared to those of the contralateral ear as another neurodiagnostic metric. Delays in absolute latency without a concomitant interpeak latency delay usually signify a peripheral versus a central or neural type of conduction block. Although absolute amplitude of individual ABR waveforms tends not to be diagnostic, the amplitude ratio between wave I and V sometimes can raise diagnostic suspicion.

In retrocochlear lesions, the effects on the ABR response, particularly the interpeak latencies and morphology of the ABR, depend upon the nature of the pathology. Some of the effects include absence of waves, prolonged interpeak latencies, or interaural wave V latency differences of more than 0.5 ms. Figure 4.22 illustrates the ABR response in a patient diagnosed with a right acoustic tumor. The *left panel* shows that the brainstem responses to click stimuli for the left ear were within normal limits for absolute and interpeak latencies. The *right panel* shows the brainstem responses for the right ear. No identifiable waves are present, a finding that is consistent with an acoustic nerve tumor affecting the internal auditory canal or a very large brainstem lesion.

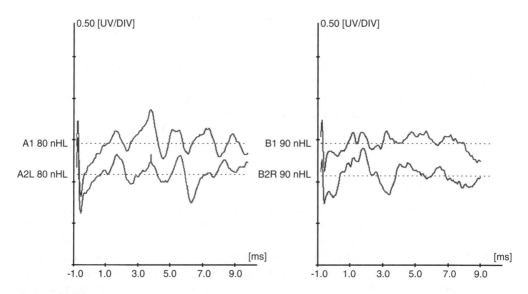

FIGURE 4.22 an ABR obtained from a 60-year-old female diagnosed with an eighth nerve tumor in the right ear. The waveform, latencies, and interpeak intervals are normal for the left ear (left panel), but not the right ear (right panel). Two ABRs are shown for each ear.

Intraoperative Monitoring

Finally, intraoperative monitoring of the ABR is used to warn a surgeon of emerging insult to the auditory nerve or brainstem during myriad surgical procedures. Examples of such surgeries include but are not limited to resection of tumor, vestibular nerve section for intractable vertigo, microvascular decompression of the trigeminal or facial nerve, and management of vertebrobasilar aneurysm. Monitoring the ABR is particularly valuable when the goal includes preservation of hearing during excision of very small acoustic nerve tumors. Severe prolongation of interpeak latencies or disruption of waveform morphology (shape) provides early warning of unintended insult during the surgery and allows for timely intervention to avoid permanent injury.

Otoacoustic Emissions

In 1978, David Kemp of the Institute for Laryngology and Otology in London reported on the discovery of OAEs, small acoustic signals in the external auditory meatus. These signals may occur spontaneously or in response to stimulation. As noted in Chapter 3, OAEs are thought to be generated in the outer hair cells of the cochlea and can be detected and recorded by small, sensitive microphones in the external auditory meatus. Importantly, these small acoustic signals are generated only when the organ of Corti is healthy, and the emissions are detected only when the middle ear system is normal. Finally, OAEs are not considered a measure of hearing; rather they reflect the status of peripheral structures that are necessary for hearing.

Chapter 3 discusses the two general classes of otoacoustic emissions, spontaneous otoacoustic emissions (SOAEs) and evoked otoacoustic emissions (EOAEs). Each is reviewed in more detail, with focus on their clinical application, in the next sections.

Spontaneous Otoacoustic Emissions

Spontaneous OAEs are continuous signals that are generated by the cochlea in the absence of auditory stimulation. They occur in more than half of normal ears, including those of infants, children, and adults. Typically, SOAEs measured in adults are concentrated in the frequency region of 1 to 3 kHz. However, spontaneous emissions have been observed at frequencies from 0.5 to 9.0 kHz. In general, SOAEs are not seen in frequency regions with sensorineural hearing loss greater than 30 dB HL. Finally, it appears that a spontaneous SOAE originates from outer hair cells corresponding to the portion of the basilar membrane tuned to that frequency.

SOAEs can be measured simply by placing a sensitive low-noise microphone housed in a soft probe tip into the external auditory meatus. The microphone is fed to a preamplifier, a filter to eliminate body or external noise, and then routed to a signal-spectrum analyzer, which provides a real-time frequency analysis of the signal. SOAEs have limited value as a clinical tool primarily because so many normal-hearing individuals fail to exhibit spontaneous emissions.

Evoked Otoacoustic Emissions

In contrast to SOAEs, EOAEs are thought to have considerable clinical value—the tests are simple, quick, reliable, informative, and objective. Chapter 3 discusses the two types of EOAEs with clinical utility. These emissions are based primarily on the stimuli that are used to evoke them. They include the transient EOAE (TEOAE) and distortion product OAE (DPOAE).

TEOAE setup

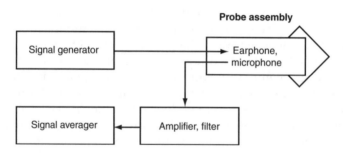

Components necessary for measuring TEOAEs.

TEOAEs were the first OAEs measured in humans, by David Kemp. These emissions have also been called Kemp echoes, cochlear echoes, and delayed evoked otoacoustic emissions. TEOAEs are broadband emissions evoked from a transient stimulus such as a click or a tone burst. A simplified diagram of the components necessary for measuring TEOAEs is shown in Figure 4.23. To measure TEOAEs a soft probe is inserted into the ear canal. Housed within the probe is a miniature sound source for delivering a click stimulus and a low-noise microphone to record the response. Responses to repeated stimuli, typically presented at moderate intensities (80–85 dB SPL), are transduced by the microphone. The signal is amplified and high-pass filtered to eliminate body or external noise before it is averaged to improve the signal-to-noise ratio. This amplification, filtering, and averaging are necessary because the EOAE is extremely low in amplitude, often less than 0 dB SPL. TEOAEs typically occur within 3 to 4 ms following the presentation of the click stimulus. An example of a TEOAE response obtained from a female subject with normal hearing is displayed in Figure 4.24. The transient OAE response waveforms shown in this figure represent an average of the emissions generated to 260 click stimuli presented at approximately 80 dB peak sound pressure level (peakSPL). The response was recorded in 64 seconds from the right ear of a young female. The signal-to-noise ratio (SNR) is the level or amplitude of the response (signal) over the noise floor (noise) for each of the frequency bands displayed. For example, for the frequency band centered at 1 kHz, the signal level is 5.8 dB SPL and noise level is −9.4 dB SPL, yielding an SNR of 15.2 dB. This is illustrated in the bar graph at the bottom of this figure labeled *Half octave band OAE power* (noise = black, emission = gray). Since OAEs are believed to originate in the outer hair cells of the organ of Corti, the presence of OAEs, or in this example, gray bars exceeding the black bars, indicates functioning outer hair cells. As noted previously, however, presence of functioning outer hair cells does not mean presence of hearing. Any dysfunction from the inner hair cells to the auditory centers of the cortex, if present, could impair hearing and go undetected by OAEs. Furthermore, to be recorded by the microphone in the ear canal, the stimulus to the cochlea and the OAE generated in the cochlea must pass through the middle ear. As a result, absence of the OAEs (e.g., gray bars not exceeding black bars in bar graph of Fig. 4.24), in and of itself does not indicate cochlear dysfunction.

The nature of DPOAEs was discussed in Chapter 3. To recap briefly, DPOAEs are the consequence of the nonlinear nature of the cochlea. When a sound signal composed of two pure tones close in frequency and intensity is presented to the ear, that

Response waveform

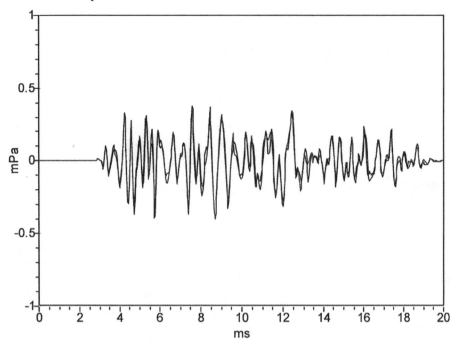

Half octave band OAE power

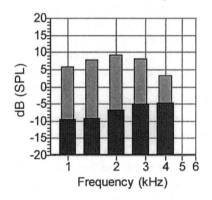

Freq (kHz)	Signal (dB SPL)	Noise (dB SPL)	SNR (dB)
1.0	5.8	-9.4	15.2
1.4	7.9	-9.1	17.0
2.0	9.2	-6.6	15.8
2.8	8.2	-5.1	13.3
4.0	3.4	-4.7	8.1

FIGURE 4.24   TEOAE response obtained in a normal-hearing adult.

signal is reliably transduced within the cochlea, but energy at frequencies not in the original signal is also produced. Of the two-tone stimulus, f_1 is the lower-frequency component; f_2 is the higher-frequency component. The most common distortion product measured by DPOAE systems is the $2f_1 - f_2$ distortion product, because in most cases it has the greatest amplitude. To illustrate this concept, if f_1 is 1000 Hz and f_2 is 1300 Hz, the difference tone or distortion product would be 700 Hz ($2f_1 - f_2$). Because the DPOAE is generated using two pure tones close in frequency, it has a frequency-specific origin. A simplified schematic for measuring DPOAEs is shown in Figure 4.25.

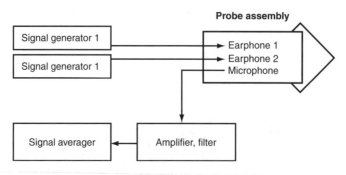

DPOAE setup

FIGURE 4.25 Components necessary for measuring DPOAEs.

Two separate channels of signal generation and transduction are needed to generate the primary tones. The eliciting tones are presented to the ear through a probe microphone assembly similar to those used in measuring other types of emissions, except there are two stimulus delivery ports. Pairs of tones are typically presented across the frequency range to elicit distortion products ranging from roughly 1000 to 6000 Hz. The tone pairs are at fixed frequency and intensity relationships. As each pair is presented, measurements are made at the $2f_1 - f_2$ frequency to determine the amplitude of the DPOAEs and also at a nearby frequency to provide an estimate of the noise floor at that moment. An example of a DPOAE obtained in a normal-hearing adult is shown in Figure 4.26. The DPOAE response shows the amplitude of the emission as a function of frequency between 1 and 8 kHz. The emission is generated in response to two input tones (f_2, f_1) with a fixed frequency ratio of $f_2/f_1 = 1.2$. For example, when $f_2/f_1 = 1.2$, the f_2 tone is at 1200 Hz when the f_1 tone is at 1000 Hz. Likewise, when the f_1 tone is at 2000 Hz, the f_2 tone is at 2400 Hz. The stimulus intensity was 55 dB SPL for the higher-frequency tone (f_2) and 65 dB SPL for the lower-frequency tone (f_1). Test duration was 33 seconds. The SNR is the difference between the signal and the noise in each of the seven frequency bands over which emissions were measured. The *black shaded region* in the lower portion of the DPOAE response graph from 1 to 3 kHz represents noise. Emission response amplitudes are displayed by *open circles*. In the *half octave band OAE power* bar graph at the bottom of this figure, noise is again shown in *black* and the emission is displayed in *gray*. The presence of DPOAEs is again signified by the *gray bars* being visible above the *black bars*. If DPOAEs are present, the outer hair cells of that cochlea are functioning appropriately. Again, the ramifications of this finding alone can be interpreted only in the broader context of other audiologic measures.

Clinical Applications of Otoacoustic Emissions

OAEs provide valuable clinical information. OAEs are present in listeners with normal hearing who have a normally functioning outer and middle ear. If the outer hair cells of the cochlea are damaged, OAEs may not be present. Specifically, if an individual exhibits an OAE, hearing thresholds are better than 30 dB HL; if, however, the OAE is absent, the hearing threshold is poorer than 30 dB HL.

DPOAE response

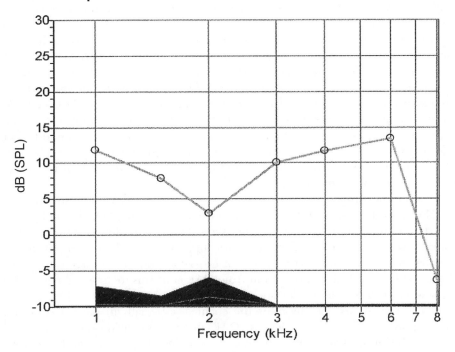

Half octave band OAE power

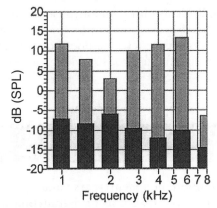

Freq (kHz)	Signal (dB SPL)	Noise (dB SPL)	SNR (dB)
1.0	11.8	-7.2	19.0
1.4	7.9	-8.5	16.4
2.0	3.0	-5.9	8.9
2.8	10.0	-9.7	19.7
4.0	11.7	-12.0	23.7
6.0	13.4	-10.0	23.4
8.0	-6.2	-14.5	8.2

FIGURE 4.26 DPOAE response obtained in a normal-hearing adult.

The OAE is a versatile measure that can be used in a number of ways. The most common applications of this test include newborn hearing screening, assessment of young infants, and monitoring the function of the cochlea. Perhaps the greatest clinical application for OAEs has been universal screening of newborn hearing. This topic is briefly introduced in Chapter 3 (Vignette 3.3) and again in Chapter 6. The use of TEOAEs as a screening tool for newborn screening has received widespread acceptance, and virtually thousands of hospitals throughout the United States have incorporated OAEs into their newborn screening programs. In fact, as discussed in Chapter 6, the National Institutes of Health developed a consensus statement with regard to newborn screening and recommended that TEOAEs be used as the first-stage screen in any such program. Clinical research has demonstrated that this tool is very effective for screening young newborns in the nursery. The test is simple, acceptable, reliable, cost effective, and practical. One limitation to the use of emissions as a screening tool is that they do not reveal middle ear disease. As noted earlier, middle ear problems result in an absent response to click stimuli. Hence, an absent response to an OAE test could be due to an outer ear problem, a middle ear problem, an inner ear problem, or perhaps some combination of these. Nevertheless, the OAE test has been effective as a screening tool and has received widespread usage in the United States and abroad.

Another important application of OAE testing is the use of this tool to supplement behavioral data in the assessment of young children. Because the OAE is an objective measure that requires no voluntary responses and because the test is simple, quick, and noninvasive, it has become a first choice for supplementing the findings from the basic test battery. That is, the test is useful for cross-checking the results of the basic audiologic test battery. If the information from OAE confirms the possibility of some hearing loss, more elaborate testing, such as ABR, can be conducted.

OAEs can also be used to monitor the cochlea, especially in patients who are being treated with ototoxic drugs. Because OAEs depend primarily on outer hair cell function and the biomechanical properties of the cochlea, they are vulnerable to toxic and physical agents. Hence, OAEs can be used to monitor the status of the ears of individuals who are receiving medical intervention or medical therapies that are potentially ototoxic.

Finally, OAEs can be used for evaluating individuals with pseudohypoacusis; that is, individuals who exhibit audiometric evidence of hearing loss with is no organic basis to explain the impairment. Once again, an objective test that does not require voluntary responses serves as an excellent supplemental test for examining subjects with suspected nonorganic hearing loss.

EVALUATION OF CHILDREN WITH AUDITORY PROCESSING DISORDERS: A COMMENT

Finally, an area that has received much attention in recent years, much of it controversial, especially in school-age children, is the diagnosis of dysfunction in the auditory portions of the central nervous system. These problems have generally been labeled as auditory processing disorders (APD) or central auditory processing disorders (CAPD). The reliability and validity of many of the tests developed to identify CAPD, both in children and adults, are still being investigated. One of the challenges is to demonstrate that such tests are truly measuring auditory abilities and not more general cognitive function. Until such tests are developed and norms using them established, however, the diagnosis and treatment of such disorders are likely to remain controversial. (Vignette 4.9 addresses the importance of test reliability and validity.) Additional information on APD is presented in Chapter 5.

VIGNETTE 4.9   The importance of test reliability and validity

The reliability and validity of a test are essential information that must be known before the widespread use of that test. Unfortunately, because of the pressures of solving problems for patients today, audiologists often don't feel that they have the time to wait for the needed research to be completed before the use of a newly developed test. The testing of auditory processing disorders (APD) in children (sometimes called CAPD, or central auditory processing disorders) is clearly an area that exemplifies this problem. Often, tests have been pressed into use before clearly establishing their reliability or validity as tests of APD.

In general, the reliability of the test refers to its accuracy or stability. Ideally, if the same test were administered to the same individual under identical conditions on 10 successive occasions, with no memory, learning, or fatigue involved, we'd like all 10 scores to be identical. For behavioral testing of humans, especially children, however, this ideal is seldom achieved. Rather, the scores vary from test to retest because of a wide variety of factors. The greater the variation in test scores in this hypothetical scenario, the poorer the reliability of the test. Many tests of APD have been found to have unacceptable reliability. For some of the proposed APD tests, the scores can be expected to vary from test to retest such that the diagnostic disposition will likely vary from normal to abnormal (or vice versa). Clearly, such tests are unacceptably unreliable for widespread clinical use.

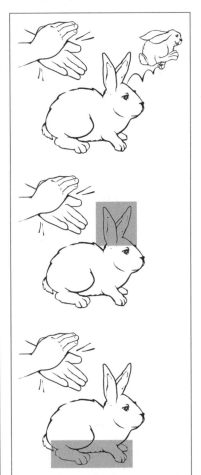

Perhaps an even thornier issue, though, has to do with establishing the validity of a test. There are many kinds of test validity, but in all cases, evaluation of a test's validity attempts to determine how well the proposed test measures what it was designed to measure. In the case of APD, is the proposed test measuring central auditory processing? First, it must be demonstrated that poor performance on the test cannot be attributed to peripheral auditory deficits. Although this has been an infrequent problem when APD was studied in children, it has been a very common problem when APD was studied in the elderly. Second, it must be demonstrated that the test is sensitive to an auditory deficit and not representative of a more general cognitive problem that can affect multiple sensory modalities. Often, in this regard, clinical researchers have taken the approach that a similarity in responses implies similarity in causality. Several tests of APD, for example, make use of tasks that were validated on cases of surgically or radiologically confirmed central auditory lesions (for example, stroke patients or patients with tumors in the central pathways). When audiologists observed similar (but usually not identical) trends in performance on proposed APD tests in individuals with no known central auditory lesions, they concluded that the locus of the dysfunction had to be central because the response pattern was similar to that obtained from patients with known central lesions.

A key problem with such reasoning is shown with the fictitious handclap test of hearing illustrated here. First, the researcher establishes that normal-hearing rabbits

(continued)

> **VIGNETTE 4.9** The importance of test reliability and validity *(Continued)*
>
> will hop away in response to a clap of the hands (*top*). Next, a rabbit's ears are surgically destroyed. (Relax! This is just a hypothetical experiment.) The experimenter then demonstrates that the rabbit fails to hop away in response to a clap of the hands (*middle*). Thus, the test has been validated as being sensitive to the presence of a hearing loss.
>
> Now another rabbit's legs are surgically removed, and the experimenter again claps. The rabbit fails to hop away, and the experimenter, noting the same response as from rabbits without ears, concludes that rabbits without legs can't hear. Clearly, the faulty reasoning in this analogy is apparent. Similarity or even equivalence of responses does not confirm similarity (or equivalence) of the underlying causal factors.
>
> In recent years, researchers have realized the need for reliable and valid measures of APD in both children and adults. Several tests are under development and evaluation at present, and it is hoped that these tools will be available for widespread clinical use in the near future.

SUMMARY

This chapter reviews the basic components of the test battery used in the measurement of auditory function. This includes the measurement of pure-tone threshold by air and bone conduction, speech audiometry, and immittance measurements. The results from these various approaches, when used as a battery, give the audiologist good insight into the nature and extent of the auditory disorder.

References and Suggested Readings

American Speech-Language-Hearing Association. Guidelines for audiometric symbols. ASHA 32(Suppl 2):25–30, 1990.

American Speech-Language-Hearing Association. Guidelines for determining threshold level for speech. ASHA 30(3):85–90, 1988.

American Speech-Language-Hearing Association. Short Latency Auditory Evoked Potentials. Rockville, MD: Audiologic Evaluation Working Group (2):335–370, 1987.

Bench J, Koval A, Bamford J. The BKB (Bamford-Koval-Bench) sentence lists for partially-hearing children. Br J Audiol 13:108–112, 1979.

Bess FH. Clinical assessment of speech recognition. In Konkle DF, Rintelmann WF, eds. Principles of Speech Audiometry. Baltimore: University Park, 1982.

Bess FH. The minimally hearing impaired child. Ear Hear 6:43–47, 1985.

Bess FH, Chase PA, Gravel JS, et al. Amplification for infants and children with hearing loss—1995 position statement. Am J Audiol 5:53–68, 1996.

Bluestone CD, Beery QC, Paradise JL. Audiometry and tympanometry in relation to middle ear effusions in children. Laryngoscope 83:594–604, 1963.

Burkard, RE, Manuel D, Eggermont JJ. Auditory Evoked Potentials: Basic Principles and Clinical Application. Baltimore: Lippincott, Williams & Wilkins, 2007.

Carhart R. Future horizons in audiological diagnosis. Ann Otol Rhinol Laryngol 77:706–716, 1968.

Carhart R, Jerger JF. Preferred method for clinical determination of pure-tone thresholds. J Speech Hear Disord 24:330–345, 1959.

Clifton RA. Development of spatial hearing. In Werner LA, Rubel EW, eds. Developmental Psychoacoustics. Washington: American Psychological Association, 1992.

Cox R, Alexander G, Gilmore C, Puskalich KM. Use of the Connected Speech Test (CST) with hearing-impaired listeners. Ear Hear 9:198–207, 1988.

Diefendorf AO. Pediatric audiology. In Lass NJ, McReynolds LV, Northern JL, Yoder DE, eds. Handbook of Speech-Language Pathology and Audiology. Philadelphia: BC Decker, 1988.

Egan J. Articulation testing methods. Laryngoscope 58:955–991, 1948.

Gorga JP, Neely ST, Widen JE. Otoacoustic emissions in children. In Kent, RD, ed. MIT Encyclopedia of Communication Disorders. Cambridge: Massachusetts Institute of Technology, 2004:515–517.

Haskins HA. A phonetically balanced test of speech discrimination for children. Master's thesis. Evanston, IL: Northwestern University, 1949.

Hirsh IJ, Davis H, Silverman SR, et al. Development of materials for speech audiometry. J Speech Hear Disord 17:321–337, 1952.

Hood JD. The principles and practice of bone conduction audiometry: A review of the present position. Laryngoscope 70:1211–1228, 1960.

House AS, Williams CE, Hecker MHL, Kryter KD. Articulation testing methods: Consonantal differentiation in a closed-response set. J Acoust Soc Am 20:463–474, 1965.

Jerger S. Speech audiometry. In Jerger J, ed. Pediatric Audiology. San Diego: College Hill, 1984.

Jerger S, Lewis S, Hawkins J, Jerger J. Pediatric speech intelligibility test I. Generation of test materials. Int J Pediatr Otorhinolaryngol 2:217–230, 1980.

Kalikow DN, Stevens KN, Elliott, LL. Development of a test of speech intelligibility in noise using sentence materials with controlled word predictability. J Acoust Soc Am 61:1337–1351, 1977.

Katz J. Handbook of Clinical Audiology. 6th ed. Baltimore: Lippincott Williams & Wilkins, in press.

Katz DR, Elliott LL. Development of a new children's speech discrimination test. Paper presented at the convention of the American Speech-Language-Hearing Association, November 18–21, Chicago, 1978.

Levitt H, Resnick SB. Speech reception by the hearing impaired: Methods of testing and the development of new tests. In Ludvigsen C, Barfod J, eds. Sensorineural Hearing Impaired and Hearing Aids. Scand Audiol Suppl 6:107–130, 1978.

Lonsbury-Martin B. Otoacoustic emissions. In Kent RD, ed. MIT Encyclopedia of Communication Disorders. Cambridge: Massachusetts Institute of Technology, 2004:511–514.

Martin FN. Minimum effective masking levels in threshold audiometry. J Speech Hear Disord 39:280–285, 1974.

Northern JL. Acoustic impedance in the pediatric population. In Bess FH, ed. Childhood Deafness: Causation, Assessment and Management. New York: Grune & Stratton, 1977.

Northern JL, Downs MP. Hearing in Children. 5th ed. Philadelphia: Lippincott Williams & Wilkins, 2001.

Olsen WO, Matkin ND. Speech audiometry. In Rintelmann WF, ed. Hearing Assessment. Baltimore: University Park, 1979.

Owens E, Schubert ED. Development of the California consonant test. J Speech Hear Res 20:463–474, 1977.

Robinette MS, Glattke TJ. Otoacoustic Emissions: Clinical Applications. New York: Thieme, 1997.

Ross M, Lerman J. A picture identification test for hearing impaired children. J Speech Hear Res 13:44–53, 1970.

Sanders JW. Masking. In Katz J, ed. Handbook of Clinical Audiology. 2nd ed. Baltimore: Williams & Wilkins, 1978:124.

Sanders JW. Diagnostic audiology. In Lass NJ, McReynolds NJ, Northern JL, Yoder DE, eds. Handbook of Speech-Language Pathology and Audiology. Philadelphia: BC Decker, 1988.

Schow RL, Nerbonne MA, eds. Introduction to Audiologic Rehabilitation. 5th ed. Boston: Pearson Education, 2007.

Schwarz D, Morris M, Jacobson J. The normal auditory brainstem response and its variants. In Jacobson, J. ed. Principles and Applications in Auditory Evoked Potentials. Boston: Allyn & Bacon, 1994:123–153.

Schwartz D, Josey AF, Bess FH, eds. Proceedings of meeting in honor of Professor Jay Sanders. Ear Hear 8:4, 1987.

Shanks JE, Lilly DJ, Margolis RH, et al. Tympanometry. J Speech Hear Disord 53:354–377, 1988.

Studebaker GA. Clinical masking in air- and bone-conducted stimuli. J Speech Hear Disord 29:23–35, 1964.

Tharpe AM, Ashmead DH. A longitudinal investigation of infant auditory sensitivity. Am J Audiol 10:104–112, 2001.

Tillman TW, Olsen WO. Speech audiometry. In Jerger J, ed. Modern Developments in Audiology. New York: Academic, 1973.

Tillman TW, Carhart R. An Expanded Test for Speech Discrimination Using CNC Monosyllabic Words. Northwestern University Auditory Test No. 6. Technical Report SAM-TR–66–55, USAF School of Aerospace Medicine, Brooks Air Force Base, Texas, 1966.

Pathologies of the Auditory System

After completion of this chapter, the reader should be able to:

- Understand the system used to classify auditory disorders.
- Discuss the most common disorders affecting the external ear and middle ear.
- Be familiar with typical disorders affecting the cochlea.
- Identify the most common disorders affecting the auditory central nervous system.
- Develop an appreciation and an understanding of the physical symptoms and audiologic manifestations associated with most of these disorders.

A variety of disorders, both congenital and acquired, directly affect the auditory system. These disorders can occur at the level of the external ear, the external auditory canal, the tympanic membrane, the middle ear space, the cochlea, the auditory central nervous system, or any combination of these sites. The following review offers a discussion of some of the more commonly seen disorders that can impair the auditory system.

CLASSIFICATION OF AUDITORY DISORDERS

All auditory disorders can be divided into two major classifications: exogenous (outside the system) and endogenous (within the system). Exogenous hearing disorders are those caused by inflammatory disease, toxicity, noise, accident, or injury that inflicts damage on any part of the auditory system. Endogenous conditions originate in the genetic characteristics of an individual. An endogenous auditory defect is transmitted from the parents to the child as an inherited trait. However, not all congenital (present at birth) hearing disorders are hereditary, nor are all hereditary disorders

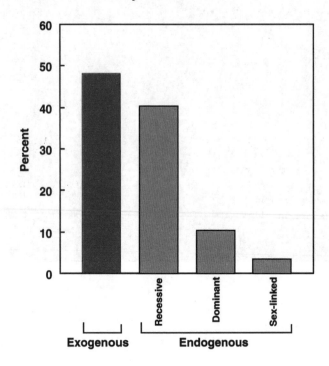

FIGURE 5.1 Percentage of individuals who exhibit exogenous and endogenous types of hearing loss.

congenital. For example, the child whose hearing mechanism is damaged in utero by maternal rubella is born with a hearing loss. This hearing loss is congenital but not hereditary. On the other hand, some hereditary defects of hearing may not manifest themselves until adulthood. A breakdown of the estimated percentage of individuals with exogenous and endogenous types of hearing loss is shown in Figure 5.1.

Genetic Transmission of Hearing Loss

As Figure 5.1 shows, hearing loss resulting from hereditary factors is thought to make up approximately 50% of auditory disorders. It is estimated that there are more than 400 genetic syndromes in which hearing loss is a regular or occasional feature (Table 5.1). In addition, at least 20 types of genetic deafness are known to occur without any other associated anomalies. Whether occurring as one manifestation of a particular syndrome (group of signs and symptoms that characterize a disorder or condition) or with no other abnormalities, hereditary hearing loss is usually governed by the Mendelian laws of inheritance. According to these genetic laws, genetic traits may be dominant, recessive, or X-linked (sex linked). Genes are located on the chromosomes, and with the exception of genes on the sex chromosomes of males, they come in pairs. One member of each gene pair (and the corresponding member of a chromosome pair) is inherited from each parent. Humans have 22 pairs of autosomes, or non–sex-determining chromosomes, and one pair of sex-determining chromosomes. The sex chromosome pair for females consists of two X chromosomes, and for males, one X and one Y chromosome. In human reproduction, each egg and each sperm cell carries half the number of chromosomes of each parent. When the egg is fertilized, the full complement of chromosomes is restored, so that half of a child's genes are from the mother and half are from the father.

TABLE 5.1 Examples of Autosomal Dominant, Recessive, and Sex-Linked Syndromic Forms of Hereditary Hearing Loss

Disorder	Prevalence	Clinical Characteristics	Hearing Loss
Autosomal dominance			
Waardenburg syndrome	1/4000; 3% of childhood hearing loss	Pigmentary anomalies (white forelock, blue irises, premature graying, partial albinism); craniofacial anomalies (**hypertelorism***, high nasal bridge, **synophrys**)	20–50% exhibit SNHL** depending on expression of syndrome
Branchio-oto-renal syndrome	1/40,000; 2% of children with profound hearing loss	Branchial abnormalities (ear pits and tags, cysts and fistulae); renal abnormalities	75% exhibit hearing loss; 30% conductive, 20% SNHL, 50% mixed
Treacher Collins syndrome	Unknown	Craniofacial anomalies (poorly developed malar bones, notching of eyelids, malformations of the external ear or canal, **micrognathia**, cleft palate)	30% exhibit conductive hearing loss; SNHL may be present
Recessive			
Usher syndrome	3.5/100,000; 10% of childhood hearing loss	SNHL and **retinitis pigmentosa**	Type 1, congenital, bilateral, profound hearing loss and absent vestibular function Type 2, moderate bilateral SNHL and normal vestibular function Type 3, progressive bilateral SNHL, variable vestibular dysfunction—found primarily in Norwegian population

(continued)

TABLE 5.1 Examples of Autosomal Dominant, Recessive, and Sex-Linked Syndromic Forms of Hereditary Hearing Loss *(Continued)*

Disorder	Prevalence	Clinical Characteristics	Hearing Loss
Pendred syndrome	Unknown; 5% of congenital childhood hearing loss	**Thyroid goiter** and SNHL	Severe to profound SNHL; 15% may be progressive
Jervell and Lange-Neilsen syndrome	Unknown (rare)	SNHL and **syncopal episodes**	Profound bilateral SNHL
Sex-Linked			
Norrie syndrome	Unknown	SNHL, congenital, or rapidly progressive blindness, **pseudoglioma**, **opacification**, and ocular degeneration	One-third exhibit progressive SNHL beginning in 2nd or 3rd decade of life
Alport syndrome	Unknown (predilection for males)	SNHL and **nephritis**	Bilateral progressive SNHL

*Terms in boldface appear in glossary at the end of text.
**SNHL, sensorineural hearing loss.

Autosomal Dominant Inheritance

In autosomal dominant inheritance, the trait is carried from one generation to another. The term *autosomal* implies that the abnormal gene is not on one of the two sex chromosomes. Typically, one parent exhibits the inherited trait, which may be transmitted to 50% of the offspring. This does not mean that half the children in a given family will necessarily be affected. Statistically, there is a 50% chance that any given child, whether male or female, will be affected (Vignette 5.1). Autosomal dominant inheritance is believed to account for approximately 20% of cases of genetically caused (endogenous) deafness. Because of the interaction of a number of genes, some traits may manifest themselves only partially; for example, only a very mild hearing loss may be observed despite a genetic structure indicating profound hearing loss.

Autosomal Recessive Inheritance

In contrast to autosomal dominant inheritance, both parents of a child with hearing loss of the autosomal recessive type are clinically normal. Appearance of the trait in the offspring requires that an individual possess two similar abnormal genes, one from each parent. The parents themselves are often heterozygous carriers of a single abnormal recessive gene. This means that each carries two genes, one normal and one abnormal with respect to a particular gene pair. Offspring carrying two of either the normal or the abnormal type of gene are termed *homozygotes*. Offspring may also be heterozygotes like their parents, carrying one of each gene type. If no abnormal gene is transmitted,

VIGNETTE 5.1 **Illustration of Mendelian law**

For this demonstration, you will need two paper cups and five poker chips or checkers (three chips of one color and two of another). For the first illustration, select one chip of one color and three of the other color. We will assume that you have one red chip and three white ones. Divide the four chips into two pairs, each pair representing a parent. The black chip represents a dominant gene for deafness. Whenever it is paired with another black chip or a white chip, it dominates the trait for hearing, resulting in deafness in the person with the gene. In this example, we have one deaf parent (one red chip, one white chip) and one normal-hearing parent (two white chips).

Each parent contributes one gene for hearing status to each offspring. When the deaf parent contributes the gene for deafness (red chip), the offspring will always be deaf. This is because the normal-hearing parent has only recessive genes for normal hearing (white chips) to contribute to the offspring. Separate the black chip from the deaf parent and slide it toward you. Slide each of the white chips from the other parent toward you, one at a time. For both of these possible offspring, the child will be deaf (a red chip paired with a white one). Now return the chips to the parents and slide the white chip from the deaf parent close to you. Slide each of the white chips from the normal parent closer to you, one after the other. When the deaf parent contributes a gene for normal hearing (white chip), the offspring will have normal hearing. This is true for pairings of each gene from the normal-hearing parent. For these two possible gene pairings, the offspring would have normal hearing.

In total, there were four possible gene pairings for the offspring. Of these, two were predicted to produce deafness and two were predicted to result in normal hearing. In this illustration of autosomal dominant deafness, the odds are that 50%, or half, of the offspring from these two parents will be deaf.

Now remove one of the white chips and replace it with a red one. Form two pairs of chips in front of you, each having one red and one white chip. In this case, the red chip represents the gene for deafness again, but it is recessive. The gene for normal hearing (white chip) is dominant. There will again be four possible pairings of the chips in the offspring, one from each parent. Examine the various combinations of genes by first sliding one chip closer to you from the parent on the left. Examine two possible pairings for each gene from the parent on the right. Now repeat this process by sliding the other chip from the parent on the left closer to you. When you have finished, you should have observed the following four pairs of chips for the offspring (red-white, red-red, white-red, and white-white). In this case of autosomal recessive deafness, only one of the possible combinations would produce a deaf offspring (red-red). The probability of a deaf child is one in four, or 25%. Two of the three normal-hearing offspring, however, will carry a gene for deafness (red-white chip pairs). These offspring are carriers of the trait.

It is sometimes difficult to understand that the Mendelian laws of hearing are only probabilities. In the case of autosomal recessive deafness, for example, one might think that if the parents had four offspring, they would have one deaf child. That is only the probability. They could very well have four normal-hearing children or four deaf children. To see how this occurs, place one red and one white chip in each of the two paper cups. Shake up the left cup and draw a chip. Repeat the process with the right cup. Examine the two chips (genes) selected, one from each cup (parent). Record the outcome (deaf or normal hearing) and replace chips in the cups. Do this 20 times, representing five families of four offspring each. When you're finished, you will likely find some families of four that had two, three, or four deaf offspring. If you did this an *infinite* number of times, however, 25% of the offspring would be deaf, as predicted by Mendelian laws for autosomal recessive deafness.

(continued)

VIGNETTE 5.1   Illustration of Mendelian law *(Continued)*

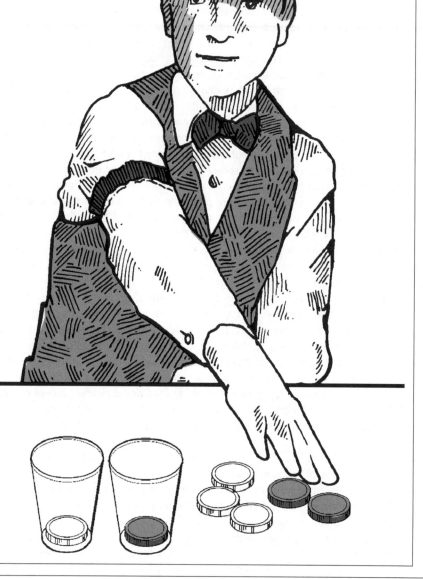

the offspring is normal for that trait. If there is one abnormal gene, the child becomes a carrier for the trait. If two abnormal genes, one from each parent, are transmitted, the offspring is affected and becomes a homozygous carrier. The probability that heterozygote parents will bear an affected homozygous child is 25% in each pregnancy on the basis that each child would inherit the abnormal gene from both the father (50% chance) and the mother (50% chance). Because the laws of probability permit this type of hearing loss to be transmitted without manifestation through several generations, detection of the true origin is often quite difficult. Recessive genes account for most cases of genetic hearing loss and can account for as much as 80% of childhood deafness.

X-Linked Inheritance

In the X-linked type of deafness, affected males are linked through carrier females. In this pattern, inherited traits are determined by genes on the X chromosome. As noted earlier, normal females have two X chromosomes, whereas males possess one X and one Y chromosome. Sons receive their Y chromosomes from their father; their X chromosomes are inherited from their mother. Daughters receive one X chromosome from their father and the other from their mother. In an X-linked trait, a carrier female has a 50% probability that each of her sons will be affected and a 50% probability that each of her daughters will be a carrier. All daughters of an affected male are carriers, but there is never a father-to-son transmission of the trait itself. Approximately 2 to 3% of deafness occurs as a result of X-linked inheritance. Examples of autosomal dominant, recessive, and sex-linked syndromic forms of hereditary deafness are shown in Table 5.1.

Advances in Hereditary Deafness

The progress made in genetic research during the past 20 years has been truly remarkable, and it is continually changing our understanding of hereditary deafness. Through gene mapping (identifying the chromosomal location of the gene) and localization (isolating the gene responsible for a disorder), it is now possible to identify genes responsible for deafness. At this writing, the chromosomal locations of approximately 70 genes for nonsyndromic deafness have been mapped. For example, in 1997, a specific gene was identified that appears to be the cause of hearing loss in many individuals. The gene is known to function in the inner ear. By testing for this gene, it is possible to identify the cause of deafness in as many as 20 to 40% of individuals in whom the cause of deafness was previously unknown. Identifying the genes that cause hearing loss may ultimately lead to therapeutic or preventive intervention in persons who exhibit genetic hearing loss. Moreover, the possibility of genetic screening to determine the diagnosis after identification of hearing loss is now a topic of widespread discussion. Genetic screening may have important benefits for both the child and the parents. Genetic testing and counseling can assist families to learn more about the cause of hearing loss to determine the probability of recurring risks and to accept a diagnosis of deafness.

Site of Lesion

Also important in the classification of an auditory disorder is the location of the lesion. Lesions in the outer or middle ear cause conductive hearing loss that is frequently amenable to medical treatment. If the damage is to the nerve endings or to the hair cells in the inner ear, the hearing loss is sensorineural. Hearing losses resulting from damage to the auditory nerve after it leaves the cochlea are sometimes designated neural. When damage is to the nerve pathways within the auditory central nervous system (see Chapter 3), the resulting condition is often known as central auditory impairment.

One other variable that can be used in the classification of auditory disorders but that does not require detailed explanation here is time of onset. Typically, the hearing loss is described in part by when the impairment was thought to occur (i.e., before delivery or after birth). Time of onset is discussed in more detail later in this chapter.

DISORDERS OF THE OUTER EAR AND MIDDLE EAR

Conductive hearing losses occur when there is a complication somewhere between the outer ear and the middle ear. A person with a conductive hearing loss exhibits normal threshold sensitivity by bone conduction measurements and decreased threshold values via air conduction. Chapter 4 introduces the term *air-bone gap* to describe this phenomenon.

A variety of disorders can produce a conductive hearing loss. All of them result in alteration of the mechanics of the external ear or the middle ear system. Some of these mechanical changes include blockage of the external or middle ear, an increase in the stiffness of the tympanic membrane or middle ear system, or an increase in the mass of the middle ear. These alterations in the mechanics of the outer and middle ear produce varying degrees and configurations of hearing loss. Recall from Chapter 2 that increasing the stiffness of a mechanical system has its greatest effect at low frequencies. Similarly, changing the mass of a mechanical system primarily affects the high frequencies. The specific configuration of the audiogram depends on the specific mechanical alterations produced by the disorder. Although the conductive loss might make it difficult to hear conversational speech, the ability to understand spoken messages is usually not impaired when speech is presented at comfortably loud levels.

Outer Ear Disorders

Deformities of the Pinna (Auricle) and External Ear Canal

A wide variety of external ear malformations or anomalies can take place; most are a result of an inherited trait. Such anomalies of the external ear can occur in isolation or as part of a complex that produces a variety of other alterations to the skull and face (called craniofacial defects). Pinna deformity can range from very mild malformations, which are difficult for the lay person to identify, to the more severe forms of the condition, such as total absence of the pinna or complete closure of the ear canal.

The most severe form of pinna deformity is *microtia*, or a very small and deformed pinna. Microtia is often associated with *atresia*, the absence or closure of the external auditory meatus. Importantly, atresia can occur without significant pinna abnormalities or as part of a constellation of other craniofacial defects. Figure 5.2 shows various pinna deformities.

Microtia and atresia are bilateral in 15 to 20% of cases, are known to affect the right ear more frequently than the left, and are slightly more prevalent in males than in females. The severity of the pinna deformity will sometimes offer an indication of the corresponding status of the middle ear space. A patient with microtia, for example, can also exhibit malformations of the middle ear ranging from minor deformities of the ossicles to a total absence of the middle ear cavity. Generally speaking, the more severe the deformation of the outer ear, the greater the conductive hearing loss. Figure 5.3 shows a conductive hearing loss seen in a severe case of microtia.

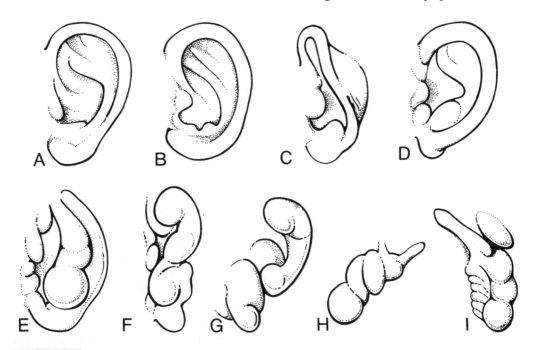

FIGURE 5.2   Variations in pinna deformities. **A** to **D**. Mild deformities. **E** to **I**. Severe deformities.

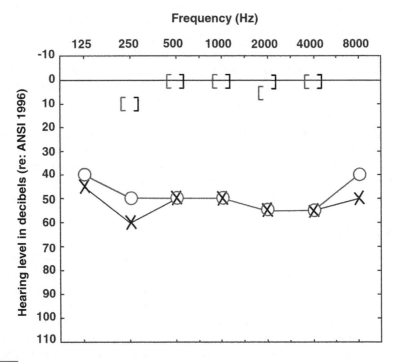

FIGURE 5.3   Audiometric hearing loss seen in a severe case of bilateral microtia with atresia.

External Otitis

A number of diseases can cause acute external otitis, which originates from viruses or bacteria. One of these diseases, called herpes simplex, invades the pinna or ear canal. The disease resembles the herpes seen on the face or other parts of the body. Another inflammatory disease is viral bullous myringitis, a complication that involves the outer layer of the tympanic membrane and then spreads laterally to the external canal. In rare instances, these diseases can produce severe swelling of the canal and subsequent hearing loss.

Collapsed Canal

An occasional clinical finding is the collapse of an ear canal brought about by the pressure that results from earphone placement. The pressure of the earphones against the side of the head moves the pinna forward and thus causes the soft cartilaginous part of the ear canal to close. This condition is thought to occur in approximately 3% of a clinical caseload and affects both children and adults. There is a tendency, however, for this condition to occur more frequently in adults, especially in the elderly population. Importantly, the collapsed canal has also been reported to occur in neonates. A collapse of the ear canal can produce a conductive hearing loss on the order of 15 to 30 dB HL, with the greatest loss occurring at 2000 Hz. The use of insert earphones, described in Chapter 4, eliminates the problem of collapsing ear canals.

Cerumen and Foreign Bodies

In some individuals, the ear canal generates excessive amounts of cerumen (earwax). If not removed on a periodic basis, this can accumulate and block the transmission of sound to the middle ear. The ear canal is also sufficiently large to accept foreign objects such as matches, paper clips, and pencil tips. Portions of these objects inserted by either children or adults can be lost in the ear canal and remain there for many years. This can result in mild forms of conductive hearing loss. Audiologists who plan to specialize in the pediatric population should recognize that children have been known to insert seeds or beans into the ear canal. The ear canal is warm and moist and provides an excellent growing environment. When the seed or bean expands, the child has pain and loss of hearing.

Finally, sharp objects inserted into the ear canal can pierce or tear the tympanic membrane. Such trauma can also cause disruption of the ossicular chain. Self-induced perforations of the tympanic membrane and/or separation of the ossicles can result in a mild to moderate conductive hearing loss. The audiologist should make a practice of inspecting the ear canal with an otoscope before conducting an audiologic examination.

Cysts and Tumors

The external ear and ear canal can serve as a site for both cysts and tumors. A cyst is a closed cavity or sac that lies underneath the skin and is often filled with a liquid or semisolid material. A cyst is primarily of cosmetic importance unless it becomes infected. If swollen from infection, a cyst can cause hearing loss.

Tumors, both benign and malignant, can arise from the pinna or ear canal. Benign tumors can have a vascular origin or can simply be an outgrowth of bone. Malignancies more frequently arise from the pinna but in rare circumstances arise in the ear canal. Occasionally these lesions become quite large and close off the ear canal.

Middle Ear Disorders

The Problem of Otitis Media

An important middle ear disorder frequently seen by the audiologist is otitis media, one of the most common diseases of childhood. Otitis media refers to inflammation of the middle ear cavity. It is considered an important economic and health problem because of its prevalence, the cost of treatment, the potential for secondary medical complications, and the possibility of long-term nonmedical consequences. The clinical audiologist must be familiar with this middle ear disorder and have a grasp of such important topics as the classification of otitis media, its natural history and epidemiology, its cause, its management, and its potential complications.

Classification of Otitis Media

Otitis media is often classified on the basis of the temporal sequence of the disease. In other words, the disease is categorized according to the duration of the disease process. For example, acute otitis media (AOM) typically runs its full course within a 3-week period. The disease begins with a rapid onset, persists for a week to 10 days, and then resolves rapidly. Some of the symptoms commonly associated with AOM include a bulging, reddened tympanic membrane, pain, and upper respiratory infection. If the disease has a slow onset and persists for 3 months or more, it is called chronic otitis media (COM). Symptoms associated with COM include a large central perforation in the eardrum and discharge of fluid through the perforation. Subacute otitis media persists beyond the acute stage but is not yet chronic.

Otitis media is also classified according to the type of fluid in the middle ear cavity. If the fluid is purulent or suppurative, like the fluid found most often in AOM, it will contain white blood cells, some cellular debris, and many bacteria. AOM is sometimes called acute suppurative otitis media or acute purulent otitis media. A fluid that is free of cellular debris and bacteria is described as *serous*, and the term *serous otitis media* is used to describe this condition. Sometimes the fluid is mucoid, having been secreted from the mucosal lining of the middle ear. This fluid is thick and contains white blood cells, few bacteria, and some cellular debris. When mucoid fluid is present, the disease may be called mucoid otitis media or secretory otitis media. Table 5.2 summarizes the most commonly employed descriptions of otitis media and their associated synonyms. In addition, Figure 5.4 illustrates a normal tympanic membrane along with several pathologic conditions including serous otitis media, otitis media with bubbles in the fluid, and acute otitis media.

TABLE 5.2 **Clinical Classification of Otitis Media and Commonly Used Synonyms**

Classification	Synonyms
Without effusion	Myringitis
Acute	Suppurative OM, purulent OM, bacterial OM
With effusion	Secretory OM, nonsuppurative OM, serous OM, mucoid OM Suppurative OM, purulent OM

OM, otitis media

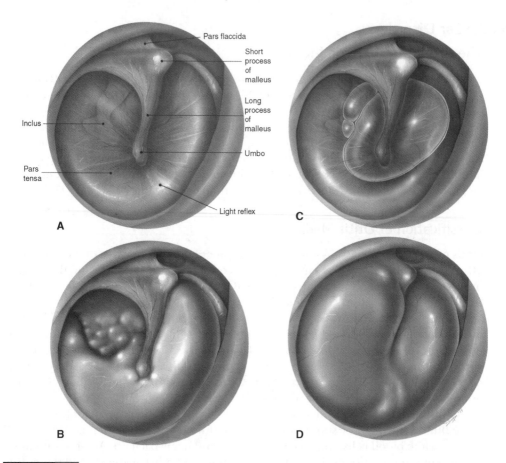

FIGURE 5.4 Normal tympanic membrane **A.** and three pathologic conditions. **B.** Serous otitis media. **C.** Serous otitis media with air bubbles. **D.** Acute otitis media. (Adapted from English GM. Otolaryngology. Hagerstown, MD: Harper & Row, 1976.)

Natural History and Epidemiology of Otitis Media

To understand fully the nature of otitis media, one must appreciate the natural history and epidemiology of the disease. *Natural history* and *epidemiology* are terms used to denote the study of the relations of various factors that determine the natural frequency and distribution of a disease. It has already been stated that otitis media with effusion is one of the most prevalent diseases in childhood (Vignette 5.2). Depending on the study reviewed, 76 to 95% of children have at least one episode of otitis media by 6 years of age. In addition, the prevalence of the disease peaks during the early years of life. The prevalence of otitis media is typically greatest during the first 2 years of life and then decreases with age. Importantly, there appears to be a relationship between the age of onset and the probability of repeated episodes. Most children who appear to be prone to middle ear disease, with five or six bouts within the first several years of life, have their first episode during the first 18 months of life. Seldom does a child become otitis prone if the first episode occurs after 18 months of age.

Otitis media varies slightly with gender, with more cases seen in males than in females. There is seasonal variation in otitis media, with highest occurrence during

VIGNETTE 5.2   Prevalence of middle ear disease in children

The prevalence of middle ear disease has reached epidemic proportions. For children below the age of 6 years, otitis media is the most common reason for a doctor visit. It is estimated that one visit in three that is made for illness results in the diagnosis of middle ear disease. According to the National Center for Health Statistics, ear infection diagnoses increased 150% between 1975 and 1990. Moreover, in 1975, there were 10 million doctor visits for earaches; by 1990, there were 24.5 million visits, costing more than $1 billion annually. Furthermore, 9 in 10 children will have at least one ear infection; most will have at least one acute ear infection by age 3, and more than one-third of children will have three acute infections. Why is the prevalence of ear infections increasing? Many authorities believe that child care is a significant factor. Children in daycare facilities have a much higher prevalence of upper respiratory infections and, subsequently, ear infections.

The extent of the management for ear infections is also substantial. For example, the most common surgery on children is myringotomy with insertion tubes (Fig. 5.9), a procedure used to drain fluid and restore hearing. In addition, the cost of antibiotics commonly prescribed for ear infections amounts to several billion dollars in annual worldwide sales. Clearly, middle ear disease has become one of the major health care problems among children in the United States.

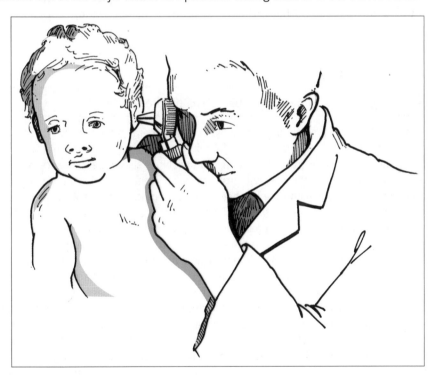

winter and spring. Some groups are more at risk for middle ear disease than others. Some of the groups considered more at risk for otitis media are children with cleft palate and other craniofacial disorders, those with Down syndrome, and those with learning disabilities. Children who reside in the inner city and children who attend daycare centers are also prone to middle ear disease, as are Native Americans.

Cause of Otitis Media

It is commonly believed that otitis media develops because of eustachian tube obstruction. As mentioned in Chapter 3, the eustachian tube is important to a healthy middle ear because it provides for pressure equalization and fluid drainage. If the pressure equalization system is obstructed, negative pressure can develop in the middle ear cavity. The negative pressure sucks the fluid from the membranous lining of the middle ear canal. The fluid that has accumulated from the mucosal lining of the middle ear has no place to escape because the eustachian tube is blocked. Vignette 5.3 shows a representation of this general process. A number of factors may produce eustachian tube obstruction, including large adenoid tissue in the nasopharyngeal area and inflammation of the mucous lining of the tube. Also, the muscular opening function of the eustachian tube is poor in children with otitis media and in children with a history of middle ear disease. In fact, in general, the muscle responsible for opening and closing the tube (tensor veli palatini) is relatively inefficient among young infants and children. Moreover, the position of the eustachian tube in children lies at an angle of only 10° in relation to the horizontal plane, whereas in adults this angle is 45° (Fig. 5.5). Furthermore, the tube is quite short in infants. Because of the angle and shortness of the tube in children, fluid is able to reach the middle ear from the nasopharyngeal area with relative ease and has difficulty escaping from the middle ear cleft.

VIGNETTE 5.3   Development of acute otitis media (AOM)

The drawings that accompany this vignette illustrate the general pattern of events that can occur in AOM. Panel A shows the landmarks of a normal middle ear system. Note the translucency and concavity of the tympanic membrane. Note also the appearance of the eustachian tube, especially at the opening in the nasopharyngeal area. Panel B shows that the pharyngeal end of the eustachian tube has been closed off by swelling because of pharyngeal infection or possibly an allergy. More specifically, the upper respiratory infection produces congestion of the mucosa in the nasopharyngeal area, the eustachian tube, and the middle ear. The congestion of the mucosa of the tube produces an obstruction that prevents ventilation of the middle ear space. Also, the tympanic membrane is retracted inward because of negative pressure caused by absorption from the middle ear. Finally, bacteria from the oropharyngeal area are drawn up the eustachian tube to the middle ear space. Panel C illustrates a full-blown condition of AOM. Fluid secretions from the goblet cells of the mucosal lining of the middle ear are trapped and have no way to leave the middle ear cavity. The bacteria drawn from the eustachian tube proliferate in the secretions, forming viscous pus. Observe also that the tympanic membrane is no longer retracted but is bulging.

Panel D shows a condition that may well result after antimicrobial treatment. The bacteria have been killed by the antibiotics, and a thin or mucoid type of fluid remains. Other possible outcomes after medical treatment might be the return to a completely normal middle ear, as in **A**, or a condition like the one shown in **B**.

The onset of otitis media with effusion, although asymptomatic, would follow a similar pattern of events. Recurrent episodes of AOM or middle ear disease with effusion are probably a result of abnormal anatomy or physiology of the eustachian tube.

VIGNETTE 5.3 Development of acute otitis media (AOM) *(Continued)*

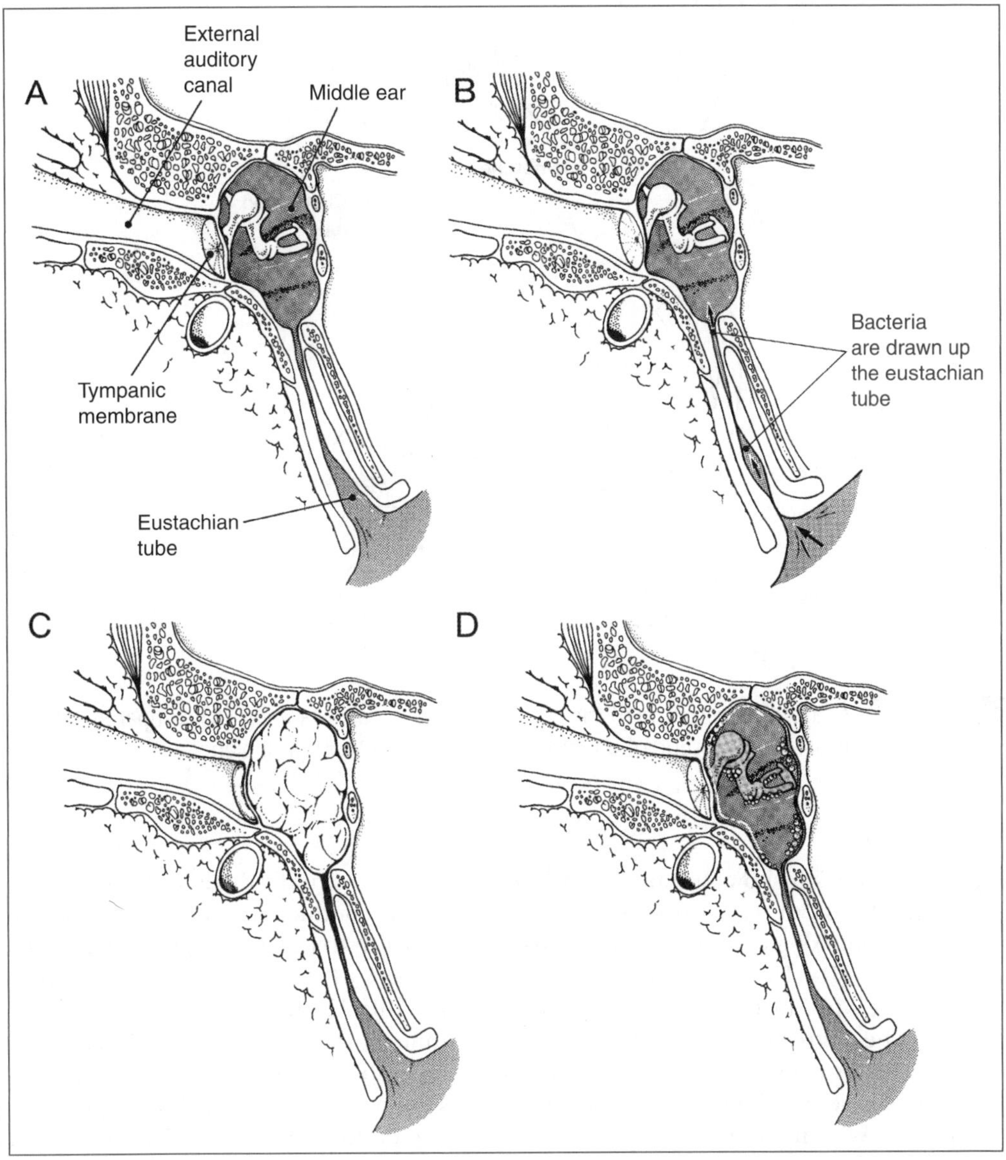

A
External auditory canal
Middle ear
Tympanic membrane
Eustachian tube

B
Bacteria are drawn up the eustachian tube

C

D

Nonmedical Complications Associated With Otitis Media

Hearing loss is considered the most common complication of otitis media. Although the nature of the loss is usually conductive, sensorineural involvement can also occur. In general, the prevalence rate depends on the criteria used to define hearing loss. Unfortunately, prevalence data are difficult to determine because of the lack of well-controlled studies in this area. Too often, there is limited information with regard to testing conditions, calibration of equipment, type of threshold procedure used, definition of hearing loss, and diagnosis of the disease.

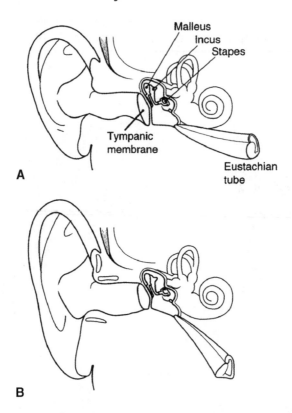

Malleus
Incus
Stapes

Tympanic
membrane

A

Eustachian
tube

B

FIGURE 5.5 Anatomic illustration of the eustachian tube in an infant ear **(A)** compared with that of the adult ear **(B)**. The tube of an infant lies more on a horizontal plane.

Figure 5.6 shows an audiometric profile typical of individuals with otitis media with effusion. It is seen that the hearing loss for air conduction is fairly flat. The average amount of air conduction loss through the speech frequency range (500–2000 Hz) is 25 dB HL. The bone conduction loss averages 3 dB HL through the speech frequencies, producing a mean air-bone gap of roughly 22 dB.

The degree of hearing loss ranges from none to as much as 50 dB HL. Figure 5.7 shows a distribution of the expected hearing loss subsequent to otitis media with effusion. These data illustrate the number of ears falling within various hearing loss categories. Within the speech frequency range, fewer than 50 ears (7.7%) showed an average loss of 10 dB HL or less, and only 5 ears showed losses of 50 dB HL or more. Most ears exhibited losses between 16 and 40 dB HL, with 21 to 30 dB HL being the most common hearing loss category.

Although otitis media is usually manifested as a conductive hearing loss, sensorineural hearing loss may be associated with the more severe forms of COM. Toxic products from the fluid are believed to pass through the round window and damage the cochlea. The damage to the inner ear produces high-frequency sensorineural hearing loss. The longer the fluid remains in the middle ear, the greater the potential for sensorineural involvement.

Another complication that may result from long-standing middle ear disease with effusion is deficiency in psychoeducational and/or communicative skills. It is widely

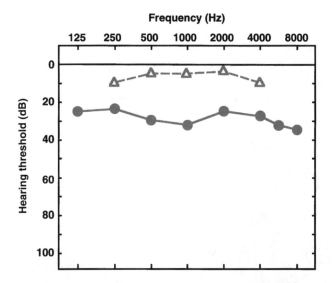

FIGURE 5.6 Audiometric profile of otitis media with effusion. *Solid circles*, air conduction thresholds. *Open triangles*, bone conduction thresholds. Standard audiometric symbols are not used because the data are mean values for a mix of left and right ears.

suspected that otitis-prone children are particularly susceptible to delays in speech, language, and cognitive development and in education. The research findings in this area, however, are inconclusive, and as yet a cause-and-effect relationship cannot be assumed.

Medical Complications Associated With Otitis Media

A number of medical complications are associated with otitis media. The most common are cholesteatoma, perforations or retraction pockets of the tympanic membrane, tympanosclerosis, adhesive otitis media, and facial paralysis.

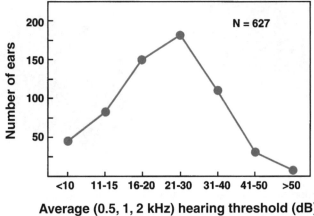

FIGURE 5.7 Distribution of degree of hearing loss in middle ear disease with effusion.

Cholesteatoma

Cholesteatoma refers to keratinizing (to become calluslike) epithelium and the accumulation of shedding cellular debris in the middle ear or other portions of the temporal bone. Although cholesteatoma can be congenital, the acquired forms of this sequela of otitis media are most common. Acquired cholesteatomas typically develop from a retraction pocket or small perforation in the superior portion of the tympanic membrane.

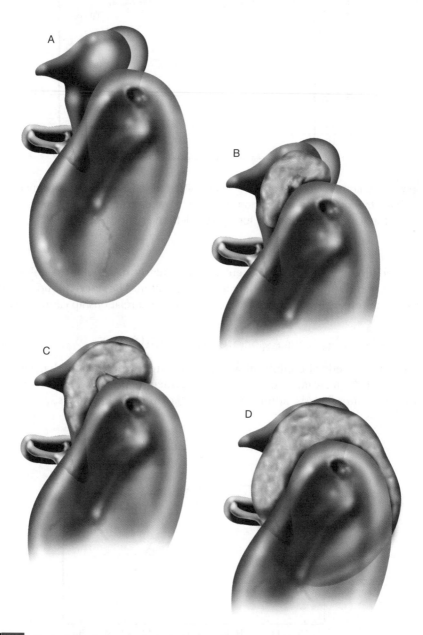

FIGURE 5.8 Evolution of an acquired cholesteatoma. **A.** Small retraction pocket. **B.** Narrow sac developing. **C.** Enlargement of the sac with erosion of ossicles. **D.** Large full-blown cholesteatoma occupying the middle ear cleft. (Adapted from Bluestone CD, Stool SE, Alper CM, et al. Pediatric Otolaryngology, vol 1. 4th ed. Philadelphia: Saunders, 2003.)

The cholesteatoma can occur without infection or it can be associated with AOM or COM. The typical evolution of an acquired cholesteatoma is shown in Figure 5.8. In the more advanced stages of the condition the cholesteatoma can erode one or more of the ossicles and/or invade other regions of the temporal bone. No typical audiometric configuration is associated with cholesteatomas—the loss may vary from 15 to 55 dB HL and will depend on the extent and duration of the condition. In most instances the hearing loss is conductive; however, if COM is present, sensorineural hearing loss is possible.

Perforation of the Tympanic Membrane

Spontaneous perforations usually are subsequent to acute infections but may also be associated with COM. Perforations of the tympanic membrane produce mild to moderate hearing deficits, provided there are no ossicular defects. The hearing loss is a result of reduction in the areal ratio between the tympanic membrane and oval window and the direct coupling of sound waves to the round window. (See Chapter 3 for a discussion of these mechanisms.) Figure 5.9 illustrates several perforations of the tympanic membrane.

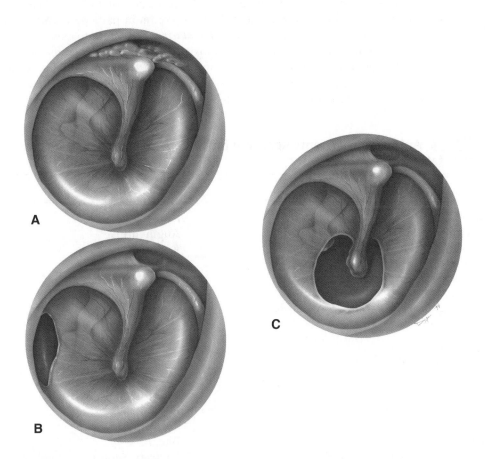

FIGURE 5.9 Perforations in three tympanic membranes. **A.** Attic perforation and associated cholesteatoma. **B.** Marginal perforation. **C.** Large central perforation. (Adapted from English GM. Otolaryngology. Hagerstown, MD: Harper & Row, 1976.)

Tympanosclerosis

Tympanosclerosis is characterized by white shalelike plaques on the tympanic membrane and deposits on the ossicles. It occurs most often after COM, which, when resolved, leaves a residual material. The plaques stiffen the tympanic membrane and the ossicular chain, producing conductive hearing loss in the low frequencies.

Adhesive Otitis Media

Adhesive otitis media is the aftereffect of chronic inflammation of the middle ear cleft and mastoid. In essence, it is a thickening of the mucous membrane lining the middle ear cavity. It can cause fixation of the ossicles, ossicular discontinuation, and hearing loss.

Facial Paralysis

Facial paralysis may occur in the course of AOM or COM. The facial nerve passes through the middle ear area in a bony tube called the fallopian canal. It is possible for the fallopian canal to become eroded and expose the facial nerve to the toxic effects of the infection.

Management of Otitis Media

A common means of treating AOM is routine administration of antimicrobial agents. These antibiotics are designed to combat the most common pathogens (*Streptococcus pneumoniae, Haemophilus influenzae,* and *Moraxella catarrhalis*) thought to exist in the middle ear fluid. Such pharmaceutical agents as amoxicillin, erythromycin, and amoxicillin-clavulanate (Augmentin) are frequently administered in the management of AOM. (Table 5.3 has a complete listing of approved antimicrobial agents.) The selection of a given drug for AOM depends on acceptability (e.g., taste), lack of toxicity or side

TABLE 5.3 **Antimicrobial Agents Approved for Therapy of Acute Otitis Media: United States, 2000**

Drug	Trade Name
Amoxicillin	Amoxil
Amoxicillin-clavulanate	Augmentin
Cephalexin	Keflex
Cefaclor	Ceclor
Loracarbef	Lorabid
Cefixime	Suprax
Ceftibuten	Cedax
Cefprozil	Cefzil
Cefpodoxime	Vantin
Cefuroxime axetil	Ceftin
Cefdinir	Omnicef
Ceftriaxone IM	Rocephin
Erythromycin + sulfisoxazole	Pediazole
Azithromycin	Zithromax
Clarithromycin	Biaxin
Trimethoprim-sulfamethoxazole	Bactrim, Septra
Ofloxacin otic	Floxin Otic

Reprinted from Bluestone CD, Klein JO. Otitis Media in Infants and Children. 3rd ed. Philadelphia: Saunders, 2001.

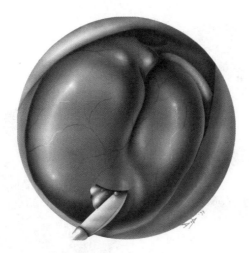

FIGURE 5.10 Myringotomy. Note the bulging appearance of the tympanic membrane. (Adapted from English GM: Otolaryngology. Hagerstown, MD: Harper & Row, 1976.)

effects, convenience, and cost. The drug is usually administered for 10 to 14 days; if the disease persists, a different antimicrobial agent is tried. Unfortunately, the overall effectiveness of antibiotic therapy in the treatment of ear disease has not been clearly established. Even when appropriate antimicrobial agents are prescribed and the fluid is sterilized, the effusion may persist for 2 weeks to 3 months. Also, antibiotic medications can produce adverse side effects, such as diarrhea, nausea, vomiting, and skin rash. Antihistamines and decongestants have also been used in the treatment of middle ear disease; however, this form of treatment has been shown to be ineffective.

A common surgical approach to the management of both suppurative and nonsuppurative otitis media is a myringotomy. Myringotomy is a surgical procedure that entails making an incision in one of the inferior quadrants of the tympanic membrane, as shown in Figure 5.10. In the acute forms of the disease, a myringotomy is performed when there is severe pain or toxicity, high fever, failure to respond to antimicrobial therapy, or some serious secondary medical complication. In secretory otitis media, a myringotomy is more commonly performed, usually to remove fluid and restore hearing sensitivity. This procedure is performed when the disease has persisted for at least 3 months. The eardrum incision can heal quickly, however, and the fluid reappears. To avoid this possibility and to ensure sustained middle ear aeration, ventilating tubes or grommets are often inserted into the eardrum (Fig. 5.11).

Tonsillectomy and adenoidectomy are also considered as management approaches to otitis media. Although tonsillectomy does not seem to be an effective treatment protocol, adenoidectomy is a common surgical procedure for the management of bilateral otitis media in children 4 years of age or older. In general, this approach is undertaken when a patient does not respond to medical therapy, large adenoids are present, and there is no evidence of nasal allergy. Under these conditions, it is assumed that the eustachian tube blockage causing the middle ear disease is a result of enlarged adenoids. The adenoids are removed to free the eustachian tube from the blockage.

A more radical surgical approach is required if chronic disease permanently impairs basic structures within the middle ear. When alteration of the middle ear structures is required, a surgical technique known as tympanoplasty is performed.

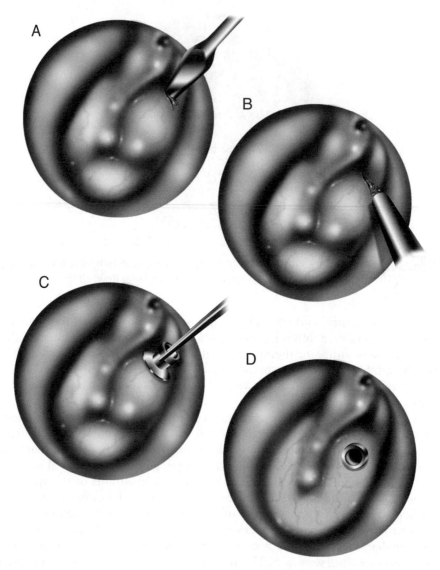

FIGURE 5.11 Insertion of a tympanostomy tube. **A.** Radial incision in the tympanic membrane. **B.** Middle ear effusion aspirated. **C.** Short tympanostomy tube inserted. **D.** Tube position. (Adapted from Bluestone, CD, Klein, JO. Otis Media in Infants and Children. 3rd ed. Philadelphia: Saunders, 2001.)

Otosclerosis

Otosclerosis, sometimes called otospongiosis, is a common cause of conductive hearing loss and is reported to affect 5 to 10% of whites. Otosclerosis means hardening of the ear; it is manifested by a buildup of spongifying bone on the osseous labyrinth, usually in the area of the oval window. The buildup of bone around the oval window immobilizes the footplate of the stapes and interferes with sound transmission to the inner ear. Although the focus of the lesion is usually limited to the region of the oval window, the growth of spongy bone can also invade the walls of the cochlea. When the cochlea becomes involved, sensorineural hearing loss may ensue, producing a condition called cochlear otosclerosis.

The disease is approximately 2.5 times as common in women as in men and may be exacerbated during pregnancy. It occurs less frequently in African-Americans and Asians than in whites and usually has its onset when the individuals are in their 20s, 30s, or 40s.

Finally, bilateral otosclerosis is much more common than unilateral disease, although the latter will be seen in 10 to 15% of cases. The cause of otosclerosis is not clearly understood. Most would agree that the disease has a genetic predisposition, because approximately 50% of affected patients report a similar condition in other family members. The mode of transmission is thought to be autosomal dominant with variable expressivity.

Audiologic Manifestations of Otosclerosis

A progressive conductive hearing loss is the primary result of otosclerosis. The affected patient typically exhibits an audiometric configuration similar to that shown in Figure 5.12. This figure depicts the air and bone conduction thresholds of a 35-year-old female patient with surgically confirmed otosclerosis. The hearing loss has progressed somewhat gradually for several years, beginning at age 25 years. Notice the moderate hearing thresholds for air conduction, with greater loss in the low-frequency region and the relatively normal bone conduction thresholds. An exception to the latter is the slight reduction of bone conduction hearing at 2000 Hz. The bone conduction loss at 2000 Hz is characteristic of otosclerosis. It is called the Carhart notch because Carhart was the first to report this notching phenomenon. Immittance measurements in otosclerotic cases are also uniquely characteristic and typically manifest absent acoustic reflexes, abnormally low compliance values, and a shallow tympanogram.

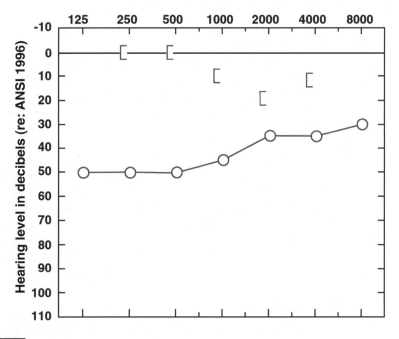

FIGURE 5.12 Audiometric example of otosclerosis.

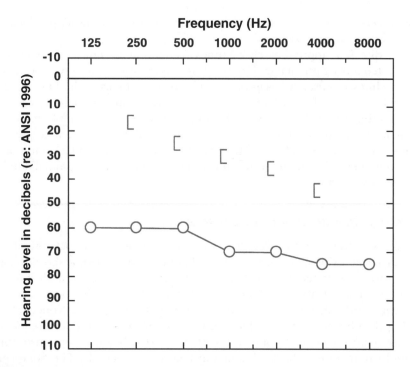

FIGURE 5.13 Audiometric example of combination of stapedial and cochlear otosclerosis.

Figure 5.13 shows an audiometric example of a patient with both stapedial and cochlear involvement from otosclerosis. A mixed hearing loss is present, representing a conductive component as a result of stapes fixation and a sensorineural component caused by the spread of the spongy bone to the cochlea.

Management of Otosclerosis

The most common approach to the management of otosclerosis is surgery of the stapes. The ideal candidates for stapes surgery are those with relatively normal bone conduction thresholds (0–20 dB HL, 500–2000 Hz) and air conduction values in the 35- to 65-dB HL range (500–2000 Hz). Surgical candidates usually exhibit an air-bone gap of at least 15 dB and have speech recognition scores of 60% or better.

One surgical approach to otosclerosis is stapes mobilization, which is simply a loosening of the stapes with a chisel-like instrument. A limitation of this technique is that in many cases fixation of the stapes and conductive hearing loss can recur. An alternative and more widely accepted approach is stapedectomy. A stapedectomy entails removal of the fixed stapes footplate and all or a portion of the stapedial arch and substitution of a prosthetic device. In cases of complete stapedectomy and the incorporation of a prosthetic device, the oval window is sealed with a graft or an absorptive sponge. Surgery usually results in complete or nearly complete restoration of hearing. Figure 5.14 shows examples of two surgical procedures.

Other Ossicular Disorders

The ossicles other than the stapes can also be partially or completely fixed. The ossicles can also be pulled apart, or disarticulated, producing a variety of different conductive hearing losses. For example, the malleus and the incus can become fixated, or

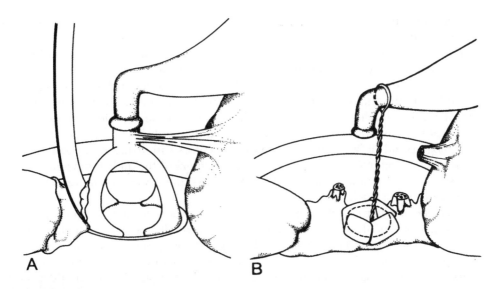

FIGURE 5.14 Two surgical procedures on the stapes. **A.** Stapes mobilization. **B.** Stapedectomy. (Adapted from Goodhill V, ed. Ear Diseases, Deafness and Dizziness. Hagerstown, MD: Harper & Row, 1979.)

there can be fixation of the malleus alone or the incus alone without any involvement of the stapes. These conditions are sometimes called pseudo-otosclerosis, and the audiologic manifestations often mock what we would expect to find in otosclerosis.

In contrast to fixation, it is possible to have discontinuity, or disarticulation, of the ossicles, again producing a significant conductive hearing loss. Discontinuity of the ossicles can be caused by a degenerative process or by trauma. For example, the introduction of a sharp object into the ear canal could pierce the tympanic membrane and cause a dislocation of the ossicles. A similar effect can result from a skull fracture, wherein the impact to the head dislodges the ossicular chain. In addition, degeneration of the ossicles is possible when a disease process (particularly cholesteatoma) is present. Under these conditions, the individual exhibits a substantial conductive hearing loss, in the neighborhood of 50 to 60 dB.

COCHLEAR AND RETROCOCHLEAR PATHOLOGY

Millions of Americans have sensorineural hearing loss as a consequence of cochlear pathology. For children, conductive hearing loss produced by middle ear pathology, as reviewed earlier in this chapter, is probably the most common type of hearing loss. For adults, however, sensorineural hearing loss resulting from underlying cochlear pathology is probably the most common type of hearing loss. Recall from the previous sections of this chapter that conductive hearing loss is usually treatable with surgery, medication, or both. With sensorineural hearing loss, however, this is usually not the case. The hearing loss is typically permanent. For individuals with significant sensorineural hearing loss, the usual course of action is to seek assistance from amplification, often a personal wearable hearing aid. Hearing aids and other types of amplification for those with hearing loss are described in detail in Chapter 7.

The description of the hearing loss produced by cochlear pathology as *sensorineural* seems particularly appropriate. Recall that a sensorineural hearing loss is one in which the threshold by bone conduction is the same as that by air conduction (within 5 dB). The threshold when the inner ear is stimulated directly through skull vibration (bone conduction) is the same as when the entire peripheral auditory system is stimulated (air conduction). If thresholds for air conduction and bone conduction are elevated to the same degree, all that can be concluded is that there is some pathology in the auditory system at or central to the inner ear. The presence of a sensorineural hearing loss does not tell us the location of the pathology along the auditory pathway; it only eliminates the outer and middle ears as possibilities. The pathology could be affecting the sensory receptors within the cochlea, the neural pathways leading from the cochlea to higher centers of the auditory system, or both the sensory and neural structures. In this context, then, *sensorineural hearing loss* is a very appropriate label.

The term *sensorineural hearing loss* is also an appropriate label for the hearing loss resulting from cochlear pathology for another reason. In cochlear pathology, the sensory receptors within the cochlea are destroyed. Exactly how this occurs depends on the specific etiology. Research suggests that the sensory destruction quickly becomes sensorineural damage. Once the hair cells within the organ of Corti are destroyed, a phenomenon known as retrograde degeneration occurs. Retrograde degeneration refers to destruction of connecting anatomic structures located more central to the structure that was destroyed. Destruction of the sensory hair cells within the organ of Corti results in the eventual degeneration of the first-order afferent nerve fibers communicating with the damaged hair cells. Most patients with sensorineural hearing loss caused by cochlear pathology, therefore, most likely have underlying damage to both the sensory (cochlea) and neural (nerve fibers) portions of the auditory system.

When a sensorineural hearing loss is observed, how do the audiologist and physician determine whether it is because of cochlear pathology or a problem lying farther up the ascending neural pathways (called retrocochlear pathology)? As mentioned in Chapter 4, several steps are involved in establishing the diagnosis. The case history taken by the audiologist or physician can provide some important clues to the location of the problem. The presence of other, frequently nonauditory, complaints, such as dizziness, loss of balance, and ringing in the ears (tinnitus), can aid the physician in establishing the diagnosis. A particular pattern of results from the basic audiology test battery may alert the physician to a probable underlying cause. The presence of a high-frequency sensorineural hearing loss in just one ear, for example, is a common audiometric configuration in some types of retrocochlear pathology. Finally, special tests can be performed on the patient at the physician's request. These tests may be auditory, in which case they will be performed by an audiologist, or they may be nonauditory. An example of a nonauditory special test is electronystagmography (ENG), which tests the vestibular system and may also be performed by an audiologist. Other tests not performed by the audiologist might include magnetic resonance imaging (MRI) and computed tomography (CT). Both MRI and CT provide visual images of the middle and inner ear structures. The most definitive auditory special test involves the measurement of the auditory brainstem response, or ABR. This test may also be administered by an audiologist. (The ABR was described in Chapters 3 and 4.)

Discussion of the special tests, auditory and nonauditory, that aid the physician in establishing the diagnosis is beyond the scope of this book. Suffice it to say that the audiologist is frequently asked to perform them. Many types of cochlear and retrocochlear pathologies, however, do produce a typical pattern of results on the basic audiologic test battery. The remainder of this chapter describes several of these pathologies and their audiologic profiles.

Cochlear Pathology

Before describing some specific causes of cochlear pathology, some general characteristics shared by most patients with cochlear pathology are noteworthy. First, for the most part, studies of human cadavers have revealed a close correspondence between the location of the damage along the length of the cochlea and the resulting audiometric configuration. For example, if postmortem anatomic studies of a patient's ear reveal damage in the basal high-frequency portion of the cochlea, a recent audiogram obtained before death would most likely indicate a high-frequency sensorineural hearing loss. Although there are exceptions, it is generally the case in cochlear pathology that the audiometric configuration provides at least a gross indication of the regions of the cochlea that were damaged by the pathology (Vignette 5.4). A high-frequency

---

VIGNETTE 5.4   Relation between location of cochlear damage and hearing loss

The three figures accompanying this vignette illustrate the correspondence between the region of the cochlea that is damaged and the resultant hearing loss. The upper portion of each figure

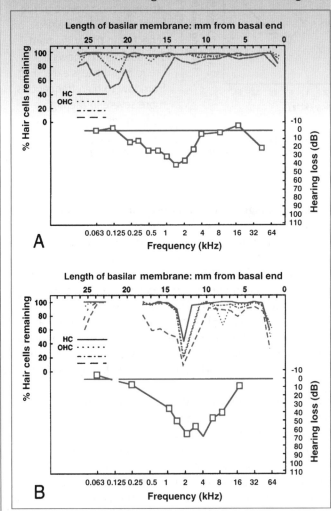

shows a cochleogram from three monkeys that were exposed to intense noise. A cochleogram depicts the percentage of hair cells (*HCs*) within the organ of Corti that remain at various locations along the length of the cochlea after noise exposure. The percentages are determined after careful microscopic examination of the cochlea.

In *Panel A*, the monkey was exposed to a low-frequency noise. This resulted in destruction of outer hair cells (*OHCs*) in the region roughly 15 to 25 mm from the base of the cochlea. Before the animal was killed to examine the type and extent of damage produced by the noise, the audiogram in the lower portion of the panel was obtained. A sensorineural hearing loss in the low and intermediate frequencies was produced.

When another monkey was exposed to a high-frequency noise (*B*), the

(continued)

VIGNETTE 5.4   Relation between location of cochlear damage and hearing loss *(Continued)*

cochleogram (*upper portion*) indicated that the damage appeared in the basal portion of the cochlea. The audiogram obtained from the same monkey after the noise exposure and just before it was killed (*lower portion*) revealed a high-frequency sensorineural hearing loss. As the damage to the sensory hair cells within the organ of Corti progressed from an apical (*A*) to a basal (*B*) region of the cochlea, the audiogram reflected the change as a shift from a low-frequency to a high-frequency sensorineural hearing loss.

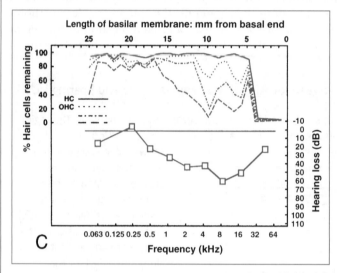

Panel C shows a cochleogram and audiogram from a monkey exposed to a broadband noise. The damage is much more extensive, affecting both the apical and basal portions of the cochlea, although most severe in the basal region. This is again reflected in the audiogram. The audiogram shows a broad hearing loss extending from low to high frequencies, more severe in the high frequencies.

Adapted from Moody DB, Stebbins WC, Hawkins JE Jr, Johnsson LG. Hearing loss and cochlear pathology in the monkey [Macaca] following exposure to high levels of noise. Arch Oto-Rhino-Laryngol 220:47–72, 1978.

---

sensorineural hearing loss reflects damage to the basal portion of the cochlea, a low-frequency sensorineural hearing loss suggests damage to the apical region of the cochlea, and a broad hearing loss extending from low to high frequencies reflects an underlying lesion along the entire length of the cochlea.

In sensorineural hearing loss caused by cochlear pathology, there is a close correspondence between the frequencies that demonstrate hearing loss and the region along the length of the cochlea that is damaged. There is a less certain correspondence, however, between the degree of hearing loss at a particular frequency and the degree of damage at the corresponding location in the cochlea. One popular conception is that mild or moderate sensorineural hearing loss is a result of destruction of the outer hair cells, whereas more severe hearing loss reflects damage to both the outer and inner hair cells.

There are also several perceptual consequences of sensorineural hearing loss caused by cochlear pathology. Except for those with profound impairments, patients with cochlear pathology most commonly complain that they can hear speech but can't understand it. This may be true especially when listening against a background of noise. The patient with cochlear pathology also frequently experiences a phenomenon known as loudness recruitment. This phenomenon is discussed in Chapter 3. The hearing loss makes low-intensity sounds inaudible. Moderate-intensity sounds that are comfortably loud to a normal-hearing person may be barely audible to the person with cochlear pathology. At high intensities, however, the loudness of the sound is the same for both a normal ear and one with cochlear pathology. Let us assume, for example, that a pure tone at 2000 Hz having a level of 110 dB SPL is uncomfortably loud for both a normal listener and a person with cochlear pathology. The person with cochlear pathology has a hearing threshold at 2000 Hz of 60 dB SPL, whereas the normal listener's threshold is 10 dB SPL. Thus, for the normal listener, the intensity of the tone has to be increased 100 dB to increase the loudness of the tone from just audible (threshold) to uncomfortable. For the person with cochlear pathology, however, an increase in intensity of only 50 dB is needed to cover the same range of loudness (from just audible to uncomfortable). Loudness increases more rapidly in the ear with cochlear pathology than in the normal ear. This is known as loudness recruitment.

Loudness recruitment makes it more difficult to fit a hearing aid on a person with cochlear pathology. Low-level sounds must be amplified to be made audible to the person with hearing loss. High-intensity sounds, however, cannot be amplified by the same amount or the hearing aid will produce sounds that are uncomfortably loud to the wearer. Possible solutions to this dilemma when fitting the patient with a hearing aid are described in more detail in Chapter 7.

Finally, the patient with cochlear hearing loss may have accompanying speech abnormalities. Depending on the severity, configuration, and age of onset of the hearing loss, the speech may be misarticulated. In addition, if the cochlear pathology produces sensorineural hearing loss in the low and intermediate frequencies, the patient will typically use speech levels that are inappropriately loud, especially while talking without wearing a hearing aid. This is because the feedback that a speaker normally receives by bone conduction is not available to assist in regulating the voice level.

The remainder of this section examines several types of pathologies. The pathologies described here are by no means an exhaustive compilation. In keeping with the general mission of this book, the pathologies described were selected because of their common occurrence either in the general population or among children.

High-Risk Factors

A number of complications that cause hearing loss can arise before, during, or soon after birth. Many of these complications are factors included in the so-called high-risk register or risk indicators. The high-risk register is a checklist of conditions known to exhibit a higher than normal prevalence of hearing loss. These conditions for newborns include an illness or condition requiring admission of 48 hours or greater to the neonatal intensive care unit (NICU), familial history of hearing loss, infections in utero (e.g., rubella or cytomegalovirus), craniofacial anomalies, and stigmata or other findings associated with a syndrome known to include a sensorineural and/or conductive hearing loss.

Some of these risk indicators are self-explanatory (e.g., family history of hearing loss, craniofacial anomalies, and infections in utero); others, however, need further explanation. Examples of conditions requiring admission to the NICU include hyperbilirubinemia, severe depression at birth, and prolonged mechanical ventilation.

Hyperbilirubinemia occurs when the bilirubin concentration in the blood exceeds 6 to 8 mg/dL. Once this level is reached, the child's skin becomes yellowish, a condition sometimes called jaundice. Hyperbilirubinemia is a complex metabolic complication that is thought to result from the production of too much bilirubin or the inability of the system to clear the bilirubin from the blood by the liver. *Severe depression at birth*, sometimes called asphyxia, is an interruption of oxygen to the body, including the brain. In newborns, asphyxia results from an interruption of the placenta or maternal blood flow before birth. Another possible factor is a blockage of the infant's airway during delivery. Asphyxia can damage the inner ear and/or auditory regions of the brain. *Prolonged mechanical ventilation* is most often associated with infants who have severe pulmonary complications such as persistent pulmonary hypertension in the newborn (PPHN). PPHN occurs typically in near full-term or postterm infants and is characterized by hypoxemia (i.e., subnormal oxygenation of blood), which results in increased pulmonary vasoconstriction and a decrease in pulmonary circulation. Such children have a 25 times greater risk of hearing loss than other babies in the NICU. Finally, *stigmata* or other findings associated with a syndrome are simply landmarks of a syndrome that might be associated with hearing loss. A complete listing of the most recent high-risk register for both newborns and infants is summarized in Table 6.1.

Viral and Bacterial Diseases

Severe viral and bacterial infections can result in varying degrees and patterns of sensorineural hearing loss. Infectious disease can be transmitted to the child by the mother in utero, a condition called prenatal, congenital, or sometimes perinatal disease. These terms carry slightly different meanings yet are often used synonymously. The term *prenatal* refers to something that occurs to the fetus before birth. *Congenital* also implies before birth but usually before the 28th week of gestation. Finally, the word *perinatal* pertains to a condition that occurs in the period shortly before or after birth (from 8 weeks before birth to 4 weeks after). A disease can also be acquired later in life, and this is usually called a *postnatal* condition. The following discussion reviews some of the more common prenatal and postnatal infectious diseases known to cause hearing loss.

Prenatal Diseases

Many of the prenatal diseases are categorized as part of the TORCH (*t*oxoplasmosis, *o*ther, *r*ubella, *c*ytomegalovirus, *h*erpes simplex) complex, an acronym used to identify the major infections that may be contracted in utero. Some use the mnemonic (S)TORCH, where *S* is for syphilis. Any disease of the (S)TORCH complex is considered a high-risk factor for hearing loss, and therefore, it is important for the audiologist to have some general knowledge of these infectious conditions. Table 5.4 lists the (S)TORCH diseases and describes the expected hearing loss with each. In addition, Figure 5.15 illustrates the audiometric patterns known to occur with most of the (S)TORCH agents. Let us now briefly review these conditions.

Syphilis

Syphilis is transmitted to the child by intrauterine infection from the mother. Syphilis may manifest itself anytime from the first to the sixth decade of life. When the age of onset is early (before 10 years), the sensorineural hearing loss is profound and bilateral, with sudden onset. With adult onset, the hearing loss is fluctuating and asymmetric and may appear either suddenly or gradually. Dizziness is also commonly associated with this condition. Figure 5.15*D* illustrates just one possible audiometric configuration associated with adult-onset syphilis.

Toxoplasmosis

Toxoplasmosis is a disease caused by an organism (*Toxoplasma gondii*) that is transmitted to the child via the placenta. It is thought that the infection is contracted by eating

TABLE 5.4 Clinical Manifestations of the (S)Torch Complex

Disease	Primary Symptoms	Prevalence of Hearing Loss (%)	Type and Degree of Hearing Loss
Syphilis	Enlarged liver and spleen, snuffles, rash, hearing loss	35	Severe to profound bilateral SNHL; configuration and degree vary
Toxoplasmosis	Chorioretinitis, hydrocephalus, intracranial calcifications, hearing loss	17	Moderate to severe bilateral SNHL; may be progressive
Rubella	Heart and kidney defects, eye anomalies, mental retardation, hearing loss	20–30	Profound bilateral SNHL—cookie-bite audiogram is common; may be progressive
CMV	Mental retardation, visual defects, hearing loss	17	Mild to profound bilateral SNHL; may be progressive
Herpes simplex	Enlarged liver, rash, visual abnormalities, psychomotor retardation, encephalitis, hearing loss	10	Moderate to severe unilateral or bilateral SNHL

SNHL, sensorineural hearing loss.

uncooked meat or by making contact with feces of cats. As noted in Table 5.4, approximately 17% of infected newborns exhibit sensorineural hearing loss. The hearing loss is typically moderate and progressive (Fig. 5.15*B*).

Rubella

Rubella is perhaps the best-recognized disease of the (S)TORCH complex. Rubella, sometimes called German measles, infects the mother via the respiratory route. The virus is carried by the bloodstream to the placenta and to the fetus. If the mother contracts the virus during the first month of pregnancy, there is a 50% chance that the fetus will be infected; in the second month, there is a 22% chance; and in subsequent months, there is approximately a 6 to 10% chance. Table 5.4 lists some of the more frequently encountered symptoms. One of the symptoms is a severe to profound bilateral sensorineural hearing loss (Fig. 5.15*C*). The child will display a trough- or bowl-shaped configuration or a corner-type audiogram. Children with **maternal** rubella have been known to exhibit both conductive and mixed-type hearing losses, although such instances are rare.

Cytomegalovirus

Cytomegalovirus (CMV) is easily the most common viral disease known to cause hearing loss. Approximately 33,000 infants are born each year with CMV. Of the symptomatic children who survive (approximately 20% die), 90% exhibit complications. One of the common complications is sensorineural hearing loss that ranges from mild

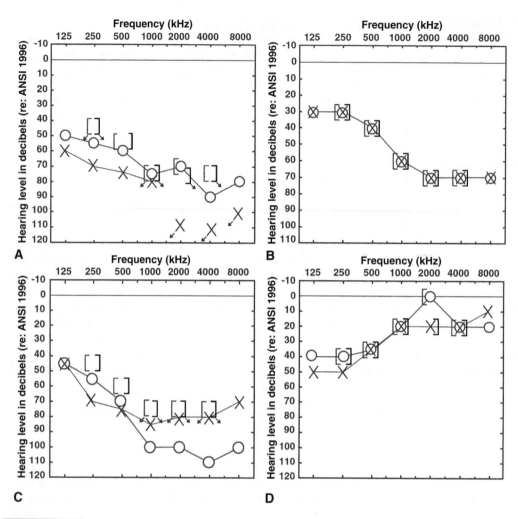

FIGURE 5.15 Audiometric examples of CMV **(A)**; toxoplasmosis **(B)**, rubella **(C)**, and syphilis **(D)**.

to profound and can be progressive. Figure 5.15*A* shows an example of a severe to profound hearing loss. The virus is passed from the mother to the fetus via the bloodstream.

Herpes Simplex Virus

Herpes simplex virus (HSV) is a sexually transmitted disease, and the acquired virus is passed on to the fetus in utero or during birth. Only 4% of infected infants survive without complication. Some of the complications of the disease include central nervous system involvement, psychomotor retardation, visual problems, and hearing loss. Sensorineural hearing loss occurs when HSV is contracted in utero.

Postnatal Infections

Several postnatal infections produce sensorineural hearing loss. The cochlear damage produced by these viral or bacterial infections appears to result from the infecting

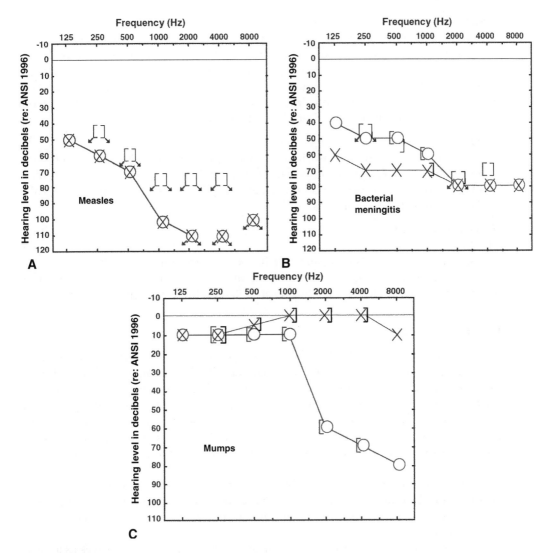

Audiometric examples of measles **(A)**, bacterial meningitis **(B)**, and mumps **(C)**.

agent entering the inner ear through the blood supply and nerve fibers. Figure 5.16 shows sample audiometric patterns for several postnatal conditions. The following is a brief review of diseases encountered most frequently by the audiologist.

Bacterial Meningitis

Hearing loss is the most common consequence of acute meningitis (Fig. 5.16*B*). Although the pathways used by the organisms to reach the inner ear are not altogether clear, several routes have been suggested. These include the bloodstream, the auditory nerve, and the fluid supply of the inner ear and the middle ear. The prevalence of severe to profound sensorineural hearing loss among patients with this disorder is approximately 10%. Another 16% exhibit transient conductive hearing loss. Interestingly, some patients with sensorineural hearing loss exhibit partial recovery, although such a finding is rare.

Mumps

Mumps is recognized as one of the common causes of unilateral sensorineural hearing loss. The hearing loss is usually sudden and can vary from a mild high-frequency impairment to profound loss. Figure 5.16C illustrates a case of unilateral severe high-frequency hearing loss. Both children and adults are affected. Because it is uncommon for this disease to be subclinical, children with hearing loss resulting from mumps are not usually identified until they first attend school.

Measles

Measles is another cause of sensorineural hearing loss. Hearing loss affects 6 to 10% of measles patients. A typical audiometric configuration is a severe to profound bilateral high-frequency sensorineural impairment (Fig. 5.16A). Patients with measles also can show conductive hearing loss.

Herpes Zoster Oticus

The first symptom associated with herpes zoster oticus is a burning pain close to the ear. Shortly thereafter, vesicles (small saclike bodies) erupt in the ear canal and sometimes on the face, neck, or trunk. Common symptoms include facial paralysis, hearing loss, and vertigo. The loss is usually a severe bilateral high-frequency hearing loss.

Ménière Disease

Ménière disease is typically defined as a symptom complex affecting the membranous inner ear. It is characterized by progressive or fluctuating sensorineural hearing loss, episodic vertigo, and frequently tinnitus (ringing or buzzing in the ear) that varies in both degree and type. Some have added the symptoms of a feeling of fullness and pressure in the ear to the classic signs associated with this disorder. The most commonly reported etiologies of Ménière disease include allergies, adrenal-pituitary insufficiency, vascular insufficiency, hypothyroidism, and even psychologic disorders.

Vertigo is considered the most characteristic symptom of Ménière disease. It can occur in attacks that are extremely severe, lasting anywhere from a few minutes to several days. In its severe form, the vertigo can be accompanied by extreme nausea and vomiting.

Tinnitus, or ringing in the ears, often precedes an episode and serves as a warning signal for an impending attack. The tinnitus usually increases as the hearing loss associated with the disease increases. Most patients with Ménière disease describe their tinnitus as a low-pitched narrow band of noise, much like a roaring sound.

The audiologic manifestation associated with this disease is most often characterized by a low-frequency sensorineural hearing loss that often fluctuates (Fig. 5.17). Although it has long been assumed that the disease is most often unilateral, estimates of bilateral involvement range from approximately 5 to 60%. In the later stages of the disease, the fluctuation in the hearing loss decreases, and the high frequencies become more involved. Typically, one sees good word recognition scores and special auditory test results consistent with a cochlear lesion.

Although uncommon, Ménière disease can occur among young children. Similar to what is seen in adults, children demonstrate fluctuating hearing loss, tinnitus, vertigo, aural pressure, and occasionally nausea. Ménière disease in children can be a serious disabling auditory disorder that can significantly influence personal behavior and daily living activities. The dramatic and unpredictable shifts in the symptom complex can produce such complications as fear, anxiety, depression, and agitation. The

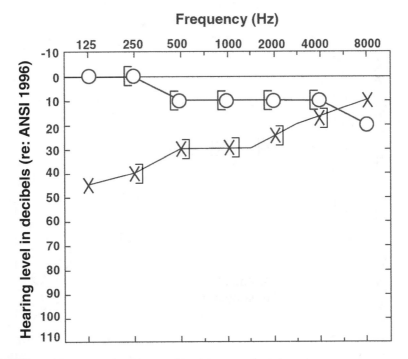

FIGURE 5.17 Audiometric example of hearing loss caused by Ménière disease.

fluctuating nature of the hearing loss in and of itself can result in confusion, embarrassment, and annoyance. The management of these children requires a coordinated effort among physician, audiologist, school, and parent.

Ototoxic Drugs

A negative side effect of some antibiotic drugs is the production of severe high-frequency sensorineural hearing loss. The aminoglycoside antibiotics are particularly hazardous. This group, also commonly called the mycin drugs, includes streptomycin, neomycin, kanamycin, and gentamicin. A variety of factors can determine whether hearing loss is produced in a specific patient. These factors include the drug dosage, the susceptibility of the patient, and the simultaneous or previous use of other ototoxic agents.

Ototoxic antibiotics reach the inner ear through the bloodstream. The resulting damage is greater in the base of the cochlea, and outer hair cells are typically the primary targets, with only limited damage appearing in other cochlear structures. As shown in Figure 5.18, this results in an audiometric pattern of moderate to severe high-frequency sensorineural hearing loss in both ears.

Some ototoxic drugs cause a temporary or reversible hearing loss. Perhaps the most common such substance is aspirin. When taken in large amounts, aspirin can produce a mild to moderate temporary sensorineural hearing loss.

Noise-Induced Hearing Loss

Exposure to intense sounds can result in temporary or permanent hearing loss. Whether or not a hearing loss actually results from exposure to the intense sound

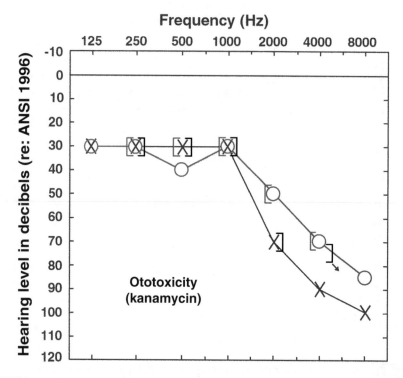

FIGURE 5.18   Audiometric example of hearing loss caused by ototoxicity.

depends on several factors. These factors include the acoustic characteristics of the sound, such as its intensity, duration, and frequency content (amplitude spectrum); the length of the exposure; and the susceptibility of the individual.

When the intense sound is a broadband noise, such as might be found in industrial settings, a characteristic audiometric pattern emerges after the exposure. This audiometric configuration is shown in Figure 5.19. It is frequently called a 4k notch, which reflects the sharp dip in the audiogram at 4 kHz. More detailed measurements of the hearing loss produced by exposure to broadband noise reveal that the notch in the audiogram is as likely to appear at 3 or 6 kHz as at 4 kHz. Because 3 and 6 kHz are not routinely included in audiometric testing, however, the notch is less frequently observed at these two frequencies. This same 4k notch configuration is observed both in temporary hearing loss after brief exposures to broadband noise and in permanent hearing loss after prolonged exposure to such noise.

Many theories attempt to explain why the region around 4 kHz seems to be particularly susceptible to the damaging effects of broadband noise. One theory is that although the noise itself may be broadband, with roughly equal amplitude at all frequencies, the outer ear and ear canal resonances (see Chapter 3) have amplified the noise in the 2- to 4-kHz region by the time the noise reaches the inner ear. Thus, this region shows the greatest hearing loss. Other theories suggest that the region of the cochlea associated with 4 kHz is vulnerable to damage because of differences in cochlear mechanics, cochlear metabolism, or cochlear blood supply. Whatever the underlying mechanism, damage is greatest in the region of the cochlea associated with

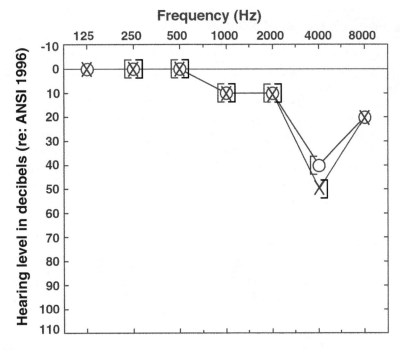

FIGURE 5.19 Audiometric pattern associated with noise-induced hearing loss.

4 kHz. The damage again seems to be most marked in the outer hair cells, although this can vary with the acoustic characteristics of the noise.

Given the permanent nature of the resulting noise-induced hearing loss, it is crucial to prevent it. Hearing conservation programs have been developed by employers to protect the hearing of employees. At least part of the employer's motivation is avoidance of hefty fines for noncompliance with federal standards regarding industrial noise levels. The primary components of an industrial hearing conservation program include surveys of noise levels and durations to which employees are exposed, regular (at least annual) monitoring of hearing thresholds for all employees, and provision of hearing protection devices, such as earmuffs and earplugs. Another key component of such hearing conservation programs is education of employees regarding the risk of permanent hearing loss from noise exposure and instruction in the effective use of hearing protection devices.

The world is increasingly noisy. Exposure to high noise levels is not confined to work environments. Many recreational sources of noise exist today, and the risk of hearing loss from prolonged exposure to high sound levels is the same whether it involves a 110-dB SPL machine-generated noise or an exposure to 110-dB SPL from loudspeakers at a rock concert (see Vignette 5.5). The biggest difference in these two cases, however, is that an employee might be exposed to the high-level machine-generated noise on a daily basis for many years, whereas the audience member at a rock concert will most likely be exposed to this same high noise level much less frequently. Of course, if one considers the rock musician, as well as both practices and performances, the differences in exposure duration, and the subsequent risk of hearing loss, might be minimal (see Vignette 5.6).

VIGNETTE 5.5   Recreational sources of noise

We live in a noise-filled society in which many recreational activities make use of devices or equipment that generates high levels of sound. In many cases, those making use of these devices may not consider the sound to be noise, but it is nonetheless high-intensity sound. The following is a listing of several recreational sources of noise. In each case, the range of maximum sound levels in dBA reported in various studies is shown.

Instruments used to measure noise have three weighting networks (A, B, and C) that are designed to respond differently to noise frequencies. The A network weighs (filters) the low frequencies and approximates the response characteristics of the human ear. The B network also filters the low frequencies, but not as much as the A network does. The C scale provides a fairly flat response. The federal government recommends the A network for measuring noise levels.

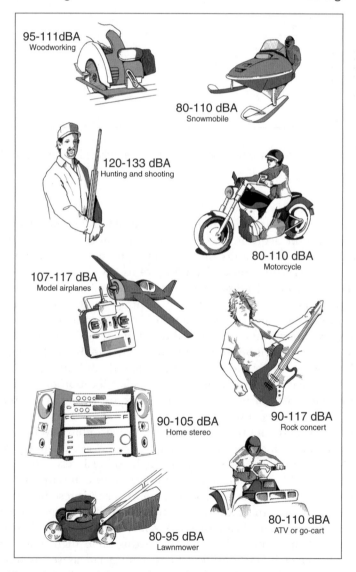

95-111dBA
Woodworking

80-110 dBA
Snowmobile

120-133 dBA
Hunting and shooting

80-110 dBA
Motorcycle

107-117 dBA
Model airplanes

90-105 dBA
Home stereo

90-117 dBA
Rock concert

80-110 dBA
ATV or go-cart

80-95 dBA
Lawnmower

Figure adapted with permission from Clark WW, Bohne BA. The effects of noise on hearing and the ear. Med Times 122:17–22, 1984.

VIGNETTE 5.6 Noise-induced hearing loss and iPods

There was much in the news media in 2005 and 2006 regarding the risk of noise-induced hearing loss from Apple iPods or similar portable MP-3 music playback devices. Unpublished reports have indicated that sound levels from such devices can be as high as 100 to 115 dB SPL. Over the past 20 to 25 years many published reports have documented such high sound levels for other personal portable music players, such as Walkman-like cassette and CD players. It is not clear that the sound levels produced by portable MP-3 players are more hazardous than these earlier devices.

One thing that is different, however, is that it is possible with most portable MP-3 players to listen to music for much longer periods, often uninterrupted. For noise-induced hearing loss, the combination of the sound level and the duration of the exposure is critical. For example, many national and international guidelines for hearing hazard suggest most individuals could spend a lifetime listening to sound levels below 85 dB SPL for 8 hours a day and not undergo a hearing loss greater than that which would occur by aging alone. Many of these same national and international guidelines indicate that as the sound level increases 3 dB, the safe duration of exposure must be cut in half. So, for example, most individuals could safely be exposed to sound levels of 88 dB SPL for 4 hours each day or 91 dB SPL for 2 hours per day throughout their lives without any noise-induced hearing loss. Thus, the new danger with portable MP-3 players, compared to earlier predecessors like portable CD players, is not necessarily in the sound levels that they produce, but in the potential for extended, uninterrupted periods of use.

Most of the research conducted on noise-induced hearing loss that forms the basis for the national and international guidelines is for continuous exposures (8 hours per day, typically with brief breaks every 2 hours) to steady-state industrial noise, not fluctuating music, over many years. In addition, most of these exposures occurred with open ears in sound-field industrial conditions, not with sound delivered in sealed ear canals by ear bud–style earphones. Additional research is needed to determine the impact of these and other factors on guidelines for safe exposures. In the interim, limiting the use of high volume control settings (less than two-thirds of full-on, for example) and length of listening each day would be the best way to minimize the risk for eventual *permanent* noise-induced hearing loss.

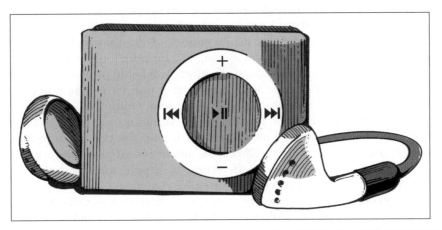

Presbycusis

Beyond approximately age 50 years, hearing sensitivity deteriorates progressively, especially in the high frequencies. The progression is somewhat more rapid for men than for women. Figure 5.20 shows the progression of hearing loss in both men and women as a function of age. The more rapid decline of hearing with age in men may not reflect differences in aging per se but may reflect their more frequent participation in noisy recreational activities such as hunting, snowmobiling, or operating power tools (e.g., lawn mowers, chain saws, and table saws).

The data in Figure 5.20 suggest that aging results in a sloping high-frequency sensorineural hearing loss that gets more severe with advancing age. However, audiometric configurations other than sloping ones can be observed in the aged. The sloping high-frequency audiogram is typical of the most common types of presbycusis, known as sensory and neural presbycusis. At least two other types of presbycusis have been described. These are called metabolic and mechanical presbycusis and are generally associated with flat and very gradually sloping audiometric configurations, respectively. As already mentioned, however, these configurations are much less common.

As shown in Figures 5.17 to 5.19, the audiometric configurations associated with ototoxic antibiotics, noise-induced hearing loss, and sensory or neural presbycusis are all very similar. In all three cases, bilateral high-frequency sensorineural hearing loss is usually observed. The underlying cochlear damage is also very similar: the basal high-frequency region of the cochlea is the main area of destruction and the outer hair cells are primarily affected. Accompanying retrograde destruction of first-order afferent nerve fibers is also typically observed, as is usually the case in cochlear pathology.

Degenerative changes associated with aging have also been observed in the brainstem and cortical areas of the ascending auditory pathway in some cases. These central changes can seriously compound the communicative impairment of the elderly person with sensorineural hearing loss. Approximately 5 to 15% of elderly persons may have central auditory deficits affecting their ability to communicate.

Retrocochlear Pathology

Retrocochlear pathology refers to damage to nerve fibers along the ascending auditory pathways from the internal auditory meatus to the cortex. Most often a tumor is involved, although not always, as in the case of multiple sclerosis.

In many cases, the auditory manifestations of the retrocochlear pathology are subtle. Frequently, for example, no hearing loss for pure tones is measured. The possibility that a tumor along the auditory pathway will fail to produce measurable hearing loss for pure tones can be understood when one recalls the multiple paths by which information ascends through the brainstem within the auditory system (see Chapter 3). Recall that after the first-order ascending neurons terminate in the cochlear nucleus, a variety of paths are available for the neurally transmitted information to ascend to the cortex. Thus, if the tumor is central to the cochlear nucleus, the information required for the detection of a pure tone can easily bypass the affected pathway and progress to the cortex.

For the detection of a pure tone, many of the brainstem centers along the ascending auditory pathways probably serve simple relay functions and perform little processing of the signal. For more complex signals, such as speech, however, some preliminary processing probably takes place in the brainstem before complete processing by the cortex. Still, in many brainstem and cortical disorders, speech recognition

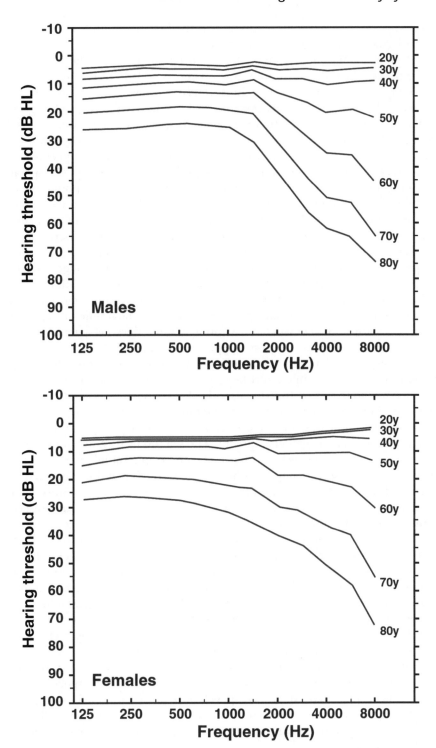

FIGURE 5.20 Hearing loss progression as a function of age in men (*top*) and women (*bottom*). (Adapted with permission from Johansson MS, Arlinger SD. Hearing threshold levels for an otologically unscreened, non-occupationally noise-exposed population in Sweden. Int J Audiol 41:180–194, 2002.)

appears normal in quiet. This seems to be caused by the multiple cues available in the speech signal that assist in its recognition.

A tumor can eliminate from the total information reaching the cortex some of the cues processed by the brainstem or a cortical center without producing a misperception of the speech signal. The patient is simply using the cues that are not affected by the tumor. If, however, the speech signal is degraded by filtering, adding noise, temporal interruption, and so forth, the cues of the speech signal become less redundant. Every cue in the speech signal is now needed for its correct recognition. Individuals with retrocochlear pathology in the brainstem or cortex typically perform poorly on speech recognition tests involving the recognition of degraded speech signals.

In recent years considerable attention has been given to a unique retrocochlear condition, central auditory processing disorders (CAPD), commonly called auditory processing disorder (APD). APD is defined by ASHA as a deficit in such central auditory processes as sound localization and lateralization, auditory discrimination, auditory pattern recognition, temporal aspects of audition, auditory performance with competing acoustic signals, and auditory performance with degraded acoustic signals. The prevalence of APD in children is 2 to 3%, whereas 5 to 15% of older adults exhibit APD. There are three main causes of APD; they include (*a*) disorganized central auditory nervous system (neuromorphologic disorders; anatomic differences in the brain), (*b*) maturational delays of the central auditory nervous system (nervous system is not as mature as that of the same-age peer without an APD), and (*c*) neurologic disorders, diseases, and insults, including neural degenerative disorders (e.g., stroke, multiple sclerosis, Alzheimer, and head injury). APD can occur at any age and can range from mild to severe. Individuals with APD are not always candidates for medical treatment, but many can benefit from therapy and compensatory strategies. In the severe to profound cases, alternative communication styles may be recommended to help with speech-language development. The symptoms seen among individuals with APD can be similar to behaviors associated with peripheral hearing loss, learning disabilities, specific language impairment, and attention deficit disorder. That is, persons with any of these conditions can have difficulty with attention to sounds, memory and repeating sounds, localization, speech understanding in noise, and discriminating between different sounds. They may also have trouble identifying sounds in initial, middle, or ending positions; recognizing sound patterns; and recognizing degraded or distorted signals. The audiologist administers a comprehensive test battery to identify the underlying processes that may be disordered. Since APD can coexist with other conditions, identification and management become special challenges, and so a team approach (audiologist, speech-language pathologist, educator, psychologist) for working with this population is recommended. Although APD is a topic of considerable interest and concern, a great deal is still unknown. More research is needed to improve on the ability to detect and manage this population.

A detailed description of the many retrocochlear disorders and the tests developed for their detection is beyond the scope of this book. Many special speech recognition tests making use of degraded speech have been developed for this population. In addition, as mentioned previously, the ABR and other auditory evoked potentials are also of tremendous assistance to the physician in establishing a diagnosis of retrocochlear pathology.

Retrocochlear pathology that occurs at the first-order afferent nerve fibers, unlike that occurring at higher centers along the ascending auditory pathway, typically results in abnormal performance on the basic audiologic test battery. These tumors, called acoustic schwannomas, acoustic neurinomas, acoustic neurilemomas,

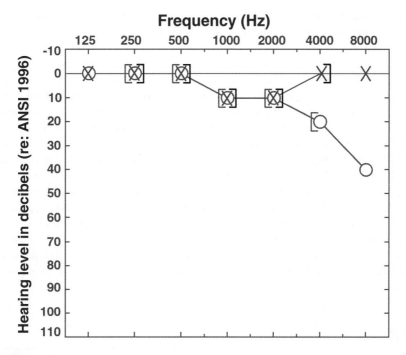

FIGURE 5.21 Audiometric pattern associated with acoustic schwannoma.

or acoustic neuromas, typically produce a high-frequency sensorineural hearing loss that is either unilateral or asymmetric between the two ears (Fig. 5.21). Most patients also complain of tinnitus on the affected side, and slightly more than half of these patients complain of dizziness. Speech recognition performance may range from normal to extremely poor at moderate intensities, but it typically becomes poorer as speech level increases to high intensities. Acoustic reflexes are usually absent or present at elevated levels when the affected ear is stimulated. A special test, known as acoustic reflex decay, measures the amplitude of the middle ear muscle contraction over time during stimulation by intense pure tones. Patients with acoustic schwannoma who have a measurable reflex threshold typically show pronounced reflex decay, especially when stimulated with pure tones at or below 1000 Hz. If several of these audiologic results are observed, the patient should be referred for additional testing. This will most likely involve measurement of the ABR and other special auditory and nonauditory tests.

NONORGANIC HEARING LOSS

The audiologist may obtain audiometric evidence of hearing loss when there is no organic basis to explain the impairment. Some of the terms commonly used to describe this phenomenon are nonorganic hearing loss, pseudohypoacusis, functional hearing loss, and psychogenic deafness. The cause for nonorganic hearing loss varies and is not clearly understood. Sometimes a patient feigns a hearing loss to gain a benefit (e.g., monetary compensation), or the patient offers incorrect audiometric information because of a psychologic disturbance. Whatever the reason, the audiologist must be able to determine whether a nonorganic hearing loss is present and if so, the extent of the impairment. Sometimes a nonorganic hearing loss coexists with an organic hearing loss.

A number of audiometric signs can alert the audiologist to the possibility of a nonorganic hearing loss. These signs include the source of the referral (e.g., insurance company referring because of a claim), inappropriate behavior during the interview (e.g., exaggerated effort to speech-read or to listen), and inconsistent audiologic test results (e.g., poor test-retest reliability). An obvious clue to nonorganic hearing loss is incompatibility between the pure-tone average and the speech recognition threshold (SRT). Recall from Chapter 4 that the pure-tone average and the SRT are related (within 6–10 dB). A person exaggerating a hearing loss for pure tones cannot always provide equivalent hearing loss data for speech and thus will usually exhibit an SRT that is considerably lower (softer) than the pure-tone average. Such a result should alert the audiologist to the possibility of a functional problem.

Numerous other special tests have been developed to detect nonorganic hearing loss. However, detailed discussion of these tests is beyond the scope of this book. Readers who want to learn more about these tests should refer to the suggested readings at the end of the chapter.

SUMMARY

The auditory system, marvelously complex and intricate, is nevertheless vulnerable to assault and damage from disease, trauma, genetic imperfection, extreme environmental conditions (i.e., noise), and aging. Many conditions affect both children and adults and can affect all levels of the auditory system, resulting in conductive, sensorineural, or retrocochlear hearing problems.

References and Suggested Readings

Bess FH, ed. Hearing Impairment in Children. Parkton, MD: York, 1988.

Bess FH, Gravel JS. Foundations of Pediatric Audiology: A Book of Readings. San Diego, CA: Plural, 2006.

Bluestone CD, Stool SE, Alper CM, et al. Pediatric Otolaryngology, vol 1. 4th ed. Philadelphia: Saunders, 2003.

Bluestone CD, Klein JO. Otis Media in Infants and Children. 3rd ed. Philadelphia: Saunders, 2001.

Carhart R. Clinical application of bone conduction audiometry. Arch Otolaryngol 51:798–807, 1950.

Dahl AJ, McCollister FP. Audiological findings in children with neonatal herpes. Ear Hear 9:256–258, 1988.

English GM, ed. Otolaryngology. Hagerstown, MD: Harper & Row, 1976.

Fria TJ, Cantekin EI, Eichler JA. Hearing acuity of children with otitis media with effusion. Arch Otolaryngol 111:10–16, 1985.

Goodhill V, ed. Ear Diseases, Deafness, and Dizziness. Hagerstown, MD: Harper & Row, 1979.

Jerger J, Jerger S. Auditory Disorders. Boston: Little, Brown, 1981.

Johansson MS, Arlinger SD. Hearing threshold levels for an otologically unscreened, non-occupationally noise-exposed population in Sweden. Int J Audiol 41:180–194, 2002.

Joint Committee on Infant Hearing 2000 Position Statement. Rockville, MD: American Speech-Language-Hearing Association, 2000.

Kavanaugh J, ed. Otitis Media and Child Development. Parkton, MD: York, 1986.

Lebo CP, Reddell RC. The presbycusis component in occupational hearing loss. Laryngoscope 82:1399–1409, 1972.

Moody DB, Stebbins WC, Hawkins JE Jr, Johnsson LG. Hearing loss and cochlear pathology in the monkey (Macaca) following exposure to high levels of noise. Arch Oto Rhino Laryngol 220:47–72, 1978.

Newton VE. Paediatric Audiological Medicine. Philadelphia: Whurr, 2002.

Northern JL, ed. Hearing Disorders. 4th ed. Boston: Little, Brown, 1991.

Parving A. Congenital hearing disability epidemiology and identification: A comparison between two health authority districts. Int J Pediatr Otorhinolaryngol 27:29–46, 1993.

Rodgers GK, Telischi FF. Ménière's disease in children. Otolaryngol Clin North Am 30:1101–1104, 1997.

Roeser RJ, Valente M, Hosford-Dunn H. Audiology: Diagnosis, Treatment, Practice Management. New York: Thieme Medical, 2000.

Shambaugh GE, Glasscock ME. Surgery of the Ear. 4th ed. Philadelphia: Saunders, 1990.

Shuknecht HF. Pathology of the Ear. Cambridge: Harvard University, 1974.

Tekin M, Arnos KS, Pandya A. Advances in hereditary deafness. Lancet 358:1082–1090, 2001.

http://www.boystownhospital.org/Hearing/info/genetics/syndromes/ten.asp

Screening Auditory Function

An important component of any comprehensive management strategy for those with hearing loss is an appropriate screening program. Screening is designed to separate persons who have an auditory disorder from those who do not in a simple, safe, rapid, and cost-effective manner. Screening programs are intended to be preventive measures that focus on early identification and intervention. The objective is to minimize the consequences of hearing loss or middle ear disease as early as possible so that the disorder will not produce a disabling condition.

The purpose of this chapter is to present information on screening for hearing loss and middle ear disease. The review covers the principles of screening, discusses screening procedures for hearing loss and otitis media used with different age groups, and recommends follow-up protocols for those identified as having an auditory disorder.

UNDERSTANDING THE PRINCIPLES OF SCREENING

Factors That Determine Whether to Screen

How does one know whether to screen for a particular disorder? Several criteria are used in establishing the value of screening for a specific disorder. First, a disorder should be important. If left unidentified, the disorder could significantly damage an individual's functional status. It is also essential that the program be capable of reaching those who could benefit. Another important criterion is the prevalence of the disorder, or how frequently it occurs in a given population. There should be acceptable criteria for diagnosis. Specific symptoms of a disease must occur with sufficient regularity that it can be determined with assurance which persons have the disorder and which do not. Once detected, the disease should be treatable. Diagnostic and treatment resources must also be available so that adequate medical and educational follow-up can be implemented. Finally, the health system must be able to cope with the program, and the program must be cost effective. It is generally believed by most, but not all, that hearing loss in people of all ages and middle ear disease in children satisfy many of these criteria and that screening for auditory disorders is justifiable, at least for selected populations (e.g., children at risk for hearing loss).

What Is an Acceptable Screening Test?

It is essential to select a screening test that will most effectively detect the conditions to be identified. A good screening tool should be acceptable, reliable, valid, safe, and cost effective. An acceptable test is simple, easy to administer and interpret, and generally well received by the public. A reliable test should be consistent, providing results that do not differ significantly from one test to the next for the same individual. It does little good, for example, to have a screening test that the same healthy individual passes five times and fails five times when the test is administered 10 times in succession. Furthermore, the test should allow examiners to be consistent in the evaluation of a response. Two examiners testing the same person should obtain the same results.

Validity may best be defined by asking, "Are we measuring what we think we are measuring?" Suppose a clinician who wants to identify middle ear disease selects a test to measure hearing. Such a test would not be valid, because although it might reliably measure a child's hearing loss, it cannot indicate the presence or absence of otitis media. Validity consists of two components: sensitivity and specificity. Sensitivity refers to the ability of a screening test to identify accurately an ear that is abnormal (whether from hearing loss or from otitis media); specificity denotes the ability of a screening tool to identify normal ears. Thus, a valid test is one that identifies a normal condition as normal and an abnormal one as abnormal.

Finally, a good screening test is one that is safe and cost effective in relation to the expected benefits. Because the instruments designed to screen for hearing loss and middle ear disease are considered safe and reasonable in cost, the greatest direct expense is usually the salary for personnel. Other factors should be taken into consideration in estimates of the expense of a screening program. These include the time required to administer the test, the cost of supplies, the number of individuals to be screened and rescreened, and the cost of training and supervising screeners. The following formula has been suggested to estimate the cost of a school screening program:

$$\text{Cost/child} = \frac{S}{R} + \frac{C + (M \times L)}{(N \times L)}$$

where C = cost of equipment in dollars, S = salary of the screening personnel in dollars per hour, L = lifetime of the equipment in years, M = annual maintenance cost in dollars, R = screening rate in children per hour, and N = number screened per year. This formula can also be modified for determining the cost of an adult screening program.

Calculation of the costs of any screening program should also consider indirect costs, such as the cost of the comprehensive audiologic assessment, monitoring, and intervention that would occur as a result of the screening. A special concern is the cost associated with false-positive test subjects, those who fail the screen but who have normal hearing. For children, such costs may include a parent's lost time from work, transportation to health care facilities, administration of unnecessary follow-up tests, and possibly unnecessary treatment. They may also include the more human cost of the anxiety of parents or caring others, the potential for misunderstanding, and the disturbance of family function. Finally, the possible cost savings resulting from a screening program must be entered into the equation. For example, educational costs might be reduced as a consequence of early identification and intervention.

Principles of Evaluating a Screening Test

This section covers some of the principles of assessing the usefulness of a screening test. Figure 6.1 sets the stage for understanding this process. The primary goal is to distinguish within the population at large those who exhibit an auditory disorder (A + C) from those who do not (B + D). Within the group with an auditory disorder, subgroup A are those with the disorder who test positive (true positives); subgroup C are those with the disorder who test negative (false negatives). Within the group without an auditory disorder, subgroup B is those without the disorder who test positive (false positives); subgroup D is those without the disorder who test negative (true negatives).

Any screening test must be evaluated against an independent standard, often called a *gold standard*. The results of the gold standard test are universally accepted as proof that the disease or disorder is either present or absent. In the case of hearing loss, pure-tone audiometry typically serves as the gold standard for any screening tool, whereas for middle ear disease, the gold standard is usually pneumatic otoscopy or electroacoustic immittance.

Figure 6.2 illustrates how the characteristics of a screening test can be evaluated against the gold standard. Toward this end, several terms and definitions must be understood. First is sensitivity [100A/(A + C)]. (The factor 100 is introduced to

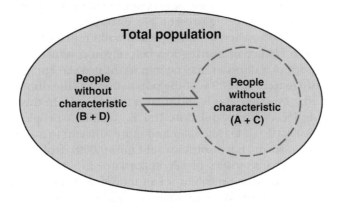

FIGURE 6.1 The screening process. The purpose is to differentiate those who exhibit an auditory disorder in the population at large from those who do not.

Gold standard test

Characteristic

		Present	Absent	Total
	Positive	A	B	A + B
	Negative	C	D	C + D
	Totals	A + C	B + D	A + B + C + D

Screening test

FIGURE 6.2 A decision matrix for calculating the operating characteristics of a screening test.

convert the result to a percentage.) We have already learned that sensitivity refers to the proportion of individuals with the characteristic correctly identified by the test. If 100 subjects have a hearing loss and the test correctly identifies 75 of them, the sensitivity of the test is 75%. Sensitivity is typically affected by the severity or duration of the characteristic. This is only logical in that the milder an impairment is, the closer it is to a normal condition and the more difficult it is to distinguish from normal. However, the measure is not affected by prevalence. Another important measure is specificity, $[100D/(B + D)]$, which refers to the proportion of individuals without the characteristic correctly identified by the test. If in a group of 100 normal subjects the test identifies 70 as normal and 30 as abnormal, the specificity is 70%. Like sensitivity, specificity is not affected by the prevalence of the disorder. The best screening tool is one that provides the highest degree of both sensitivity and specificity.

It is possible to vary the accuracy of a screening test by altering the pass-fail criteria. A cutoff on a hearing screening test, for example, might be 15 dB HL or 40 dB HL. A 15-dB HL cutoff will provide high sensitivity but lower specificity. This is because the 15-dB HL criterion will result in a larger portion of near-normal subjects being classified as having hearing loss. If a 40-dB HL cutoff is used, however, sensitivity will decrease but specificity will increase. The 40-dB HL cutoff will miss some of the mildly impaired near-normal subjects but will avoid misclassifying most of the subjects with normal hearing.

An important concept in any screening program is the prevalence of the disorder that is to be screened. Prevalence (derived from the word *prevail*) refers to the proportion of individuals in the population who demonstrate the characteristic $[100(A + C)/(A + B + C + D)]$. An important use of prevalence data is as a pretest indicator of the probability of the disorder being present. For example, if the prevalence of hearing loss in the elderly is 30%, when an older person walks into a hearing clinic, you know that there is a 30% chance of hearing loss before you conduct any tests. To illustrate how the prevalence of a disorder may be important to a screening program, consider the following two extremes. If 99% of the population has the disorder, it is easier simply to assume that everyone has it and treat it accordingly. In this case, we would be mistreating only 1% of the population. If 1 in 1 million people have the disorder (prevalence = 0.0001%), it may be safer and more efficient to assume that no one has it. Failure to screen for such a disorder would miss 0.0001% of the population.

Additional test characteristics of key importance in screening for a disorder are positive predictive value (the probability of an individual having the disorder when the test is positive) and negative predictive value (the probability of not having the disorder when the test is negative). Unlike sensitivity and specificity, predictive values are strongly dependent on the prevalence of the disorder in the population being tested. For a disorder of very low prevalence, even a highly specific test is likely to have a low positive predictive value. For example, a test that has a sensitivity of 90% and a specificity of 90% in detecting a disorder has a positive predictive value of 79.4%, and thus a false-positive rate of 20.6%, if the prevalence of the disorder is 30%. However, the positive predictive value decreases to 50% if the prevalence is only 10% and to 8.3% if the prevalence is only 1%.

In most hearing clinics, especially when screening for hearing loss, tests must yield maximum accuracy. The ideal test would be one that always gave positive results in anyone with a hearing loss and negative results in anyone without a hearing loss. Unfortunately, no such test exists. As a rule, one attempts to maximize the sensitivity and specificity of a screening test. This is done by evaluating different pass-fail criteria and test protocols in comparison to the gold standard. Vignettes 6.1 and 6.2 discuss how to apply these general principles to actual screening data.

VIGNETTE 6.1   Guidelines for calculating the operating characteristics of a screening tool

Let us go through the step-by-step procedures for calculating the characteristics of a screening tool. To assist in this process, some screening data are presented. The gold standard was pure-tone audiometry. In this example, 99 patients were screened and then tested using pure-tone audiometry. Of the 47 patients who failed the screening test, 27 actually had a

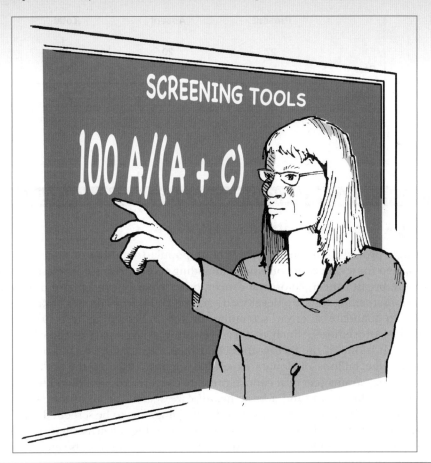

(continued)

VIGNETTE 6.1 Guidelines for calculating the operating characteristics of a screening tool *(Continued)*

---

hearing loss and 20 did not. On the other hand, 52 patients passed the screening. Of these, the gold standard showed that three had a hearing loss and 49 did not. The prevalence of hearing loss in the population screened $[100/(A + C) (A + B + C + D)]$ is 100(30/99), or about 30%.

First, the sensitivity, or the percentage of valid positive test results, is calculated from the data. The formula for computing sensitivity is $100A/(A + C)$. When applied to our data, this gives 100(27/30) = 90%. This is excellent.

Next, compute specificity, or the percentage of valid negative test results, using the formula $100D/(B + D)$. This results in 100(49/69) = 71%. This is adequate but not excellent.

In this example, we see that the screening test appears to be a valid tool for the identification of a hearing loss, offering acceptable sensitivity and specificity values. Now, on your own, calculate the operating characteristics of a screening tool for the example in Vignette 6.2.

| | Gold standard test Hearing impairment characteristic | | |
	Present	Absent	Total
Fail	27	20	47
Pass	3	49	52
Totals	30	69	99

(Screening test)

STATUS OF IDENTIFICATION PROGRAMS IN THE UNITED STATES

Screening: A Common Health Care Practice

No single procedure in health care is more popular than that of screening. Tests are performed for a variety of conditions including blood pressure, cholesterol, genetics, diabetes, breast cancer, colorectal cancer, other types of cancer, and of course, hearing. New screening tests are developed each year, and legislation is always being introduced to mandate a given screening protocol. Screening tests usually lead to additional procedures, which in turn constitute a large part of today's health care practice. It is one of the factors that contribute to the high costs of health care. For example, the billions of dollars expended for just three of the widely recognized screening programs (cervical cancer, prostate cancer, and high blood levels of cholesterol) are sufficient to fund a basic health care system for all of the poor and uninsured. Today's health care system actively encourages us to be screened for a variety of conditions. Vignette 6.3 highlights a typical screening advertisement published in a local newspaper and illustrates how such screening advertisements can sometimes mislead the consumer.

VIGNETTE 6.2   Computing the characteristics of a screening tool using hypothetical screening data

Now compute the characteristics of a screening tool for the example. For this example, compute prevalence, sensitivity, and specificity.

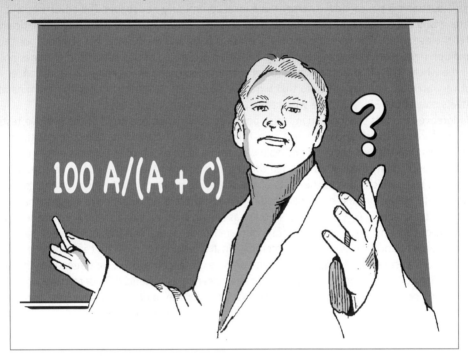

Example:

| | | Gold standard test | | |
| | | Hearing impairment characteristic | | |
		Present	**Absent**	**Total**
Screening test	Fail	160	20	180
	Pass	40	180	220
	Totals	**200**	**200**	**400**

How did you do? You can find the answers in the back of the chapter.

Hearing Screening Programs for Children

Identification programs for hearing loss have been implemented in the United States for various age groups including the neonate, the infant, the preschooler, and the school-age child. Despite the importance of early identification, most screening has occurred at the school-age level. Only within the past few years has newborn hearing

VIGNETTE 6.3   Screening: a popular procedure in today's health care environment

Screening is one of the most popular procedures in health care, and health care facilities aggressively promote the need to be screened for a variety of conditions. The accompanying figure illustrates a typical advertisement in a local community newspaper. The advertisement states, "One out of every 11 men will develop prostate cancer, with the risk rising dramatically after the age of 40." The message is clear, the risk is high, and we'd better get screened for this condition right away. Unfortunately, the information presented in this advertisement does not tell the whole story. That is, the digital rectal examination used for screening prostate cancer is not very accurate. Studies illustrate that when we screen asymptomatic males, the examination detects only about 33% of those with cancer; the test misses most cases.

Moreover, the test produces many false positives. Fewer than one-third of the positive tests actually turn out to be cancer, whereas two-thirds or more of the failures are false-positives. This means that the test suggests probable cancer in a large group of individuals who are normal. Hence, many individuals who fail the test but do not have cancer will be referred for additional tests, which adds to the costs of the screening program; not to mention the cost of fear, anxiety, confusion, and misunderstanding. Finally, there is no evidence to suggest that the digital rectal screening is worthwhile. No one has shown that individuals who are screened for this problem are any better off than those who are not screened. This lack of evidence has caused some national groups to recommend against screening for prostate cancer. The lesson—just because a screening procedure is popular and we are encouraged to be screened by health care facilities does not necessarily mean that the screening is beneficial. To determine whether a screening procedure is beneficial, we must first consider the principles of screening discussed earlier in this chapter and apply these principles to the available evidence.

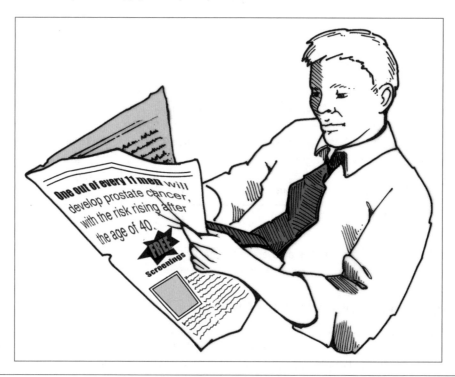

screening become widespread; in fact, because of the undaunted efforts of Marion Downs (see Vignette 6.4) and others, more than 40 states now mandate universal newborn screening.

Interestingly, many pediatricians do not recognize the importance of screening very young infants for hearing loss. It has been estimated, for example, that only 3% of children from 6 months to 11 years of age receive a screening test at their primary health care source. Although it is true that more reliable responses can be obtained from infants and young children than from neonates, there is the problem of locating all of the groups of older youngsters for the hearing test. Once newborns leave the hospital, it is not until age 5 years, at the kindergarten level, that these children are available for testing at one common location. The few screening programs that do exist are conducted in day care centers, well-baby clinics, and Head Start programs. These programs, however, attract only a specific segment of children, primarily those

---

VIGNETTE 6.4 **Marion P. Downs (1914–), advocate for early identification for hearing loss in infants**

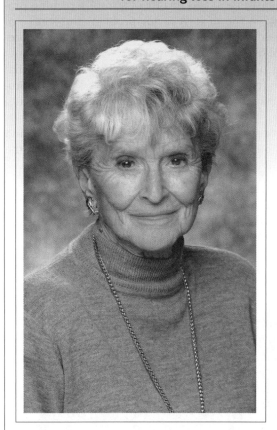

Throughout her professional career Marion Downs championed the early identification of hearing loss in very young infants. Having recognized the value of early auditory stimulation, while teaching at the University of Denver in the early 1950s she introduced the concept of early identification. After entering the faculty of the University of Colorado Medical School in 1959 she was able to implement the concept by developing a comprehensive early identification program for all newborns in the Denver area and screened more than 10,000 babies using the arousal test, which was later judged to be impractical. Consequently, Downs proposed to the American Speech-Language-Hearing Association the formation of the National Joint Committee on Infant Hearing and chaired the committee in its first few years. The committee continues to be instrumental in promoting the concept of universal newborn hearing screening.

Downs served as an advocate for early identification and habilitation throughout the world as a consultant to foreign governments and by presenting workshops and lectures in some 18 countries. In 1997, Downs was honored by having a national center on hearing and infants named after her. The center promotes her lifelong dream of achieving early intervention for newborns not only in Colorado but throughout the country. Now over 90, Downs continues to advance her long ideal of newborn hearing screening and early intervention.

from lower socioeconomic levels. Even if a massive national effort were made to screen all preschoolers at these various centers, a large percentage of children would be missed. Yet screening the preschool child has several distinct advantages over the screening of newborns:

1. Children become easier to test as age increases.
2. Children with a progressive hearing loss and those whose hearing loss was not detected at the newborn screening would stand a good chance of being identified.
3. Children with hearing loss who have recently moved into the community would have a chance of being identified.

Under our present system, children whose hearing loss was not detected at the newborn identification program or who moved into a community at preschool age are not identified until screening occurs in kindergarten. There is a critical need for a national effort directed at infant and preschool hearing screening programs in every state.

Hearing screening programs using pure-tone audiometry are most often conducted in the school system because it affords easy access to the children. However, the availability, accessibility, comprehensiveness, and quality of school screening programs vary significantly from one state to the next. A major problem and source of frustration for audiologists involved in school screening programs is the lack of appropriate follow-up services offered to children who fail the screen.

The use of immittance screening programs is not universal. It is estimated that about half of the states use immittance (tympanometry) as part of their screening procedures. Some of the problems associated with mass immittance screening are discussed later in this chapter.

Figure 6.3 shows the percentage of school programs that conduct pure-tone and immittance screening. The emphasis on pure-tone and immittance screening in the

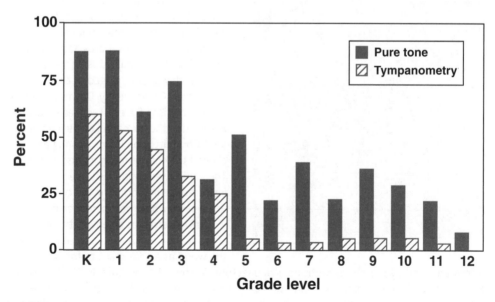

FIGURE 6.3 Percentage of school programs conducting pure-tone and immittance screening by grade level. (Adapted from Roush J. Screening school-age children. In Bess FH, Hall JW, eds. Screening Children for Auditory Function. Nashville: Bill Wilkerson Center, 1992.)

schools is at the elementary level, and few programs screen in the secondary grades. Moreover, a much larger percentage of school programs use pure-tone screening than immittance screening.

Hearing Screening Programs for Adults

There are almost no formal hearing screening programs in the United States for adult populations. Screenings do occur, however, in the armed forces, and most communities conduct health fairs where individuals can have their hearing tested. Adult screening programs are also known to take place at community health centers, retirement communities, and nursing homes. Interestingly, evidence suggests that the primary-care physician typically does not screen for hearing loss even if the patient complains of a hearing loss. There is a critical need for audiologists to educate both consumers and health care professionals about the importance of hearing health care, including early identification and intervention.

Audiologists and other health professionals have failed to sensitize both the lay public and the educational and medical communities to the effects of auditory impairment on total development and quality of life. The importance of early detection of hearing loss and the effectiveness of the screening methods available are two concepts that have not been presented well to the educational or medical community. Until we begin to educate these other professional groups, we cannot hope to improve the identification programs.

IDENTIFICATION OF HEARING LOSS

Screening the Neonate

The advantages of detecting sensorineural hearing loss as early in life as possible are important enough to encourage the implementation of newborn screening programs. It has now been demonstrated that children who receive intervention from age 3 years or younger show significantly better speech and language outcomes later in life. Early identification and intervention (one definition of *intervene* is to *come in and modify*) also result in substantial cost savings. For example, a deaf infant who receives educational and audiologic management during the first years of life has a better than 50% chance of being mainstreamed into a regular classroom.

Historically, the screening procedures advocated for the newborn nursery have been controversial. Audiologists have not agreed on the most effective and appropriate techniques. The National Joint Committee on Infant Hearing Screening (a committee of representatives from the American Academy of Otolaryngology, the American Academy of Pediatrics, the American Academy of Audiology, the American Speech-Language-Hearing Association [ASHA], the Council on Education of the Deaf, and the directors of speech and hearing programs in state and welfare agencies) endorsed universal newborn screening. If universal hearing screening was not available, the committee recommended, at a minimum, screening infants who were considered at high risk for hearing loss. Table 6.1 lists the joint committee's neonatal intensive-care criteria (risk indicators) for both newborns and infants. Infants who pass a newborn screen but possess risk factors for hearing loss or speech-language delay should receive periodic audiologic monitoring, medical surveillance, and ongoing observation of communication development, especially if the risk indicators are associated with progressive forms of

TABLE 6.1   Indicators or Risk Factors Associated With Sensorineural or Conductive Hearing Loss

Neonates (birth–28 d)	Infants (29 d–2 y)
1. Illness or condition requiring admission ≥48 h to NICU (Cone-Wesson et al., 2000) 2. Stigmata, other findings associated with syndrome known to include sensorineural, or conductive hearing loss 3. Family history of permanent childhood sensorineural hearing loss 4. Craniofacial anomalies, including morphologic abnormalities of pinna and ear canal 5. In utero infection, e.g., CMV, herpes, toxoplasmosis, rubella	1. Parent or caregiver concern for hearing, speech, language, and/or developmental delay 2. Family history of permanent childhood hearing loss 3. Stigmata, other findings associated with syndrome known to include sensorineural or conductive hearing loss or eustachian tube dysfunction 4. Postnatal infection associated with sensorineural hearing loss, including bacterial meningitis 5. In utero infection, e.g., CMV, herpes, rubella, syphilis, toxoplasmosis 6. Neonatal indicators, specifically hyperbilirubinemia requiring exchange transfusion, persistent pulmonary hypertension with mechanical ventilation, conditions requiring ECMO 7. Syndromes associated with progressive hearing loss such as neurofibromatosis, osteoporosis, Usher syndrome 8. Neurodegenerative disorders, e.g., Hunter syndrome; sensorimotor neuropathies, e.g., Friedreich ataxia, Charcot-Marie-Tooth syndrome 9. Head trauma 10. Recurrent or persistent otitis media with effusion for at least 3 mo

CMV, cytomegalovirus; ECMO, extracorporeal membrane oxygenation.
Adapted from the American Speech-Language-Hearing Association Joint Committee on Infant Hearing 2000 Position Statement. A new position statement will be published in late 2007; however, the statement was not available when this book went to press.

hearing loss. Unfortunately, studies have demonstrated that although the use of a high-risk register can identify some infants with hearing loss, many children with hearing loss do not have any of the risk factors listed in the register.

Behavioral Observation Audiometry

A number of behavioral techniques have been advocated in the neonatal intensive-care unit (NICU) for screening for hearing loss. These techniques make use of a high-intensity broadband stimulus, or a band of noise centered around 3000 Hz. The stimuli are presented while the infant is at rest in a crib. The child's behavioral responses to these stimuli are observed or recorded. A common behavioral technique of this type once used in neonatal nurseries is the Crib-O-Gram. This test uses a motion-sensitive transducer placed under the crib to detect the infant's responses to the high-level noise presentations. Even subtle respiratory movement can be identified with this device. Behavioral techniques, however, have a number of limitations. They generally identify only children with severe forms of hearing loss. In addition, because of the sound-field approach, it is possible that unilateral sensorineural hearing loss will not be detected. Finally, concern has been expressed about the sensitivity and specificity of this approach, because the response depends as much on the infant's motor state as it does on sensory ability.

Auditory Brainstem Response

The auditory brainstem response (ABR) (See Chapters 2 and 4) has been suggested as a reliable indicator of hearing sensitivity in infancy. The advantages of the ABR for newborn screening include (a) the use of less intense, near-threshold stimuli, making it possible to detect milder forms of hearing loss, (b) the ability to detect both unilateral and bilateral hearing losses, and (c) the use of a physiologic measurement that depends entirely on a sensory response. Limitations to the technique include the cost and sophisticated nature of the instrumentation, the use of an acoustic click that makes the ABR primarily sensitive to only high-frequency hearing loss, and the fact that the ABR is not a conscious response at the level of the cortex (presence of an ABR does not mean the individual can hear). Nevertheless, the ABR is thought to provide a good estimate of hearing status when used carefully, especially when one considers the limitations of the alternative procedures. A child who fails an ABR screening in the intensive-care nursery must be retested later under more favorable conditions.

Several ABR-based screening systems with automated response collection and evaluation have been designed for use with neonates. These portable automatic devices are based on microprocessors. Their primary function is to screen for handicapping hearing loss in newborn infants. These simple and cost-effective systems use various automated algorithms to determine whether an infant passes or fails. These devices are generally preferred for screening because they do not require test interpretation, they reduce the possible influence of tester bias, and they ensure test consistency.

Otoacoustic Emissions

As noted in Chapter 2 and Chapter 4, evoked otoacoustic emissions (OAEs) have been used as a screening tool to identify hearing loss in neonates. There is some disagreement as to the details of such a screening protocol, including (a) whether transient-evoked OAEs (TEOAEs) or distortion-product OAEs (DPOAEs) or both should be used and (b) the appropriate stimulus parameters to optimize screening efficiency. However, the scientific and clinical communities have recommended that OAEs become an integral part of a universal neonatal hearing screening program for the United States. It has generally been recommended that either OAEs or ABR be used for the initial screening, with all screening failures retested with the alternative measure. Many of the advantages and disadvantages described for the use of ABR as a screening tool also apply to the use of OAEs as a screening measure. One important limitation to OAE is that the test will not identify individuals with neural complications; hence, infants with auditory neuropathy (see Chapter 5) will not be detected with OAEs.

National Institutes of Health Consensus Statement

Interest in the early identification of hearing loss among newborns and young infants has increased. Several professional organizations have developed position statements concerning the need for early identification in addition to proposing recommended screening protocols. In 1993, the National Institute on Deafness and Other Communication Disorders sponsored a national meeting on early identification of hearing loss in infants and young children. A task force composed of members of several disciplines developed a consensus statement on early identification after presentations and discussions at the conference. The task force supported universal hearing screening within an infant's first 3 months of life, preferably before hospital discharge. A two-stage screening protocol was recommended. First, all infants would be screened with OAEs; those who failed the OAE test would receive an ABR screen at 40 dB nHL (0 dB nHL represents normal hearing for these systems, just as 0 dB HL does for the audiogram). Failure at this second stage would lead to a comprehensive diagnostic hearing assessment within 6 months. Periodic infant hearing screening throughout early childhood was also recommended.

The National Institutes of Health (NIH) consensus recommendation was met with some controversy. Some advocates of early identification believed that implementation of a universal screening program was premature because of the limited data on screening healthy newborns in well-baby nurseries (most screening had been conducted in NICUs) and because there was limited information on the performance of the two-tier screening protocol. Other major concerns with the recommendation of universal newborn screening were the overall costs of such programs and the practicability of implementing identification programs in remote and rural communities—communities in which 25% of the births in the United States take place. Many of these concerns have been addressed since the NIH statement was published, and more and more hospitals in the United States are initiating successful screening programs for healthy newborns or high-risk babies using the protocol recommended by the NIH or some modification of it.

The New York State Universal Newborn Hearing Screening Project has shown that successful implementation of universal newborn hearing screening can occur in a state with a high annual birth rate and geographic and socioeconomic diversity. In fact, this project highlights both the feasibility and practicability of a large newborn screening program. The New York state project investigated outcome measures of a multicenter statewide hearing screening program—eight hospitals across the state participated in the 3-year project. An acceptable 72% of the infants who failed the in-hospital screening returned for outpatient testing. The percentage of in-hospital fails returning for retesting was significantly higher than the percentage of in-hospital misses returning for retesting. An important result of this project was that program improvement occurred over time (although considerable variation was noted across hospitals). Program improvement was particularly evident for the percentage of in-hospital fails that returned for outpatient retesting. Despite a concentrated follow-up effort, however, the number of in-hospital misses that returned for retesting was somewhat disappointing (31%). The overall prevalence of hearing loss was 1.96/1000—in the NICU prevalence was 8/1000; in the well-baby nursery, 0.9/1000. The positive predictive value for permanent hearing loss based on in-patient screening was an acceptable 4%. For outpatient rescreening the positive predictive value was 22%. This project has demonstrated that with adequate funding and a well-coordinated effort, an effective universal newborn hearing screening program can be implemented in a large, diverse state. Also, the project illustrates the need for more research, especially in the areas of minimizing inpatient misses and compliance with follow-up testing.

Screening the Infant and Preschool-Age Child

Identification Tests and Procedures

Selection of screening techniques depends on the age, maturity, and cooperation of the child. Generally speaking, a test using sound localization in the sound field will be required for children aged 4 months to 2 years. Conventional audiometric screening using earphones can usually be used with children aged 3 years or older. Children aged 2 to 3 years are the most difficult group for whom to select an appropriate test. Some of these children can be conditioned for traditional screening techniques with earphones, whereas others necessitate a test based on sound localization.

Infant and Pre–Nursery School Child (4 Months to 3 Years)

Certainly, OAEs or ABRs may be used to screen infants and toddlers for hearing loss. Too often, however, these devices are not available where infants and preschool age children are typically screened.

The use of calibrated acoustic stimuli (e.g., narrowband noise) is often suggested for eliciting a localization (head turn) response in a sound field setting. The child is placed on the parent's lap and the acoustic stimulus is presented about 2 feet from either ear. If the child fails to localize the signal, a rescreening is recommended. A second failure results in a third test a week later. If the child again fails the test, a complete diagnostic examination is conducted. Unfortunately, this technique does not offer ear-specific information, and a child with unilateral hearing loss will probably be missed.

Sometimes, delays in speech and language development are the most sensitive and valid indicators of hearing loss among preschool children. It has been suggested that primary-care physicians and other allied health personnel screen young children for hearing loss simply by asking the parent three basic questions: (*a*) How many different words do you estimate your child uses? Is it 100 words, 500 words, or what? (*b*) What is the length of a typical sentence that your child uses? Is it single words, two words, full sentences, or what? (*c*) How clear is your child's speech to a friend or neighbor? Would they understand 10%, 50%, 90%, or what? Table 6.2 presents a general guide for referring children with a speech delay.

A more formal test that probes for delays in speech and language development is known as the Early Language Milestone Scale (ELM). The ELM was designed primarily

---

TABLE 6.2 **Referral Guidelines for Children With "Speech" Delay**

---

12 Months
  No differentiated babbling or vocal imitation
18 Months
  No use of single words
24 Months
  Single-word vocabulary of ≤10 words
30 Months
  Fewer than 100 words, no evidence of two-word combinations, unintelligible
36 Months
  Fewer than 200 words, no use of telegraphic sentences, clarity <50%
48 Months
  Fewer than 600 words, no use of simple sentences, clarity <80%

From Matkin ND. Early recognition and referral of hearing-impaired children. Pediatr Rev 6:151–156, 1984.

for physicians and other health care professionals. It is considered a simple, rapid, cost-effective means of screening for communication disorders in children from birth to 36 months of age; however, it is most sensitive at 24 months of age and higher. The test combines parental report, direct testing, and incidental observation. Important for the primary-care physician is the fact that the test takes only 1 to 5 minutes to administer. Sensitivity values as high as 97% and specificity values as high as 93% have been reported for use of the ELM with preschool-age children. More representative values for sensitivity and specificity of the ELM are 65 to 70% and 65 to 75%, respectively. Nevertheless, asking parents specific questions about speech-language development seems to be a viable option for determining the presence of hearing loss among young children.

Preschooler (3 to 6 Years)

When the child reaches 3 years of age, the more traditional hearing test with earphones can be used for screening. By means of a portable pure-tone audiometer, signals may be presented at various frequencies at a fixed intensity level. The child merely indicates to the examiner, usually by raising a hand, when a tone is perceived. The ASHA has recommended that 1000, 2000, and 4000 Hz be used as test frequencies. If immittance testing is not part of the program, 500 Hz should also be tested (assuming background noise levels in the test area are acceptable). The ASHA further recommends a screening level of 20 dB HL for all frequencies tested. A lack of response at any frequency in either ear constitutes a test failure. Children who fail should be screened again, preferably within the same test session, but no later than 1 week after the original test. Rescreening can significantly reduce the overall number of test failures. Figure 6.4 illustrates the value of rescreening. Children who also fail the second screen should be referred for a complete audiologic evaluation.

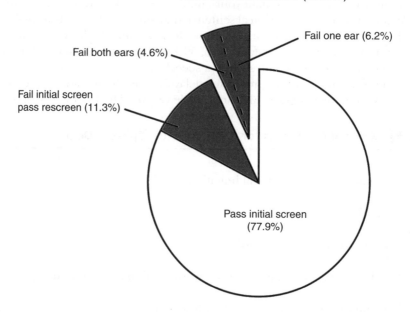

FIGURE 6.4 The value of rescreening for pure-tone audiometry. (Adapted from Wilson WR, Walton WK. Public school audiometry. In Martin FN, ed. Pediatric Audiology. Englewood Cliffs, NJ: Prentice-Hall,)

Procedural Considerations for Preschool-Age Children

In developing a screening program at the preschool level, special attention should be directed toward the groundwork and orientation before the screening. The success of any screening program largely depends on the cooperation of the teachers, the children, and the parents. All three of these parties must be familiarized with the screening process that is to take place.

First, a letter should go to the teacher outlining the need for and the purpose of the screening program. The letter should also review the teacher's responsibilities in preparing the children for the screening. Table 6.3 outlines some suggested prescreening activities with which the teacher can orient the children to the listening task. Such activities performed before the identification program can help avoid wasted time during the actual screening. It is also most helpful to provide the teacher with a

TABLE 6.3 Recommended Prescreening Activities

I

Objective	To introduce children to wearing earphones in hearing testing.
Materials	Old set of earphones (if possible) or set of earmuffs.
Procedure	Let each child examine and wear the earphones. Talk about headband and muff.
Variation	Allow children to put earphones on each other's ears.

II

Objective	To prepare children for hearing test.
Materials	Blocks, shoe boxes.
Procedure	Put a shoe box on the table. Demonstrate holding a block up to your ear. Have one child stand behind you and clap hands. Drop the block in the box when you hear the clap. Have each child take a turn standing in front of the box with the child's back toward you. Tell the children to listen very carefully and drop the blocks into the box when they hear the clap.
Variation	Let the children be the hand clappers.
Note	If a child does not seem to understand, guide the child through the activity until he or she can hold the block to the ear and drop it in the box without help.

III

Objective	To prepare children for hearing test.
Materials	Blocks, shoe boxes, bell.
Procedure	Put a shoe box on the table. Demonstrate holding a block up to your ear. Have one child stand behind you and ring a bell. Drop the block in the box when you hear the bell. Have each child take a turn standing in front of the box with his or her back to you. Tell the children to listen very carefully and drop the blocks in the box when they hear the bell.
Variation	Repeat activity and ring bell softly. Have the children take turns being bell ringer.
Note	Encourage children to listen for soft or little sound of bell as preparation for hearing test sounds, which will be very soft.

TABLE 6.4 Sequence of Screening Responsibilities

Agency Providing Screening	Program Receiving Screening
Appoint a person to coordinate all screening activities.	Appoint a program representative to coordinate screening activities.
Procure the list of all program centers or children needing to be screened.	List all program centers or children to be screened.
Establish personnel needs according to number of children to be screened. Secure necessary personnel to implement successful screening.	
Organize a training session in use of screening materials, test forms, test protocol for screeners.	
Establish schedules, including dates and times, allowing ample time for necessary prescreening activities.	Establish schedules, including dates and times, allowing ample time for necessary prescreening activities.
Assist in screening site selection, if needed.	Choose screening sites.
Mail screening materials and preschool record forms to recipients. Materials should be in teachers' hands 3 weeks prior to screening date to allow ample time for completion of forms, mailing of parent release forms, and training in the classroom.	Inform teachers of dates, times, sites, personal responsibilities. All pertinent information should be in writing and given to teachers approximately 2 wk prior to screening date.
Conduct screening according to schedule.	Assist in screening as needed.
Assist in contacting resource agencies for follow-up or serve as resource.	Contact resource agencies for necessary follow-up for children failing the screen. Obtain comprehensive speech and language evaluations, therapeutic management, and in-service teacher training assistance.
Type and mail a preschool screening summary report indicating results of screening by individual names grouped by classrooms. This report should be complete within 2 weeks of the screening.	Receive and review the preschool screening summary report with teachers and staff.
Provide ongoing monitoring of follow-up activities on all children failing the screening.	Actively pursue follow-up management of all children failing the screening.

list of the screening responsibilities of those who will be conducting the screening and of those who will be receiving the screening. This list will serve as an excellent guide and provide the teacher and/or administrator with a better understanding of the entire process from start to finish (Table 6.4). Finally, a sample letter to the parents of each child should be included in the packet of materials. The letter should explain the screening program so that the parents will understand the value of screening and support the process (Fig. 6.5).

The person who will be responsible for conducting the screening program should visit the facility and meet with the appropriate teachers and administrators. Together they should review carefully the sequence of the screening program and discuss any

Dear Parent,

Special arrangements have been made for your child and the others in your child's class to be tested for hearing. This test is a wonderful opportunity and we want to be sure that every parent knows all about it.

Certain learning problems don't ordinarily show up until later school years, when they are harder to remedy. If these special needs can be found early in the school years, the problem can often be solved before it really gets started.

We are very fortunate to have trained, qualified people who will be testing our children during school hours one day in the near future. The testing is provided without any cost to you. Your child will enjoy the "games" that check the ability to listen. There is everything to gain...and nothing to lose.

Because of the large number of children to be tested, the procedure will have to be speedy. Therefore, our children will be taking what is called a screening test, which doesn't draw any conclusions—it just finds the children who may need more careful testing.

The majority of the children will pass with flying colors (and have an enjoyable day doing it). If any problem areas are discovered, someone from the center (school) will get in touch with you to make arrangements to check out the problem completely.

None of us likes to think that our child could have anything that stands in the way of learning. By taking advantage of this screening test, we can make sure. The earlier a problem is found, the less a problem it becomes.

If you have any questions, please contact us.

Teacher

FIGURE 6.5 Sample letter for teacher to send parents before the screening test.

concerns. This is also an excellent opportunity to review with the program officials the sites available for the screening. Needless to say, a quiet room is essential. Other considerations in selecting a testing site have been identified by others:

1. The site will need appropriate electrical outlets (only grounded three-prong outlets should be used) and lighting.
2. The site should be away from railroad tracks, playgrounds, heavy traffic, public toilets, and cafeterias.

3. The site should be relatively free of visual distractions.
4. Ideally, the site should have carpet and curtains to help reduce the room noise.
5. The site should have nearby bathroom facilities to accommodate the needs of the children and screeners.
6. The site should have chairs and tables appropriate for small children.

Some other suggestions and hints for screening preschool children include the following:

1. One person should be individually responsible for ensuring that the children move through the screening process smoothly and that all children receive the test.
2. Arrangements should be made for the children to have name tags showing their legal names and nicknames.
3. All forms should be accurately completed before the screening date. Each child should have his or her own individual preschool record form.
4. When screening children aged 3 to 6 years, it is wise to alternate age groups during the screening day; for example, 3-year-olds should be followed by 5-year-olds. This is because 3-year-olds are much harder to test and take more time. Another factor to keep in mind is that younger children tire more easily than older children and need to be screened earlier in the day.
5. Screening activities should run from 8:30 or 9:00 A.M. until 3:00 or 3:30 P.M. each day. Schedule a full day, even if it means adjustments of schedules and bus runs and special notes of explanation for parents.
6. At all costs, avoid changing screening sites in the middle of the day. Each time you must dismantle a screening site in one center, move, and reassemble in another site, you lose approximately 1 hour plus travel time.
7. If the children are to be away from their own building during their regular lunch period, make arrangements for them to have lunch at the screening site, if possible.
8. If the agency at which the screening is taking place has a speech clinician on staff, ask to have that person available to assist in the screening effort.

Screening the School-Age Child

The practice of screening in school-aged children is more than 50 years old, and all states conduct some form of hearing screening in the schools. The Joint Committee on Health Problems in Education (consisting of members of the National Educational Association and the American Medical Association) has described the following primary responsibilities to be met by a screening program: awareness of the importance of early recognition of suspected hearing loss, especially in the primary grades; intelligent observation of pupils for signs of hearing difficulty; organization and conduct of an audiometric screening survey; and a counseling and follow-up program to help children with hearing difficulties obtain diagnostic examinations, needed treatment, and such adaptations of their school program as their hearing condition dictates.

Who Is Responsible for the Audiometric Screening Program?

Health and education departments are the agents primarily responsible for coordinating audiometric screening programs. Ideally, the state department of education should coordinate the periodic screening of all school-aged children and provide for the necessary educational, audiologic, and rehabilitative follow-up. The state department of health should coordinate the activities of identification audiometry, threshold measurement, and medical follow-up for students who fail the screening tests.

Personnel

The personnel designated to conduct the screening tests have been nurses, audiologists, speech-language pathologists, graduate students in speech and hearing, and even volunteers and secretaries. To ensure quality programs, only professionals trained in audiology should be used to coordinate and supervise hearing screening programs. Volunteers and lay groups can best be used for support, such as in the promotion of screening programs. Certified audiologists or speech-language pathologists should administer screening programs and use trained audiometrists or technicians to perform the screening. Public health nurses may serve as organizers and supervisors but can be of most value in the follow-up phase of the program. A nurse's responsibilities might include (a) counseling parents and children about the child's needs for medical diagnosis and treatment, (b) using all available facilities for diagnosis and treatment, and (c) coordinating information about the child and family with specialists in health and education.

Who Should Be Screened?

It is not economically feasible to screen all children in the schools. A target population must be identified. Most programs have concentrated their annual screening efforts on children of nursery school age through grade 3. In fact, the ASHA guidelines recommend screening in all of these grades. After grade 3, children may be screened at 3- to 4-year intervals. Concentrating the screening efforts on the first 3 or 4 years allows careful observation of other special groups of schoolchildren. The following groups of children require more attention than is provided by routine screening:

1. Children with pre-existing hearing loss
2. Children enrolled in special education programs
3. Children with multiple handicaps
4. Children with frequent colds or ear infections
5. Children with delayed language or defective speech
6. Children returning to school after a serious illness
7. Children who experience school failure or who exhibit a sudden change in academic performance
8. Children referred by the classroom teacher
9. Children who are new to the school

Equipment, Calibration, and the Test Environment

An important component of any identification program is the audiometric equipment used in the screening. The equipment needed for individual pure-tone screening should be simple, sturdy, and portable. Most screening audiometers are portable and weigh as little as 2 or 3 lb. The performance characteristics of these instruments must remain stable over time. An audiometer that does not perform adequately could produce a higher-than-normal false-positive or false-negative rate. Care should be taken to

TABLE 6.5 Approximate Allowable Octave-Band Ambient Noise Levels (dB SPL re: 20 μPa) for Threshold Measurements at 0 dB HL (ANSI, 1991) and for Screening at the ASHA-Recommended Value of 20 dB HL

Octave band levels	Test Frequency (Hz)			
	500	1000	2000	4000
For testing with ears covered by earphone mounted in MX-41/AR cushion (ANSI 3.1-1987)	19.5	26.5	28.0	34.5
Plus ASHA screening level re: ANSI-1989	20.0	20.0	20.0	20.0
Resultant maximum ambient octave-band noise level allowable for ASHA screening	39.5	46.5	48.0	54.5

ensure that all of the equipment used in screening satisfies the national performance standards. Unfortunately, this is not always done. Audiometers used in the schools often fail to meet calibration standards. School audiometers should receive weekly intensity checks with a sound level meter and daily listening performance checks. All aspects of the audiometer should be thoroughly calibrated each year. It is also suggested that spare audiometers be available in case of a malfunction during a screening.

Older audiometers are most subject to instability and malfunction and should receive careful checking. Clinical audiologists who use these instruments for threshold measurement (after a screen failure) should know that the masking stimuli generated by many of these portable audiometers are often inadequate.

Once again, screening must be conducted in a quiet environment to ensure accurate measurements. Although some modern schools have sound-treated rooms or mobile units with testing facilities, most do not. Screening programs must be conducted in a relatively quiet room designed for some other purpose. Some helpful guidelines for selecting an appropriate room for screening have been outlined in the section on preschool screening. Table 6.5 shows the allowable octave-band ambient noise levels for each test frequency recommended by the ASHA. These ambient noise levels are measured using a sound-level meter with an octave-band filter (see Chapter 2).

Identification Tests and Procedures

During the more than 50-year history of identification audiometry in the schools, tests have been developed for screening the hearing of young school-age children. These tests may be classified as either group or individual screening tests. Most of the group tests were designed in earlier years to save time by testing large numbers of children at once. These techniques have never achieved wide acceptance. Most screening programs in this country use individual tests. Group screening, as it exists today, has only historical significance.

Individual Screening Tests

It is generally accepted that the individual pure-tone screening test is the most effective approach to screening hearing. In 1961, the National Conference on Identification Audiometry (NCIA) wrote a comprehensive monograph on general guidelines for individual pure-tone screening. These guidelines recommended that screening be conducted at frequencies of 500, 1000, 2000, 4000, and 6000 Hz and that the screening occur in a sound-treated environment.

More recently, the ASHA developed its own set of guidelines for pure-tone screening in the schools. The ASHA procedures recognize that sound-treated environments are not readily available in the schools. The ASHA guidelines differ from the NCIA recommendations in that (*a*) it is not recommended that screening occur in sound-treated rooms, (*b*) test frequencies of 500 and 6000 Hz are not included in the recommendations, and (*c*) rescreening of all failures is recommended.

Screening Adult Populations

With the increased awareness of hearing loss in the elderly population, we have witnessed an increased interest in the hearing screening of adult populations. Unfortunately, in primary-care medical practices wherein most older adults are seen regularly, we find that they are seldom screened and referred for audiologic evaluation. There seem to be several reasons for this.

First, the elderly accept their hearing loss as part of getting older and believe that there is simply no recourse for improvement. Second, it is found that primary-care physicians often fail to recognize a hearing loss. Even when hearing loss is suspected or is reported to the physician, more than half of the patients are not referred for follow-up audiologic services. It seems that the primary-care physician looks upon hearing loss in the elderly in the same way that our society at large does. Deafness is viewed as a common byproduct of aging, and little value is seen in rehabilitating the individuals affected by it. Physicians who do screen for hearing loss rely on such techniques as the case history, or whisper or watch-tick tests, approaches whose validity and reliability have not been tested. Recent studies have shown, however, that primary-care practitioners will indeed screen for hearing loss if provided with appropriately validated screening tools and if they are convinced that hearing loss is important to the life quality of their patient. Again, just as with preschoolers, the task confronting the audiologist is to educate and inform the public and the health care community.

Pure-Tone Screening

There is no accepted standard or guideline for identification of hearing loss in the adult population. Some clinicians have suggested that a pure-tone screening level of 20 or 25 dB HL be used for frequencies of 1000 and 2000 Hz and that 40 dB HL be used for 4000 Hz. ASHA recommends that a 25-dB HL level should also be used for all frequencies including 4000 Hz. Unfortunately, there are limited data to support the validity of a 20- or 25-dB HL criterion at any frequencies for screening adults. We do not know with certainty the sensitivity, specificity, and test accuracy of pure-tone screening when using 20 or 25 dB HL as the cutoff point. Some have suggested that hearing screening in the aged should be done at the test frequencies 1000 and 2000 Hz, with a level of 40 dB HL serving as the pass-fail criterion. Failure for two test conditions (one frequency in each ear or both frequencies in one ear) constitutes a test failure. Data using this guideline are presented later in this section. Regardless of the test protocol, it is advisable to rescreen those who fail. The recommendations related to environment, calibration, personnel, and procedural setup discussed previously regarding the screening of children can be followed with some modifications for screening the adult population.

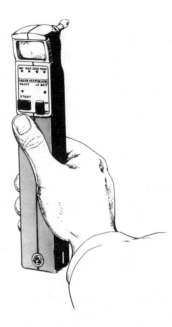

FIGURE 6.6   An audioscope. (From Lichtenstein MJ, Bess FH, Logan SA. Validation of screening tools for identifying hearing impaired elderly in primary care. JAMA 259:2875–2878, 1988.)

Several tools have been advocated for screening the older adult population. One of these is the Welch-Allyn Audioscope, a handheld otoscope with a built-in audiometer that delivers a tone at 25 or 40 dB HL for 500, 1000, 2000, and 4000 Hz (Fig. 6.6). To use the audioscope, the clinician selects the largest ear speculum needed to achieve a seal within the ear canal. A tonal sequence is then initiated, with the subject indicating the tone was heard by raising a finger. The audioscope is found to perform very well against the gold standard of pure-tone audiometry with use of the 40-dB HL signal at 1000 and 2000 Hz. The sensitivity of the audioscope has been reported to be 94%, and its specificity is between 72% and 90% for identifying a hearing loss. In addition, the test has been found to have excellent test-retest reliability.

Communication Scales

Communication scales are another type of screening tool that can be used efficiently with the older adult population. A popular scale at present is the Hearing Handicap Inventory for the Elderly–Screening Version (HHIE-S). This screener is a self-report test that contains 10 items, 5 dealing with the social aspects and 5 with the emotional aspects of hearing loss. Figure 6.7 lists the test questions and the instructions for scoring. The test has been reported to identify most elderly persons with high-frequency hearing losses exceeding 40 dB HL in the better ear. Again, this tool yields acceptable sensitivity and specificity values. Using a cutoff score of 8, one finds a sensitivity value of 72% and a test specificity of 77%. Although these values are not as high as those reported for the audioscope, they are acceptable values for a screening tool. The pencil-and-paper format and the low number of test items are additional advantages of the HHIE-S.

Even though the audioscope and the HHIE-S provide acceptable sensitivity and specificity values, the best test result is obtained when these two tools are used in

Enter 4 for a "yes" answer, 2 for a "sometimes" answer, 0 for a "no" answer.	
1. Does a hearing problem cause you to feel embarrassed when you meet new people?	
2. Does a hearing problem cause you to feel frustrated when talking to members of your family?	
3. Do you have difficulty hearing when someone speaks in a whisper?	
4. Do you feel handicapped by a hearing problem?	
5. Does a hearing problem cause you difficulty when visiting friends, relatives, or neighbors?	
6. Does a hearing problem cause you to attend religious services less often than you would like?	
7. Does a hearing problem cause you to have arguments with family members?	
8. Does a hearing problem cause you to have difficulty when listening to television or radio?	
9. Do you feel that any difficulty with your hearing limits/hampers your personal or social life?	
10. Does a hearing problem cause you difficulty when in a restaurant with relatives or friends?	

TOTAL _____

HHIE-S scores may be interpreted as shown below. (Hearing loss is defined as [a] the inability to hear a 40-dB HL tone at 1000 Hz or 2000 Hz in each ear or [b] the inability to hear both frequencies in one ear.)

HHIE-S score	Probability of hearing loss (%)
0–8	13
10–24	50
26–40	84

FIGURE 6.7 The Hearing Handicap Inventory for the Elderly—Screening Version (HHIE-S). (Adapted from Ventry IM, Weinstein BE. Identification of elderly people with hearing problems. ASHA 25:37–42, 1983; and from Lichtenstein MJ, Bess FH, Logan SA. Validation of screening tools for identifying hearing impaired elderly in primary care. JAMA 259:2875–2878, 1988.)

combination. Table 6.6 lists the screening characteristics of the audioscope and the HHIE-S when used in combination. This table shows the sensitivity and specificity for each of the screeners alone and for the two instruments used in combination. Two specific pass-fail criteria seem to afford the most favorable outcome. These criteria are (*a*) audioscope—fail and HHIE-S score above 8 and (*b*) audioscope—pass and HHIE-S score above 24. When these criteria are used, it is seen that the sensitivity is 75% and the specificity is 86%. Although there is some loss of sensitivity compared with that

TABLE 6.6 Sensitivity and Specificity of Screening Tests in Diagnosis of the Hearing-Impaired Elderly

Screening Test	Sensitivity (%)	Specificity (%)
Audioscope	94	72
HHIE-S Score		
>8	72	77
>24	41	92
Combined scores: audioscope fail and HHIE >8, or audioscope pass and HHIE >24	75	86

seen when either of the screeners is used alone, there is considerable improvement in specificity. This reduces the potential for overreferrals—an important factor when one is screening on a large-scale basis. Once again, as with most screening protocols, it is recommended that one retest before referral is made.

Another commonly used self-report communication scale is the Self-Assessment of Communication (SAC). Similar to the HHIE-S, the SAC is a 10-item questionnaire that queries an individual regarding perceptions of communication problems resulting from hearing loss. The SAC was standardized on a sample of adults over age 18 years; the posttest probability of hearing loss is similar to that of the HHIE-S. Figure 6.8 lists the test questions for the SAC.

Identification of Middle Ear Disease in Children

Electroacoustic Immittance

There is considerable interest in using electroacoustic immittance measures to identify middle ear disease among children. Several factors have contributed to the interest in using immittance as a screening tool. Some factors relate to immittance in particular, and others relate to screening for middle ear disease in general. These factors include the ease and rapidity with which immittance measurement can obtain accurate information, the relative ineffectiveness of pure-tone audiometry in detecting a middle ear disorder, the high prevalence of otitis media, and the growing awareness of the medical, psychologic, and educational consequences that may result from middle ear disease. Today this popular technique is used routinely, not only in audiology centers but also in public health facilities, pediatricians' and otologists' offices, and schools.

In 1977, a special task force studied the use of immittance measures in screening for middle ear disease. The task force recognized the potential value of immittance screening but concluded, after reviewing the available data, that mass screening with immittance was premature. The task force also recommended screening of special groups of children, such as Native American children, those with sensorineural hearing loss, developmentally delayed or mentally impaired children, and children with Down syndrome, cleft palate, or other craniofacial anomalies. The task force did not oppose immittance screening as such, but only universal (mass) screening on a routine basis. In fact, recognizing that many screening programs were already in operation and that others were soon to be implemented, the task force developed procedural guidelines to be used in the screening of preschool- and school-age children.

Name _____   Date _____

Raw Score ___X 2 =___-20 =___ X 1.25___%

Please select the appropriate number ranging from 1 to 5 for the following questions. Circle only one number for each question. If you have a hearing aid, please fill out the form according to how you communicate when the hearing aid <u>is not</u> in use.

Various Communication Situations

1. Do you experience communication difficulties when speaking with one other person (for example, at home, at work, in a social situation, with a waitress, a store clerk, with a spouse, boss)?

   | 1) almost never (or never) | 2) occasionally (about ¼ of the time) | 3) about half of the time | 4) frequently (¾ of the time) | 5) practically always (or always) |

2. Do you experience communication difficulties when conversing with a small group of several persons (for example, with friends or family, co-workers, in meetings or casual conversations, over dinner or while playing cards)?

   | 1) almost never (or never) | 2) occasionally (about ¼ of the time) | 3) about half of the time | 4) frequently (¾ of the time) | 5) practically always (or always) |

3. Do you experience communication difficulties while listening to someone speak to a large group (for example, at a church or in a civic meeting, in a fraternal or women's club, at an educational lecture)?

   | 1) almost never (or never) | 2) occasionally (about ¼ of the time) | 3) about half of the time | 4) frequently (¾ of the time) | 5) practically always (or always) |

4. Do you experience communication difficulties while participating in various types of entertainment (for example, movies, TV, radio, plays, night clubs, musical entertainment)?

   | 1) almost never (or never) | 2) occasionally (about ¼ of the time) | 3) about half of the time | 4) frequently (¾ of the time) | 5) practically always (or always) |

5. Do you experience communication difficulties when you are in an unfavorable listening environment (for example, at a noisy party, where there is background music, when riding in an auto or bus, when someone whispers or talks from across the room)?

   | 1) almost never (or never) | 2) occasionally (about ¼ of the time) | 3) about half of the time | 4) frequently (¾ of the time) | 5) practically always (or always) |

6. Do you experience communication difficulties when using or listening to various communication devices (for example, telephone, telephone ring, doorbell, public address system, warning signals, alarms)?

   | 1) almost never (or never) | 2) occasionally (about ¼ of the time) | 3) about half of the time | 4) frequently (¾ of the time) | 5) practically always (or always) |

Feelings About Communication

7. Do you feel that any difficulty with your hearing limits or hampers your personal or social life?

   | 1) almost never (or never) | 2) occasionally (about ¼ of the time) | 3) about half of the time | 4) frequently (¾ of the time) | 5) practically always (or always) |

8. Does any problem or difficulty with your hearing upset you?

   | 1) almost never (or never) | 2) occasionally (about ¼ of the time) | 3) about half of the time | 4) frequently (¾ of the time) | 5) practically always (or always) |

Other people

9. Do others suggest that you have a hearing problem?

   | 1) almost never (or never) | 2) occasionally (about ¼ of the time) | 3) about half of the time | 4) frequently (¾ of the time) | 5) practically always (or always) |

10. Do others leave you out of conversations or become annoyed because of your hearing?

   | 1) almost never (or never) | 2) occasionally (about ¼ of the time) | 3) about half of the time | 4) frequently (¾ of the time) | 5) practically always (or always) |

FIGURE 6.8   The Self-Assessment of Communication. (Adapted from Schow RL, Nerbonne MA. Communication screening profile; use with elderly clients. Ear Hear 3:135–147, 1982.)

A problem with immittance screening has been the difficulty of developing appropriate pass-fail criteria. The pass-fail criteria developed by the ASHA and the special task force mentioned earlier have resulted in unacceptably high referral rates (32 to 36%). The screening criteria known as the Hirtshal program seem to produce a better result. The program uses only tympanometry and does not include the acoustic reflex. At the first screen, all children with normal tympanograms are cleared. The remaining children receive a second screen in 4 to 6 weeks, and all cases with flat tympanograms are referred. Children still remaining receive a third screen 4 to 6 weeks later. Children with normal tympanograms or tympanograms having peaks in the range of −100 to −199 daPa are cleared. Children with flat tympanograms or tympanograms with peaks below −200 daPa at the third screen are referred. With the Hirtshal screening approach, sensitivity and specificity values are 80% and 95%, respectively. Moreover, the program yields an acceptable referral rate of only 9%.

The ASHA developed a new guideline for screening children that involves the use of case history, visual inspection of the ear canal and eardrum, and tympanometry with a low frequency (220 or 226 Hz) probe tone. The ASHA recommended that children be screened as needed or if an at-risk condition existed. Children 7 months of age to 6 years should be screened if they present with any of the following conditions:

1. A first episode of acute otitis media before 6 months of age
2. Bottle feeding
3. Craniofacial anomalies, stigmata, or other syndromic conditions
4. Ethnic populations known to have a high prevalence of middle ear disease (Native American and Eskimo populations)
5. Family history of middle ear disease with effusion
6. Residence in day care or in crowded conditions
7. Exposure to cigarette smoke
8. Diagnosis with sensorineural hearing loss, learning disabilities, or other developmental complications

Typically, the first scheduled screening program should occur in the fall in conjunction with screening for hearing loss. A second scheduled screening is recommended for those who failed or were missed in the fall.

For history, the protocol simply considers recent evidence of otalgia (earache) or otorrhea (discharge from the ear). Visual inspection via otoscopy is performed to identify gross abnormalities; the use of a lighted otoscope or video-otoscope is recommended. A child is referred for medical observation and/or audiologic evaluation if (*a*) ear drainage is observed; (*b*) structural defects or ear canal abnormalities are seen in the ear; (*c*) tympanometry reveals a flat tympanogram and equivalent ear canal volume outside normal range; and (*d*) tympanometric rescreen results are outside test criteria listed in Table 6.7. Data pertaining to the performance of this protocol are limited.

Acoustic Reflectometry

Another approach for detecting middle ear disease with effusion is known as acoustic reflectometry. This is a noninvasive, objective method and reportedly is useful even if a child is crying or if there is partial obstruction of the ear canal.

The handheld otoscope-like instrument generates an 80-dB SPL probe tone that begins at a frequency of approximately 2000 Hz and increases linearly to approximately 4500 Hz in 100 ms (0.1 s). The microphone in the device measures the combined amplitude of the probe tone and any sound waves reflected off the tympanic

TABLE 6.7 **Recommended Initial Tympanometric Screening Test Criteria**

Infants[a]	1 y–School Age[b]
Y_{tm} <0.2 mmho or TW >235 daPa	Y_{tm} <0.3 mmho[c] or TW >200 daPa

Mmho-millimho; daPa, dekapascal; TW, typanometric width; Y_{tm}- peak admittance.
[a]Infants: Roush, Bryant, Mundy, et al., 1995.
[b]Older children: Nozza, Bluestone, Kardatzke, and Bachman, 1992, 1994.
[c]For children more than 6 years of age, when using ±400 daPa for compensation of ear canal volume,
    Y_{tm}<0.4 mmho is the recommended criterion.
From American Speech-Language-Hearing Association Audiologic Assessment Panel 1996. (1997). *Guidelines for audiologic Screening*. Rockville, MD.

membrane (Fig. 6.9). According to the developers, operation is based on the consideration of one-quarter wavelength resonances. Briefly, an acoustic wave traveling in a tube will be completely reflected when it impinges on the closed end of that tube. The reflective wave will completely cancel the original one at a distance one-quarter wavelength from the closed end of the tube, resulting in zero sound amplitude at this point. Accordingly, the level of reflected sound is inversely proportional to the total sound. Greater reflection produces a reduced sound level at the microphone and suggests that middle ear impedance is high, as in otitis media with effusion. The degree of reflectivity is numerically displayed on the otoscope. A reading of 0 to 2 denotes a clear ear, and a reading above 5 implies higher impedance, as with effusion.

Studies of the acoustic reflectometer have reported mixed results; approximately half of the studies report excellent sensitivity and specificity values, and half report unacceptable values. Research on this device is limited, however. More research is needed before this screening instrument can receive widespread acceptance.

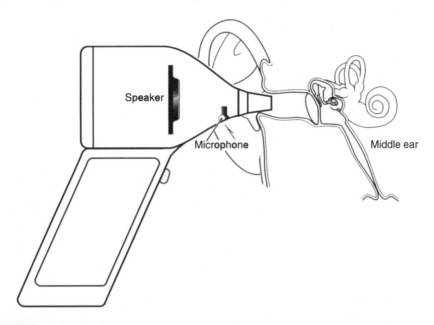

FIGURE 6.9 An acoustic reflectometer.

Handheld Tympanometers

Small portable handheld immittance screening tympanometers have been developed for screening programs. These otoscope-like units typically run on rechargeable batteries and incorporate a small printer to record a hard copy of the data. The tip of the tympanometer is placed into the ear, and when a pneumatic seal is obtained, a microcomputer initiates the miniature pump that varies pressure to the ear canal from 1200 daPa to 2300 daPa with a 226-Hz probe tone at 85 dB SPL. These instruments record data recommended by the ASHA Immittance Screening Guidelines. Hence, the data are reported in terms of equivalent ear canal volume, static admittance, and tympanometric width. Although these handheld instruments appear to have significant potential in screening programs, additional research is needed to determine the usefulness of these systems with various age groups of children.

FOLLOW-UP

Follow-Up Programs for Children

Screening is of little value if follow-up is not provided for the appropriate management of children who fail the screen. This aspect of the conservation program takes as much planning and effort as any other phase of the screening program. Noncompliance has been one of the principal problems of hearing screening programs for newborns. In some studies, 25 to 80% of infants who failed newborn screening have been lost to follow-up despite aggressive recruiting efforts and the offering of cost-saving incentives to parents. In other studies, after early identification of hearing loss, lag times of 8 to 9 months have transpired before infants returned for intervention. Presently, there are no data on compliance in hearing screening programs for infants beyond the newborn period.

For preschool and school-age programs, the screening coordinator is responsible for the follow-up under most circumstances. A child who fails the second screen should receive a comprehensive audiologic test at the screening site as soon as possible. Within a few days after the screening, steps essential to appropriate follow-up should begin. Letters should be sent to parents indicating whether their child passed or failed the screening test. For children who failed the screening, the letter should also recommend that the child be referred for medical evaluation. Approximately 6 weeks after the screening, the parents should be asked whether the recommendations were followed.

Frequently, the public health nurse handles this phase of the follow-up program. In some states, audiologists and educators coordinate this activity. After the medical examination, the child is referred to an audiologic facility for comprehensive testing and counseling. Parent counseling is an important aspect of the follow-up process that too often is overlooked by the supervisors of screening programs. Parents must receive special assistance and guidance to understand and cope with the prospect of having a child with hearing loss. They must receive help before they can help their child.

Finally, the child should be referred to educational services for planning and placement. The follow-up is a lengthy and ongoing process requiring close coordination among all persons involved.

Follow-Up Programs for Adult Populations

A person who fails the screening protocol should receive an otologic examination and a comprehensive audiologic evaluation. Needless to say, the hearing evaluation will provide information about the extent and nature of the hearing loss and determine whether the patient could benefit from amplification. If amplification is warranted, the individual should be referred for hearing aid selection and evaluation. Procedures for this particular protocol are outlined in Chapter 7.

SUMMARY

This chapter defines and justifies screening and discusses important considerations and techniques of identification programs. Identification is an important first step in the overall hearing conservation program. The early identification of hearing loss and middle ear disease is the key to effective and appropriate management. There is still much to be learned about our screening programs for the identification of both hearing loss and middle ear disease. In particular, we need to learn more about the feasibility of universal screening of healthy newborns. Other critical issues, such as performance of screening tools, accessibility and availability of follow-up services, compliance, and costs, must be further explored. There is also a need for more research on screening with immittance and acoustic reflectometry for middle ear disease in children. There is still only limited information available about the application of the acoustic reflectometer as a screening device, and the audiologist therefore needs to keep abreast of new developments. Finally, it is important to determine the sensitivity, specificity, and test accuracy of pure-tone audiometry for the adult population when using a 20- or 25-dB HL cutoff point.

References and Suggested Readings

American Academy of Pediatrics. Newborn and infant hearing loss: Detection and intervention. Taskforce on Newborn and Infant Hearing. Pediatrics 103:527–530, 1999.

American National Standards Institute. American National Standards Specifications for Audiometers. ANSI S3.6–1989. New York: Author, 1989.

American Speech-Language-Hearing Association: Guidelines for audiologic screening. ASHA Desk Reference, Rockville, MD, 1997.

American Speech-Language-Hearing Association: Considerations in screening adults/older persons for handicapping hearing impairments. ASHA 34:81–87, 1992.

Avery C, Gates G, Prihoda T. Efficacy of acoustic reflectometry in detecting middle ear effusion. Ann Otol Rhinol Laryngol 95:472–476, 1986.

Bess FH. Children With Hearing Impairment: Contemporary Trends. Nashville: Vanderbilt Bill Wilkerson Center, 1998.

Bess FH, Gravel JS. Foundations of Pediatric Audiology: A Book of Readings. San Diego, CA: Plural, 2006.

Bess FH, Hall JW. Screening Children for Auditory Function. Nashville: Bill Wilkerson Center, 1992.

Bess FH, Penn TO. Issues and concerns associated with universal newborn hearing screening programs. J Speech-Lang Pathol Audiol 24:113–123, 2001.

Coplan J, Gleason JR, Ryan R, et al. Validation of an early language milestone scale in a high risk population. Pediatrics 70:677–683, 1982.

Downs M. Early identification of hearing loss: Where are we? Where do we go from here? In Mencher GT, ed. Early Identification of Hearing Loss. Basel: Karger, 1976.

Harford ER, Bess FH, Bluestone CD, Klein JO, eds. Impedance Screening for Middle Ear Disease in Children. New York: Grune & Stratton, 1978.

Hayes D. State programs for universal newborn hearing screening. Pediatr Clin North Am 46:89–94, 1999.

Herrmann BS, Thornton AR, Joseph JM. Automated infant hearing screening using the ABR: Development and validation. In Bess FH, Gravel JS, eds. Foundations of Pediatric Audiology: A Book of Readings. San Diego, CA: Plural, 2006.

Joint Committee on Infant Hearing 2000 Position Statement: Principles and Guidelines for Early Hearing Detection and Intervention Programs. American Speech-Language-Hearing Association, 2000.

Kileny PR. ALGO-1 automated infant hearing screener: Preliminary results. In Gerkin KP, Amochaev A, eds. Hearing in Infants: Proceedings From the National Symposium. Seminars in Hearing. New York: Thieme-Stratton, 1987.

Lichtenstein MJ, Bess FH, Logan SA. Validation of screening tools for identifying hearing impaired elderly in primary care. JAMA 259:2875–2878, 1988.

Lous J. Screening for secretory otitis media: Evaluation of some impedance programs for long-lasting secretory otitis media in 7-year-old children. Int J Pediatr Otorhinolaryngol 13:85–97, 1987.

Matkin ND. Early recognition and referral of hearing-impaired children. Pediatr Rev 6:151–156, 1984.

Northern JL, Downs MP. Hearing in Children. 5th ed. Baltimore: Lippincott Williams & Wilkins, 2002.

Nozza RJ, Bluestone CD, Kardatzke D, Bachman RN. Towards the validation of aural acoustic immittance measures for diagnosis of middle ear effusion in children. Ear Hear 13:442–453, 1992.

Nozza RJ, Bluestone CD, Kardatzke D, Bachman RN. Identification of middle ear effusion by aural acoustic admittance and otoscopy. Ear Hear 15:310–323, 1994.

Prieve B, Dalzell L, Berg A, et al. New York State Universal Newborn Hearing Screening Demonstration Project: Outpatient Outcome Measures. In Bess FH, Gravel JS, eds. Foundations of Pediatric Audiology: A Book of Readings. San Diego, CA: Plural, 2006.

Roeser RJ, Valente M, Hosford-Dunn H. Audiology: Diagnosis, Treatment, Practice Management. New York: Thieme Medical, 2000.

Roush J. Screening school-age children. In Bess FH, Hall JW, eds. Screening Children for Auditory Function. Nashville: Bill Wilkerson Center, 1992.

Roush J, Bryant K, Mundy M, et al. Developmental changes in static admittance and tympano-metric width in infants and toddlers. J Am Acad Audiol 6:334–338, 1995.

Sackett DL, Haynes RB, Guyatt, GH, Tugwell P. Clinical Epidemiology: A Basic Science for Clinical Medicine. 2nd ed. Boston: Little Brown, 1991.

Stevens JC, Parker G. Screening and surveillance. In Newton VE, ed. Paediatric Audiological Medicine. London: Whurr, 2002.

Ventry IM, Weinstein BE. Identification of elderly people with hearing problems. ASHA 25:37–42, 1983.

Walton WK, Williams PS. Stability of routinely serviced portable audiometers. Lang Speech Hear Serv Schools 3:36–43, 1972.

Weber BA. Screening of high-risk infants using auditory brainstem response audiometry. In Bess FH, ed. Hearing Impairment in Children. Parkton, MD: York, 1988.

Welsh R, Slater S. The state of infant hearing impairment identification programs. ASHA 35:49–52, 1993.

Wilson WR, Walton WK. Public school audiometry. In Martin FN, ed. Pediatric Audiology. Englewood Cliffs, NJ: Prentice-Hall, 1978.

Answers to Problem in Vignette 6.2

Prevalence, 50%;   Sensitivity, 80%;   Specificity, 90%.

PART 3

Management Strategies

Amplification and Rehabilitation

After completion of this chapter, the reader should be able to:

- List and describe the devices available to assist in the rehabilitation of those with hearing loss, including conventional hearing aids, assistive listening devices, classroom amplification, bone-anchored hearing aids, cochlear implants, and vibrotactile systems.
- Understand the basic components, function, and electroacoustic characteristics of hearing aids.
- Describe the general approaches used to select and evaluate conventional hearing aids.
- Understand some of the principles and techniques used in the management of children and adults with hearing loss.

P robably the most significant problem of adults with hearing loss is difficulty understanding speech, especially against a background of noise. Individuals with severe or profound sensorineural hearing loss also have trouble hearing their own speech. This typically results in speech production problems as well, making the overall communication process even more difficult. The intent of rehabilitation for adults with hearing loss is to restore as much speech comprehension and speech production ability as possible. For the child with congenital hearing loss, however, the problem is more complicated because the child has not yet learned the symbols of our language system. In these circumstances, the emphasis is on helping the child to acquire this complex language system and to use language appropriately so that communication skills can be gained. The focus is more on habilitation than on rehabilitation. In other words, the objective is not to restore a skill that once existed but to help the child develop a new skill, the ability to communicate.

This chapter reviews various approaches for developing and/or improving the communicative abilities of children and adults with hearing loss. This process is usually called aural rehabilitation or aural habilitation. A central core of any rehabilitation or habilitation program is the use of a hearing aid, an amplification device designed to help compensate for the hearing deficit. A substantial portion of this chapter focuses on various aspects of amplification systems.

AURAL REHABILITATION OR HABILITATION PROCESS

Aural rehabilitation has at least two phases. The first phase is identification of the problem. Before an intervention strategy can be developed, one must know about the type and degree of hearing loss and the impact of the impairment on communicative, educational, social, or cognitive function. For the adult with hearing loss, measurement of the patient's audiogram, administration of speech recognition tests, and use of self-report surveys or questionnaires can provide much of this information. Pure-tone and speech audiometry have already been discussed (see Chapter 4). Self-report surveys are often used to assess in detail the social, psychological, and communicative difficulties of those with hearing loss. The Hearing Handicap Inventory for the Elderly Screening version (HHIE-S), discussed in Chapter 6, is an example of such a survey, but in an abbreviated format.

The phase after identification of the problem is intervention. For those with hearing loss, the nature of the intervention package is determined in large part by the identification phase. Consider, for example, just the degree and type of hearing loss, ignoring other factors, such as age and social or emotional difficulties. First, regarding type of hearing loss, the most appropriate candidates for amplification are those with sensorineural hearing loss. Occasionally, individuals with chronic conductive hearing loss not amenable to medical or surgical intervention are fitted with a hearing aid. Most often, though, the individual with sensorineural hearing loss as a result of cochlear pathology is the type of patient fitted with a rehabilitative device, such as a hearing aid.

Generally, as the degree of sensorineural hearing loss increases, speech comprehension difficulties increase. The need for intervention increases in proportion to the degree of difficulty with speech comprehension. Thus, those with mild hearing loss (pure-tone average of 20 to 30 dB HL) generally have less need for intervention than do those with profound hearing loss (PTA >85 dB HL). Conventional hearing aids provide the greatest benefit to those with hearing loss whose average hearing loss is between 40 and 85 dB HL. For milder amounts of hearing loss, the difficulties and the need for intervention are sometimes not great enough for full-time use of a conventional hearing aid. Part-time use of hearing aid, or another type of device known as an assistive listening device, is usually recommended for these patients. For the profoundly impaired the difficulties in communicating and the need for intervention are great. Unfortunately, the conventional hearing aid offers limited benefit in such cases. For patients with profound impairments, alternative devices, such as vibrotactile systems and cochlear implants, are sometimes explored. Although cochlear implants are becoming a much more common option for patients with profound hearing loss, especially young children, high-powered conventional aids are probably still the rehabilitative device most commonly encountered among the profoundly impaired. Because amplification provides limited benefit for this group, though, the fitting of the hearing aid is usually accompanied by extensive training in several areas, including speech reading (lipreading), auditory training, and/or manual communication (finger spelling and sign language).

Consider also the time of onset of the hearing loss. Of course, the intervention approach is much different for a child with congenital hearing loss than for someone who acquired the hearing loss after communication developed. With a congenital onset, the emphasis focuses on such critical issues as early amplification, parental guidance, and a comprehensive habilitation package designed to facilitate communication development.

In summary, the intervention phase of aural rehabilitation or habilitation typically begins with the selection and fitting of an appropriate rehabilitative device, such as a hearing aid. This is followed by extensive training with the device in communicative situations.

Many of the procedures used in the identification phase of rehabilitation have been reviewed in earlier chapters. This chapter focuses on the intervention phase. The remainder of this chapter is divided into three sections. The first section reviews many of the rehabilitative devices available, emphasizing the conventional hearing aid. Methods of selecting and evaluating hearing aids are also reviewed in the first section. The final two sections review training methods and philosophies for rehabilitation or habilitation of children and adults.

AMPLIFICATION FOR THOSE WITH HEARING LOSS

Classification of Conventional Amplification

Today, the following six types of hearing aids are available: (*a*) body aid, (*b*) eyeglass aid, (*c*) behind-the-ear (BTE) aid, (*d*) in-the-ear (ITE) aid, (*e*) in-the-canal (ITC) aid, and (*f*) completely-in-the-canal (CIC) aid. Figure 7.1 shows five of the six types of hearing aids (*a* through *e*). The most recently introduced hearing aid type, CIC, is illustrated in Vignette 7.1. When the first electroacoustic hearing aids were developed

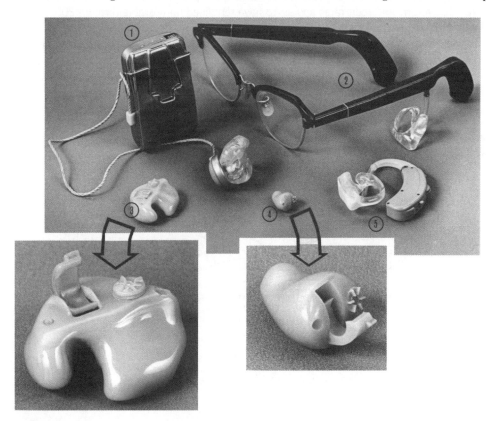

FIGURE 7.1   The different types of hearing aids. *1*, body; *2*, eyeglass; *3*, in the ear; *4*, in the canal; *5*, behind the ear.

The drawing depicts the size and position of a completely-in-the-canal (CIC) hearing aid as worn by an adult. The CIC is the smallest commercially available hearing aid and the least conspicuous visually. Its small size presents some special challenges to the audiologist, the wearer, and the manufacturer. First, for the manufacturer, the circuitry must be miniaturized so as to fit all components within this small space. In addition, given its small size and deep insertion, it is not possible to adjust its controls manually, as in other hearing aids. In most cases, manufacturers produce their CIC instruments with electronic automatic volume control (AVC). The AVC circuit monitors the input level and gradually adjusts the gain to maintain a constant output level, much as the wearer would do with a manual volume control wheel. For the audiologist, two of the major challenges with such devices are the need for deep earmold impressions, because the device is designed to fit deeper within the ear canal than most other hearing aids, and the verification of a good fit with real-ear measurements. Finally, for the user, the primary adjustment is centered on the small size of the device. It is inserted and removed with a semirigid extraction string that is very small itself. Because most hearing aid users are elderly and many have diminished manual dexterity, the insertion and removal of these tiny devices, as well as battery replacement and hearing aid cleaning, can be challenging.

Since 1994, the average price of the CIC hearing aid has been approximately twice that of the BTE and full-shell ITE hearing aids and approximately 50% higher than the ITC hearing aid for the same electronic circuitry. In 2000, the percentage of hearing aids returned to the manufacturer for credit (that is, the wearer returned the hearing aids to the dispenser within the 30-day money-back trial period) was highest for the CIC type at 23%. The return rate for ITC hearing aids was 19% in 2000, whereas the return rate for full-shell ITE hearing aids was 15%. These return-for-credit rates appear to have remained fairly stable through 2005, with an overall return rate across all hearing aid types of about 17%.

Incidentally, at one time the industry apparently considered naming these hearing aids totally-in-the-canal devices, or TIC. However, it was probably considered inadvisable to tell people that they had just paid a fair amount of money for a TIC in their ear—the industry wisely opted for CIC instead.

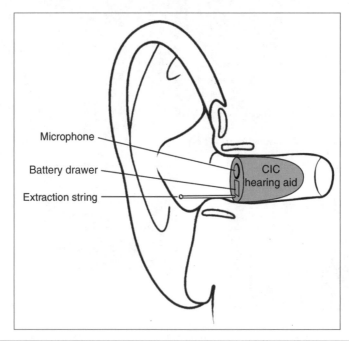

several decades ago, the body aid was the only type available. In the ensuing years, the other types of instruments were developed. In 1960, eyeglass hearing aids were the most popular, accounting for 44% of hearing aids sold, with the remaining 56% divided evenly between body and BTE instruments. As indicated in Figure 7.2, BTE hearing aids became the most common type sold in the 20 years from 1962 through 1982. Since 1983, however, the trend has been for ITE aids to capture an increasingly large portion of the hearing aid market. From about 1987 through 2000, approximately 80% of the hearing aids sold in the United States have been ITE instruments; the bulk of the remaining 20% of instruments sold have been of the BTE type. However, since 2000, the percentage of BTE hearing aids sold has steadily increased, reaching 33% in 2005 (and projected at more than 40% for 2006). Two technology-related factors appear to have spurred the increased sales of BTE instruments in the United States: (*a*) increased interest in directional microphones, which are better implemented in BTE hearing aids; and (*b*) development of open-fit coupling systems that connect the hearing aid to the ear and eliminate a plugged-ear feeling and auditory perception. Each of these factors is described in more detail later in the chapter.

The sales percentages for ITEs shown in Figure 7.2 actually represent the combination of all types of ITE hearing aids, including the ITE, ITC, and CIC types. From 1995 through 2000, approximately 43% of the aids sold were custom ITE aids, most of which were full-concha devices like the type shown as *3* in Figure 7.1. The ITC type, shown as *4*, accounted for 22.5%, and 14.5% were the CIC type, as shown in Vignette 7.1. Since 2000, the percentages for full-concha ITE instruments have steadily decreased, reflecting the increased popularity of the smaller and less conspicuous open-fit (sometimes referred to as the open-canal fitting) BTE instruments. The increasing popularity of the ITC and CIC hearing aids and of the small, open-fit BTE devices, is a result of both consumer pressures to improve the cosmetic appeal of the devices and rapid developments in electronics. High-fidelity electronic components, digital processors, and the batteries to power them have been drastically reduced in size, making smaller devices possible.

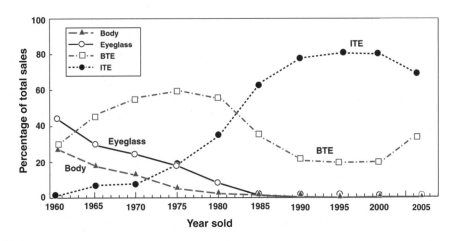

FIGURE 7.2 Sales trends for various hearing aid types since 1960. *BTE,* behind the ear; *ITE,* in the ear.

Operation of Amplification Systems

Components and Function

Although the outer physical characteristics of the types of hearing aids shown in Figure 7.1 differ, the internal features are very similar. The hearing aid, for example, is referred to as an electroacoustic device. It converts the acoustic signal, such as a speech sound, into an electrical signal. The device then manipulates the electrical signal in some way, reconverts the electrical signal to an acoustic one, and then delivers it to the ear canal of the wearer. A microphone is used to convert the acoustic signal into an electrical signal. The electrical signal is usually amplified in the hearing aid. It may also be filtered to eliminate high or low frequencies from the signal. A tiny loudspeaker, usually referred to as a receiver, reconverts the amplified electrical signal into a sound wave. Up to this point, the hearing aid could be thought of as a miniature public address (PA) system with a microphone, amplifier, and loudspeaker. Unlike a PA system, though, the hearing aid is designed to help a single person, the hearing aid wearer, receive the amplified speech. The microphone is positioned somewhere on the hearing aid wearer, and the amplified sound from the receiver is routed directly to the wearer's ear. For ITE and ITC hearing aids, the sound wave is routed from the receiver to the ear canal by a small piece of tubing in the plastic shell of the instrument. For the other types of hearing aids, an earmold is needed. The earmold (or shell for the ITE and ITC hearing aids) is made of a synthetic plastic or rubberlike material from an impression made of the outer ear and ear canal. The earmold, often custom made for the patient's ear, allows the output of the hearing aid to be coupled to the patient's ear canal. As a result, only the patient receives the louder sound and not a group of people, as with a PA system.

We previously examined recent trends in the sales of various types or styles of hearing aids (Fig. 7.2). There have also been changes in the use of various types of internal components, or circuitry, in hearing aids in recent years. A profound change in the internal circuitry of hearing aids has occurred since the mid-1990s. In 1994, analog electrical circuits were in about 95% of the hearing aids sold. There were no digital circuits, although some analog hearing aids could be programmed by a computer (called *programmable analog* hearing aids). These constituted about 5% of the hearing aids sold in 1994. Commercially viable digital hearing aids emerged in 1998, and by 2006 they accounted for almost 95% of the hearing aids sold in the United States. These trends are illustrated in Figure 7.3. Clearly, one can assume that contemporary hearing aids will most likely contain digital circuitry, rather than analog circuitry, although audiologists will continue to encounter both technologies in their clinical work for at least a few more years.

Although the internal circuitry of the hearing aids has changed dramatically in this century, the basic function as a personal PA system has remained unchanged. That is, first an ear-level microphone converts the acoustic signal to an electrical signal. Next, a digital processor manipulates that electrical signal, primarily providing amplification for soft or moderate level sounds. Finally, a receiver converts that processed electrical signal back to sound that is delivered to the wearer's ear canal. The similarity of components in the analog and digital approaches to amplification are illustrated in Vignette 7.2.

If the fundamental function of the components in analog and digital hearing aids is so similar, as suggested in Vignette 7.2, why did hearing aid manufacturers change from analog to digital technology? There were several reasons. Among these: (*a*) A move

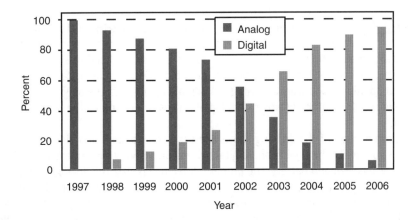

FIGURE 7.3 Percentage of hearing aids sold in the United States from 1997 (and earlier) through 2006 containing either analog (both nonprogrammable and programmable) or digital circuits.

VIGNETTE 7.2 **Basic components of an electronic hearing aid**

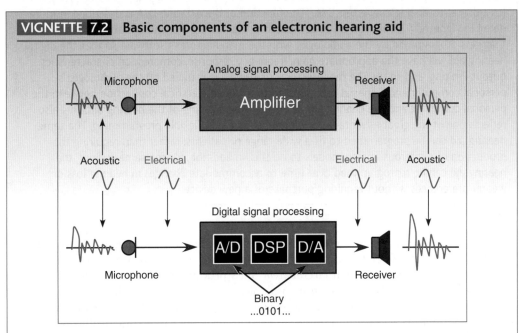

The top part of the schematic drawing shows the basic components of an analog electronic hearing aid. As illustrated here, the hearing aid is like a miniature PA system, with a microphone, amplifier, and loudspeaker (or receiver). The microphone and receiver are transducers: their primary job is to convert waveforms from one form of energy to another. The microphone converts sound waves to electrical voltage waveforms. The amplifier makes this incoming electrical waveform larger, and the receiver converts it back to a sound wave. The amplifier necessitates a portable power supply, and this is supplied by a battery. There may be other controls for the patient to adjust, such as a manual volume control (not shown). A volume control allows the user to adjust the loudness so that sound is comfortably loud in

(continued)

VIGNETTE 7.2   Basic components of an electronic hearing aid *(Continued)*

different environments. In 2005, however, only about 50% of the hearing aids sold included an adjustable volume control. Since most hearing aids sold in 2005 were digital (Fig. 7.3), this illustrates an additional potential advantage of digital hearing aids; the ability to incorporate a suitable *automatic* volume control in the digital processor eliminates the need for manual adjustment.

The bottom portion of the drawing shows the basic components of a digital hearing aid. The overall structure of the analog and digital hearing aids is very similar, each type including a microphone, receiver, and battery. The primary difference is that the analog amplifier is replaced by the digital signal processor. Although this can seem like a minor difference, swapping one red box for another, it is a very significant change in hearing aid technology. The move to digital circuitry provides manufacturers and clinicians with almost unlimited flexibility to have the signal processed or modified for the patient's benefit. The real challenge now is in determining how best to do that.

In the digital signal processor in the bottom drawing are three main modules or components: (*a*) an analog-to-digital converter (A/D); (*b*) a digital signal processor (DSP); and (*c*) a digital-to-analog converter (D/A). The function of the A/D and D/A is described in more detail in Vignette 7.3. The DSP is the computer in the hearing aid, and it is this component that gets programmed by the audiologist with the manufacturer's software so that the digital hearing aid will have the appropriate gain, frequency response, compression characteristics, output limiting, and so on. The manufacturer's software is installed on the audiologist's personal computer and a special cable is used to make an electrical connection between the personal computer and the hearing aid to enable programming of the hearing aid. This also reflects one of the great advantages of digital hearing aids: flexible programming. The same hearing aid can be programmed to fit a wide range of patients, rather than requiring the production of numerous analog models to do this. In addition, for the same patient, the hearing aid can be reprogrammed over time to accommodate changes in hearing loss or wearer preferences without requiring purchase of a new device.

---

in the broader consumer electronics markets to digital technologies improved both the availability of relatively inexpensive microchips for digital processing and battery technology to support such circuits. (*b*) Mass production of the circuitry comprising digital hearing aids became more reliable. (*c*) Improvements in software provided enhanced flexibility, with the same hardware capable of performing substantially different functions. (*d*) Certain signal-processing strategies can be practically realized only in digital form.

Regarding the latter potential advantage of digital circuitry, one point of emphasis has included reduction of the acoustic feedback that can occur in hearing aids. Feedback is typically a whistling sound generated by the hearing aid when the amplified sound coming out of the hearing aid inadvertently feeds back into the microphone, gets amplified again, feeds back into the microphone again, gets amplified again, and so on. (Most people have heard the squeal of feedback in a PA system when the speaker or performer wearing a microphone moves into the sound path of the loudspeaker presenting the amplified signal.) In the past, the solution has often been to reduce the gain or volume of the hearing aid, but this also decreases the amplification for sounds of the same frequency that *should* be amplified for the hearing aid wearer, such as speech sounds. Digital signal processing has enabled the development of more sophisticated approaches to feedback cancellation that are directed primarily at the unwanted feedback sound and not other similar sounds of interest to the wearer.

Many of the other potential advantages of digital hearing aid circuitry differ in detail but share a common objective: to decrease the level of the background noise amplified by the hearing aid. The hearing aid microphone transduces all sounds entering it, not just the wanted sounds. Speech communication often takes place in a background of other competing sounds, such as traffic, music, or other people talking. About two-thirds of the hearing aids sold in the United States are sold to individuals 65 years of age or older. It has been demonstrated repeatedly that older adults, because of their age-related sensorineural hearing loss, not only require amplification of soft and moderate level sounds (see Chapter 5) but must also have the background noise decreased to achieve sufficient benefit from hearing aids. Digital hearing aids have held great promise for reduction of the background noise level, although clear benefits to speech communication in older adults have not yet been substantiated. Although numerous approaches to the use of digital signal processing to reduce background noise levels are being pursued, the two general areas receiving the most attention to date are various directional microphone technologies and noise reduction strategies. Of these two general approaches to reducing background noise levels, various implementations of directional microphone technologies have been more promising. As noted previously, the ability to better implement directional microphone technologies in larger BTE hearing aids is one of the reasons for the recent surge in sales of this type of hearing aid. In 2005, according to the Hearing Industries Association, 35% of the hearing aids sold used directional technology, and about half of BTEs sold in 2005 included directional technology. Directional microphones are relatively sensitive to sounds coming from a specific direction and relatively insensitive to sounds coming from other directions. In general, in hearing aids, they are designed to be more sensitive to sounds coming from the front than from the rear of the wearer. Thus, if the wearer faces the sound source and is able to position competing background sounds to the rear, directional microphones will selectively decrease the background noise. Directional microphones have been around, even in hearing aids, for decades, but the pairing of directional technologies with digital signal processing holds great promise for the future in terms of noise reduction.

At present, although large reductions in background noise can be demonstrated for select listening conditions in the laboratory with some directional microphones, benefits to hearing aid wearers in everyday circumstances are much more modest. Further research is needed in the areas of directional technologies and noise reduction to demonstrate a clear benefit of digital hearing aids in everyday speech communication. Nonetheless, as enumerated previously, digital technology in hearing aids has many other advantages, and because of these factors alone, hearing aid manufacturers have almost universally moved to the use of digital circuitry in their products. Consequently, digital circuitry appears to be the circuitry of choice in hearing aids for the foreseeable future, and it is important to understand some of the fundamental concepts of digital processing. These are reviewed in Vignette 7.3.

Electroacoustic Characteristics of Hearing Aids

The primary purpose of the hearing aid is to make speech audible without causing discomfort. Modern-day conventional hearing aids have several electroacoustic characteristics that are used to describe the hearing aid's performance. Probably the two most important of these characteristics are the amount of amplification, or gain, and

VIGNETTE 7.3 Basics of digital signal processing

It seems everything is digital these days, and hearing aids are no exception. What exactly is digital signal processing? Entire textbooks have been devoted to this topic, and it is impossible to cover all the details in much depth. However, some fundamental concepts of digital signal processing can be explained without going into too much detail or assuming too much background in engineering.

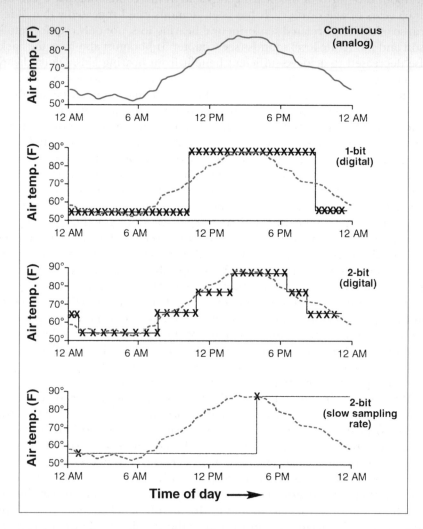

To explain these fundamental concepts, we'll make use of temperature variations during a 24-hour period, as shown in the top panel. The temperature in this particular location and on this particular day was around 50 to 60°F in the early morning and gradually increased to a peak of around 87°F by mid-afternoon before cooling again in the evening. In this *top panel* temperature is plotted as a continuous function of the time of day. There is a temperature indicated for every moment in time in the 24-hour span. This continuous function can be considered an analog representation of the daily temperature variations.

| VIGNETTE 7.3 | Basics of digital signal processing *(Continued)* |

Is it necessary to have a continuous function to capture all of the important information about daily temperature variation? Can we sample the temperature at intervals and get the same amount of information? Yes, the temperature can be measured and quantified at discrete points during the day without losing important information about the temperature changes. In fact, a mathematically derived frequency, the Nyquist frequency, indicates the lowest rate at which temperature readings could be obtained without loss of information. For this example, let's assume that by sampling the temperature at half-hour intervals we can safely capture the information in the waveform. (For audio signals, the sampling rate or frequency should be at least twice the highest frequency of interest in the signal. Generally, this means sampling frequencies of at least 10,000 Hz but preferably ≥20,000 Hz.)

In the digital world, numeric values that are sampled at each point are represented as bits of information. The word *bits* is derived from **binary digits**. Most digits with which we are familiar are from the base 10, or decimal, number system. In grade school, we learned that the decimal system organized numbers into the 1's column, the 10's column, the 100's column, and so on. Thus, in the decimal system, 752 is known to mean 7 hundreds plus 5 tens plus 2 ones. The possible numbers in each column for the decimal or base 10 system range from 0 through 9 (you can't represent a 10 *in a single column* for base 10 numbers). A more formal way of expressing this example is that 752 equals $7 \times 10^2 + 5 \times 10^1 + 2 \times 10^0$.

The binary number system, on the other hand, is a base 2 system. In this case, there is a 1's (2^0) column, a 2's (2^1) column, a 4's (2^2) column, an 8's (2^3) column, and so on. In addition, the only two digits available for use are 0 and 1 (you can't have a 2 in a base 2 system). In a system that uses only one binary digit or one bit, only two possible values exist: 1 and 0.

If we chose to code the temperatures sampled each half-hour with a one-bit system, the resulting digital representation of the temperature variations would resemble that in the second panel. Essentially, we would have only two temperature values to work with, in this case with 0 corresponding to 55° and 1 corresponding to 85°. Clearly, one bit of information is not enough to code the temperature variations. Too many temperatures between 55° and 85° are lost in this 1-bit code. If the coding is doubled to 2 bits, four values are available to quantify the temperature variation: 00, 01, 10, and 11 (or 0, 1, 2, and 3 in the decimal system). The third panel shows that the accuracy of our quantification of daily temperature variation has improved considerably with 2-bit resolution. The bottom panel illustrates the case of a sampling rate that is too low. Even though enough amplitude values (4) are available, information is lost because the temperature is not sampled often enough.

Imagine that instead of temperature variations during a 24-hour period, the waveform of interest is a sound wave transduced by a hearing aid microphone. For most audio applications, including hearing aids, 8-bit coding of amplitude variations in the sound wave is adequate, but 12- or 16-bit resolution is preferred. The device that converts the continuously varying analog waveform into a discrete series of binary numbers is called an analog-to-digital (A/D) converter. Once converted to a string of 1's and 0's, the sampled signal is in the same digital language as that used by computers to process information. The computer can be programmed to adjust the gain characteristics of the hearing aid with great precision, to enhance the speech signal or to cancel out some of the background noise. Once processed by the computer, the string of 1's and 0's representing the sound wave is reconverted to an analog signal using a digital-to-analog (D/A) converter and transduced by the hearing aid receiver (loudspeaker).

the maximum sound pressure level that can be produced, or the output sound pressure level (OSPL). These characteristics can be measured in several ways. A standard issued by the American National Standards Institute, ANSI S3.22-2003, describes a set of measurements that must be made on all hearing aids sold in the United States. It is not necessary in an introductory text such as this to review the ANSI standard in detail. Rather, the concepts underlying gain and OSPL and their importance in fitting the hearing aid to the patient are critical.

Gain is simply the difference in decibels between the input level and the output level at a particular frequency. Consider the following example. A 500-Hz pure tone is generated from a loudspeaker so that the sound level at the hearing aid's microphone is 50 dB SPL. The output produced by the hearing aid under these conditions is 90 dB SPL. The acoustic gain provided by the hearing aid is 40 dB. The gain is simply the difference between the 50-dB SPL input and the 90-dB SPL output. The gain of the hearing aid can be measured at several frequencies. Most hearing aids provide some amplification or gain over the frequency range 200 to 6000 Hz, and many have extended the high-frequency end of the range to 10,000 to 12,000 Hz. When the gain is measured across this whole frequency range by changing the frequency of the input signal and holding the input level constant, a frequency response for the hearing aid is obtained. The frequency response displays how the output or gain varies as a function of frequency. The concepts of gain and frequency response are illustrated in Figure 7.4. Because the gain is seldom constant at all frequencies, an average gain value is frequently calculated and reported. In the ANSI standard, the gain is measured at three frequencies, 1000, 1600, and 2500 Hz, and the values are averaged. These frequencies are used because of their importance to speech understanding and because the hearing aid usually has its greatest output in this frequency region.

A feature shared by many hearing aids is volume control, either on the hearing aid itself or in a handheld remote control, which allows the user to adjust the gain. The frequency response can be measured while the position of the volume control is varied. Usually at least two sets of measurements are obtained: one with the volume control in the full-on position and one designed to approximate a typical or as-worn volume setting. The volume control is designed to provide an approximately 30-dB

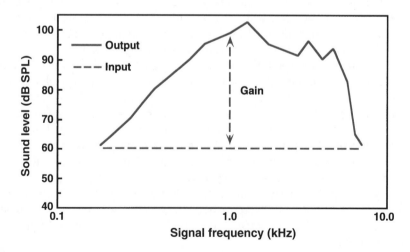

FIGURE 7.4   Calculation of hearing aid gain. The *output curve* represents the frequency response of the hearing aid for a constant 60-dB *input*.

variation in gain. It is typically assumed that a hearing aid wearer will select a volume setting somewhere in the middle of this 30-dB range, that is, approximately 15 dB below the full-on position. If the frequency response is measured with the volume control of the hearing aid in the full-on position, the gain is referred to as full-on gain. When the volume control is in the middle of the usable range, the gain approximates use gain, or as-worn gain. The ANSI standard calls this the reference test gain.

As mentioned previously, a second fundamental electroacoustic characteristic of the hearing aid is the OSPL, which is measured to determine the maximum possible acoustic output of the hearing aid. Consequently, a high-level input signal (90 dB SPL) is used, and the volume control is set to the full-on position. Under these conditions, the hearing aid is likely to be at maximum possible output. The audiologist should adjust the OSPL carefully to optimize the amount of gain available to the wearer while simultaneously minimizing the likelihood that the hearing aid will produce uncomfortably loud output (Vignette 7.4).

The gain and OSPL of a hearing aid are interrelated, as illustrated in Figure 7.5. The function shown in this figure is known as an input-output function because it displays the output along the ordinate as a function of the input level along the abscissa.

VIGNETTE 7.4 **Matching output sound pressure level (OSPL) to loudness discomfort level (LDL)**

For fitting the hearing aid to the patient, it is as important to pay attention to the maximum OSPL as to the gain, frequency response, or any other aspect of the fitting. Setting the maximum output too high can result in sounds frequently being overamplified, that is, amplified in excess of the wearer's LDL. This situation, shown in *panel A*, would likely lead to rejection of the hearing aid due to frequent loudness discomfort while using the hearing aid.

It is equally important to make sure one is making use of the full dynamic range (range from threshold to LDL) of the patient when fitting the device. If the OSPL is too far below LDL, as illustrated in *panel B*, the signal processor must compress the output much more than is necessary, and this can have undesirable perceptual consequences for the wearer.

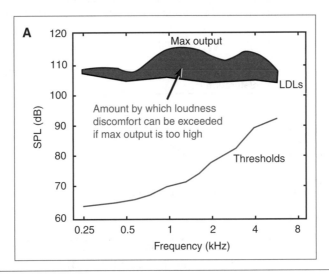

(continued)

VIGNETTE 7.4 Matching output sound pressure level (OSPL) to loudness discomfort level (LDL) *(Continued)*

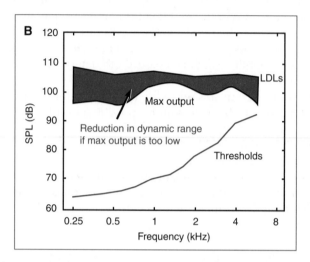

To obtain an appropriate match of the OSPL to the patient's LDL, the clinician must know the patient's LDL values at several frequencies. There are various approaches to establishing the patient's LDLs. As noted in Chapter 4, these measurements are not a routine part of the audiologic test battery in many clinics. As a result, they must either be measured directly prior to the hearing aid fitting or estimated from some other measurements available to the clinician. In fact, several formulas have been developed to allow the audiologist to estimate LDL from the pure-tone air conduction threshold at the same frequency. The errors in such estimates are great, however, and we recommend direct measurement of LDLs whenever possible, given their critical importance regarding the acceptance of the hearing aid by the wearer. With young children and in some other populations it may not be possible to obtain valid LDLs, and estimates derived from other measures, such as pure-tone thresholds, are often necessary.

Hawkins DB. Selecting SSPL90 using probe-microphone measurements. In Mueller HG, Hawkins DB, Northern JL, eds. Probe Microphone Measurements: Hearing Aid Selection and Assessment. San Diego: Singular Publishing Group, 1992:145–158.

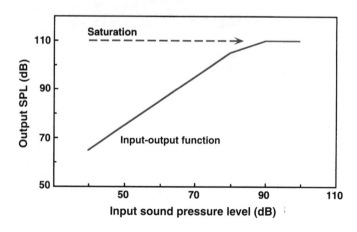

FIGURE 7.5 A linear input-output function for a hearing aid.

For this hypothetical input-output function, the volume control is assumed to be in the full-on position. Note that low input levels (50–60 dB SPL) reveal output values that exceed the input by 25 dB. The gain (output minus input) is 25 dB at low input levels. At high input levels (90 to 100 dB SPL) the output remains constant at 110 dB SPL. This is the OSPL of the hearing aid. The instrument simply can't produce an output higher than 110 dB SPL. Because the hearing aid output is limited to 110 dB SPL, the *gain* at these higher input levels is lower. The gain for the 90- and 100-dB inputs is 20 and 10 dB, respectively. Because of this interaction between gain and OSPL, gain is usually measured for input levels of 50 dB. These are also levels that approximate those of conversational speech, the input signal of greatest interest.

As noted previously, one of the major changes in hearing aids over the past several decades has been the drastic reduction in the size of the devices. In addition to making them smaller, the hearing aid industry has been striving to increase the quality of the electronic circuitry within the instruments. Through the early 1990s, most hearing aids sold in the United States had electronic circuitry that functioned just like that described in Figure 7.5. Over most of the range of input sound levels in Figure 7.5, every time the input was increased 10 dB, the output demonstrated a corresponding increase of 10 dB. This was true until the maximum output level of the hearing aid was reached. Such a circuit is generally called a linear circuit.

Most hearing aids dispensed today have intentionally nonlinear amplification circuits, often called compression circuits, which are designed to obtain a better match between the wide range of sound levels in the environment and the narrower range of listening available in the person with hearing loss. Figure 7.6 illustrates an input-output function that might be obtained for a typical hearing aid with nonlinear compression. (With the advent of digital circuitry, however, it is increasingly difficult to describe the "typical" hearing aid, as the extreme flexibility of these devices presents almost unlimited possibilities for sound processing.) Figure 7.6 shows that as the input level increases from 30 to 50 dB SPL, the output also increases 20 dB, from 60 to 80 dB SPL. The slope of this portion of the input-output function, 1 dB/dB, is characteristic of linear gain. This linear 1 dB/dB slope, extended to higher output levels by the *dashed line*, serves as a reference for the other portions of the measured input-output function. In this example, the slope of the input-output function is shallower beginning at an input level of 50 dB SPL and remains constant until the input level reaches 110 dB SPL. Above an input level of 110 dB SPL, the slope of the input-output function is very shallow (almost flat or horizontal). The region of the input-output function corresponding to input levels from 30 to 50 dB SPL is the *linear* region, that from 50 to 110 dB SPL as the *compression* or *wide dynamic range compression* (WDRC) region, and input levels of 110 dB SPL or greater as the *output-limiting* region of the input-output function. These regions are labeled in Figure 7.6.

What is the purpose of the WDRC region of the input-output function? As the input increases from 50 to 110 dB SPL in this region, the output increases only 30 dB, from 80 to 110 dB SPL. Thus, the hearing aid has taken a wide range of inputs at the microphone (60 dB) and compressed or squeezed that wide range into a narrower 30-dB range of outputs delivered into the wearer's ear canal. This is necessary, as noted previously, because the sensorineural hearing loss of the patient makes it hard to hear soft sounds while leaving the perception of very loud sounds unaltered. Thus, the wearer's perceptual dynamic range, from softest audible sound to loudest tolerable sound, is narrower than normal, and the wide dynamic range of sound levels encountered in everyday life must be squeezed into this narrower perceptual range. This is the primary purpose of WDRC. Once the compressed output reaches a high output

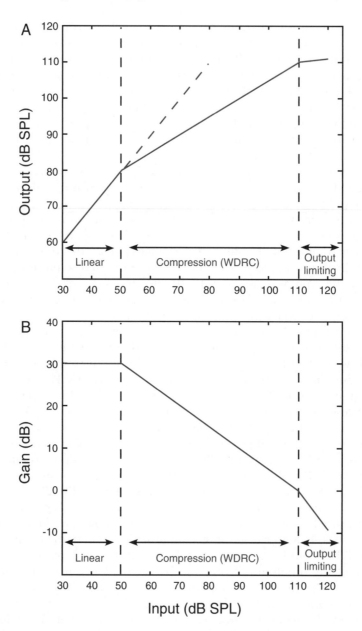

FIGURE 7.6 An input-output function for a nonlinear hearing aid with amplitude compression. **A.** The output level as a function of the input level. **B.** The gain (difference between output and input in top panel) as a function of input level. The *vertical dashed lines* represent the boundaries between the linear, compression (WDRC), and output-limiting regions of the input-output and input-gain functions. The *medium dashed line* **(A)** extends the linear portion of the function to demonstrate that the slopes of the function in the compression and output-limiting regions are much shallower than for the linear region.

level, 110 dB SPL, presumably a level slightly below the hypothetical wearer's loudness discomfort level (LDL) (Vignette 7.4), even stronger compression is provided to limit the maximum output so as not to exceed the LDL of the wearer.

It is sometimes helpful to think of the input-output function in terms of gain instead of output. The lower panel of Figure 7.6 illustrates the same input-output function as the upper panel, but in terms of gain instead of output. The gain values in the lower panel are simply the *difference* in output and input levels for each input level in the top panel of this figure. Thus, the hearing aid gain for input levels of 30 to 50 dB SPL is constant at 30 dB, followed by a gradually decreasing gain over the WRDC portion of the function, and then nearly 0-dB gain for input levels above 110 dB SPL. Thus, this two-stage compression circuit (WDRC and output-limiting compression) provides greater amounts of gain for soft sounds and no gain for loud sounds, consistent with the perceptual needs of the listener with sensorineural hearing loss.

The input-output function illustrated in Figure 7.6A is one of numerous possibilities available with digital hearing aids. In this example, the input-output function is divided into three regions: linear, WDRC, and output limiting. However, many more regions could be defined, each with its own slope for that region of the input-output function. The input levels that define the boundaries between regions of the input-output function having different slopes, such as input levels of 50 and 110 dB SPL in Figure 7.6, are *compression thresholds*, or *knee points*.

The slope of the input-output function, if shallower than 1, indicates compression, but the reciprocal of the slope is used to describe this parameter in hearing aids. For example, recall from the top portion of the Figure 7.6 that the output changed 30 dB, for a 60-dB change in input. The conventional mathematical slope would be defined as change in output (y-axis) divided by change in input (x-axis), which would be 30/60 dB, or ½. However, the reciprocal of the slope, 2/1, is used to express this parameter of compression systems in hearing aids, known as the compression ratio. (Also, 2:1 is a more common format to use for the compression ratio than 2/1.) Thus, the shallower the slope of the input-output function, the higher the compression ratio. In Figure 7.6A the compression ratio for the WDRC portion of the input-output function is 2:1, but it is 10:1 for the output-limiting portion of the input-output function (1-dB increase in output for each 10-dB increase in input above 110 dB SPL).

It is primarily the listener's dynamic range that determines the compression ratio for the WDRC portion of the input-output function, and values typically range from 1.5:1 to 5:1, with 2:1 and 3:1 being among the most common. In addition, compression thresholds for WDRC are generally lower than 50 to 55 dB SPL. Output-limiting compression is designed to ensure that the output doesn't exceed the upper limit of person's dynamic range (LDL). As a result, high compression ratios are desired, and these are typically about 10:1 or greater. In addition, although the compression threshold for the output-limiting portion of the input-output function is typically high (>90 dB SPL) and is expressed in terms of input level, the compression circuit for this region of the input-output function is most often triggered by the output level (output-dependent compression). Since we do not want the output in the patient's ear canal to exceed loudness discomfort, activation of severe compression on the basis of the output level is the most appropriate strategy. Moreover, the severe output-limiting compression will be activated at the specified output level regardless of the volume control position, and this is also desirable.

Although a detailed discussion of the temporal aspects of compression systems is beyond the scope of this text, compression circuits in typical hearing aids do not turn on or off instantaneously. The times required to turn on or turn off the compression can range from as little as 1 ms to as much as several seconds, depending on the purpose of the compression system. This is yet another parameter available to the clinician in adjusting the hearing aid and one that should vary with the purpose of the compression system. For example, for output limiting, we would like to minimize the time required to activate the compression to ensure that sounds that are too loud don't pass through the hearing aid to the wearer before the compression can be activated. For WDRC compression, it is not necessary to be as fast acting as for output-limiting compression.

Figure 7.6 illustrates the input-output and input-gain functions for just one compression channel. If this compression applies to all frequencies passing through the hearing aid, it is single-channel compression. However, single-channel compression is seldom used in contemporary hearing aids. Instead, the frequency range of interest (200–6000 Hz, for example) is often divided into several channels, each with its own channel-specific compression characteristics. Consider a simple two-channel WDRC hearing aid. The clinician could use the manufacturer's software to program one channel spanning 200 to 1500 Hz and the other spanning 1500 to 6000 Hz. The lower-frequency channel could be programmed to have input-output characteristics like the linear function in Figure 7.5, and the higher-frequency channel could be programmed to have input-output characteristics like the WDRC function in Figure 7.6A. Such a strategy might be appropriate for listeners with mild hearing loss from 250 to 1000 Hz and moderate or severe hearing loss (and narrower dynamic range) in the high frequencies. As noted in Chapter 5, this is a very common audiometric configuration for adults exposed to high levels of noise. Although some digital hearing aids have 20 or more channels, to date research has not supported a general more-is-better rule with regard to the number of channels. In fact, although there is research support for two channels being superior to one channel, at least in terms of speech communication, there is not as much support favoring further increases in the number of channels (at least above 4–8).

Clearly, one of the challenges facing the field of audiology is the pace at which manufacturers are implementing changes in the very flexible digital circuits in hearing aids. For example, imagine a 20-channel digital hearing aid with each channel having its own set of (multiple) compression thresholds, compression ratios, and temporal characteristics. The range of choices available to the clinician and the patient is almost mind boggling! As a result, clinicians have come to rely more on the manufacturers for guidance as to how to set these parameters of the circuitry to optimize the fitting of the hearing aid to the patient, but the manufacturer's guidance is not always based on evidence that the fitting parameters chosen are in fact optimal clinically. By the time researchers in the field have evaluated the clinical utility of emerging technology, the industry has moved on to another version of the technology or an entirely different approach based on engineering considerations. Nonetheless, there is little question that the less conspicuous high-fidelity digital hearing aid of today is a better product than its low-fidelity analog predecessor of many years ago and that the field, in partnership with the industry, will continue to find new ways to make use of the expanded capabilities of contemporary hearing devices to assist wearers in their daily lives.

Candidacy for Amplification

How does one know whether an individual is a good candidate for amplification? We have already indicated that the ideal candidate for amplification is one who displays a sensorineural hearing loss. Many audiologists use the degree of hearing loss as a rule

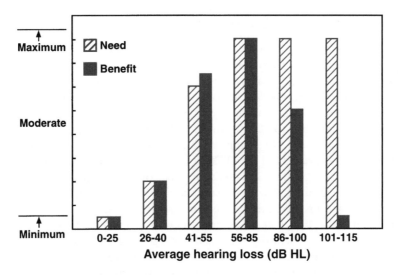

FIGURE 7.7 Need for and potential benefit from amplification as a function of degree of hearing loss.

of thumb for determining candidacy. Figure 7.7 shows a general guideline based on the average (500–2000 Hz) pure-tone hearing loss in the better ear. As hearing loss increases, the need for assistance increases, reaching a maximum for moderate amounts of hearing loss. Potential benefit from amplification is lowest at the two extremes, mild and profound impairment. Those with the mildest hearing losses and those with the most profound hearing deficits usually benefit the least from a hearing aid. There are many exceptions to this rule of thumb, which is based simply on pure-tone thresholds. Because of this, there is now a tendency to move away from these pure-tone guidelines and to consider anyone with a communicative difficulty caused by hearing loss as a candidate for amplification.

There are other considerations in determining hearing aid candidacy. Some of these factors are the patient's motivation for seeking assistance, the patient's acceptance of the hearing loss, and the patient's cosmetic concerns. Even if a significant hearing loss is present, some patients put off seeking assistance for several years. The reasons for this delay are not altogether clear, although the cost of the hearing aid and the failure of the primary care physician to refer for a hearing aid are considered contributing factors. Factors that influence individuals to pursue amplification include communication problems at home, in noisy situations, in social settings, and at work; and encouragement from a spouse.

Acceptance of a hearing loss is another consideration in determining hearing aid candidacy. Some individuals simply deny that a hearing problem exists. This is true particularly for persons with very mild losses, those who fear loss of employment, and those whose hearing loss came on gradually.

Finally, one cannot overlook cosmetic concerns when considering a patient's candidacy for amplification. Amplification is still considered a stigma. Although acceptance of hearing aids is improving, many individuals with hearing loss are concerned about the stigma associated with readily visible amplification devices. (This is discussed in more detail later in Vignette 7.10.)

Hearing Aid Selection and Evaluation

Once it has been established that an individual can benefit from amplification, an appointment for hearing aid selection and evaluation is usually scheduled. In the selection phase, some important clinical decisions must be made. For example, what type of hearing aid would be most appropriate for a given person with hearing loss? Recall from Figure 7.1 that a number of types of hearing aids are available. The audiologist and patient have to decide whether the patient will benefit most from a BTE instrument or one of the ITE systems (ITE, ITC, or CIC). As noted earlier, most hearing aids sold today are BTE, ITE, ITC, or CIC units. Importantly, very few young children wear ITE, ITC, or CIC systems because of the frequent need to recast the earpiece as the ear canal grows. Approximately 75% of hearing aids selected for children are BTE systems. Sometimes it is appropriate to use a hearing aid that includes a bone conduction transducer. Bone conduction hearing aids are used most often in patients with pinna deformities such as those discussed in Chapter 5.

Another important clinical decision that must be made in the selection phase is whether to recommend one hearing aid (monaural amplification) or two (binaural amplification). For many years, there was considerable controversy over the true benefits of binaural amplification. Although one would intuitively think that binaural amplification is superior to monaural amplification, it has traditionally been difficult to demonstrate objective advantages for two hearing aids. More recently, however, evidence in favor of binaural fittings has been mounting, and this has affected clinical practice. In 1980, 75% of patients were fitted monaurally. A decade later, approximately 50% of the hearing aid wearers in the United States were fitted monaurally. Since 2000, about 75% of hearing aids dispensed in the United States were binaural fittings. The primary reason that binaural amplification is not even more widespread is undoubtedly the added cost to the patient of buying two hearing aids rather than one. Nonetheless, there is considerable clinical evidence that failure to fit hearing aids on both ears of patients with bilateral hearing loss can result in temporary and perhaps permanent decreases in auditory function in the unaided ear. The deterioration over time of auditory perceptual function in the hearing-impaired ear left unaided has been referred to as an *auditory deprivation* effect.

In addition to avoiding these possible deprivation or adaptation effects, some of the reported advantages to binaural amplification include better sound localization, binaural summation (a sound is easier to hear with two ears than with one), and improvement in speech recognition in noise. Experienced hearing aid users often favor binaural amplification and report that two aids offer more balanced hearing, better overall hearing, improved speech clarity in noise, improved sound localization skills, and more natural and less stressful listening. Accordingly, binaural amplification is being recommended with increasing regularity. Some clinical research indicates that the benefits of binaural fittings over monaural ones increase as the amount of hearing loss increases. Monaural fittings may be appropriate for many persons with mild hearing loss.

Several other factors that must be considered in the selection process are beyond the scope of this text. Briefly, the audiologist must consider the type of microphone (directional versus omnidirectional), earmold material (soft Silastic versus hard acrylic), and type of earmold or shell (e.g., vented versus not vented). Additional choices include whether to use a remote control for adjusting volume on the hearing aid. For children, an additional consideration is the adaptability of the instrument to various classroom amplification systems.

Modern-day hearing aids provide a wide range of electroacoustic characteristics that can be tailored to the patient's individual needs. Hearing aid selection has undergone major changes in recent years. Today, most audiologists use a prescriptive approach to hearing aid selection. Using information obtained from the patient, such as the pure-tone thresholds, the appropriate gain can be prescribed according to some underlying theoretical principles. From the mid 1970s through the mid-1980s, at least a dozen prescriptive hearing aid selection methods were developed. Although they differ in detail, these methods have the same general feature that more gain is prescribed at frequencies for which the hearing loss is greatest. As an example, one of the simplest approaches makes use of the so-called half-gain rule. One simply measures the hearing threshold at several frequencies and multiplies the hearing loss by a factor of one-half. Thus, for a patient with a flat 50-dB hearing loss from 250 through 8000 Hz, the appropriate gain would be 25 dB (0.5×50 dB) at each frequency. A person having a sloping hearing loss with a 40-dB HL hearing threshold at 1000 Hz and an 80-dB HL threshold at 4000 Hz would require gains of 20 and 40 dB, respectively, using this simple half-gain rule.

Most of these earlier prescriptive methods, like the simple half-gain rule, assumed that the gain required was constant for an output level up to the patient's LDL, and no further increases in output were provided regardless of input. That is, linear input-output functions were assumed. Contemporary compression hearing aids are nonlinear, and the gain is designed to vary with input level (Fig. 7.6B). Thus, new nonlinear prescriptive approaches had to be developed to prescribe gain for low, medium, and high input levels. Regardless of the prescriptive method used, once the prescription is generated and the hearing aid arrives, the audiologist uses manufacturer-supplied software to program the hearing aid to match the prescription.

OSPL can also be prescribed for the patient. Usually, additional information is required from the patient. One common approach is to measure the LDL of the patient for tones or narrow bands of noise. The LDL is a measure of the maximum sound level that the patient can tolerate at each frequency. As noted in Vignette 7.4, it would not be desirable for the hearing aid's acoustic output to exceed the maximum tolerable level of the patient, because this might cause the patient to reject the hearing aid. The OSPL of the hearing aid is frequently adjusted to a value slightly lower than the LDL. In this way, the audiologist can ensure that the acoustic output of the hearing aid will not exceed the maximum tolerance level of the patient.

Once the appropriate prescription has been made and the hearing aid has been programmed, the next process, the fitting or verification, is conducted. In this process, the hearing aid is inserted into the patient's ear, and its acoustic performance on the wearer is verified. This is best accomplished using real-ear measurements of the sound pressure level generated in the ear canal near the eardrum, with and without the hearing aid in place. This is made possible by using a tiny microphone connected to a long, thin tube made of flexible plastic. The probe tube can be safely inserted into the ear canal, yet it is strong enough to resist being squeezed shut when the hearing aid is inserted. When sound pressure level measurements are made at several frequencies in the patient's ear canal with and without the hearing aid, the difference between these two measurements provides a measure of the real-ear insertion gain of the hearing aid (Vignette 7.5). The measured insertion gain is compared with the target gain, and the hearing aid's settings are adjusted until a reasonable match is observed. Similar adjustments should also be made in the maximum output of the hearing aid to assure that real-ear sound pressure levels measured in the aided conditions for high-level input signals (90 dB SPL) do not exceed the LDL. In fact, one of the recent trends in

---

VIGNETTE 7.5 **Measurement of real-ear insertion gain**

As noted in the text, the measurement of real-ear insertion gain is a common first step in the verification of the fit of the hearing aid. The drawing illustrates the basic arrangement of equipment needed for this measurement. A small loudspeaker is located at ear level about 1 m from the patient (either straight ahead or at a slight angle). A long, very narrow, flexible tube, the probe tube, is inserted into the ear canal. The closed end of the probe tube terminates at a microphone, and the microphone is connected to the real-ear measurement device. This device sends stimuli to the loudspeaker and records the measurements made with the microphone at the end of the probe tube. (Often another microphone is attached to the side of the patient's head to monitor and regulate the output level of the loudspeaker at the patient's ear.)

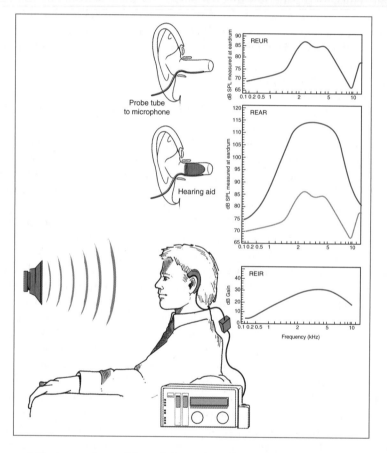

The top panel illustrates the position of the probe tube in the ear canal for the initial unaided measurements. When the sound is presented from the loudspeaker as a series of 70-dB SPL pure tones increasing in frequency from 100 to 10,000 Hz and measured in the open ear canal with the probe tube, a frequency response like that shown in the top panel is obtained. This is the real-ear unaided response (REUR). It shows the 15- to 20-dB resonant boost provided by the ear canal and pinna (see Chapter 3). The middle panel shows the next measurement, made with the hearing aid inserted and adjusted to the appropriate settings. Sound is again presented from the loudspeaker as a series of 70-dB SPL pure tones increasing in frequency from 100 to 10,000 Hz. The sound levels recorded with the probe tube microphone in the aided condition are the real-ear aided response (REAR).

VIGNETTE 7.5   Measurement of real-ear insertion gain *(Continued)*

Comparison of the aided measurement condition in the middle panel to the unaided measurement condition in the upper panel shows two noteworthy observations regarding the location of the probe tube. First, for the aided condition, the tip of the probe tube extends at least five-sixteenths of an inch beyond the canal portion of the hearing aid. When the hearing aid is inserted, it doesn't cover up or block the opening of the probe tube. Second, the location of the probe tube within the ear canal for the unaided and aided measurements is the same; the probe tube was not pulled out or pushed in significantly when moving from the unaided to the aided measurements.

The lower panel shows the difference between the REAR and REUR curves; this is the real-ear insertion response (REIR). Essentially, this curve shows how much real-ear insertion gain (REIG) was provided, in decibels, at each frequency from 100 to 10,000 Hz as a result of hearing aid insertion. If the REIR was flat at 0 dB, for example, this would imply that there was no gain provided by the hearing aid. The audiologist compares the REIR to target values generated by various prescription procedures and fine-tunes the hearing aid until the REIR demonstrates a close match to the target values. The REIR is a reliable measure, can be obtained in a matter of minutes, provides a detailed picture of the hearing aid's response on that particular patient, and requires no active participation on the part of the hearing aid wearer. It has become a very common and powerful tool for the verification of a hearing aid's performance on an individual wearer.

---

hearing aid fitting or verification has been, in principle, to measure hearing thresholds and LDLs with the probe tube microphone in the patient's ear canal and then present a range of speech intensities, from soft speech to loud speech, to verify that soft speech is audible (above threshold) across all frequencies and that loud speech does not exceed LDL at any frequency (Vignette 7.6).

After fine-tuning the gain and maximum output of the hearing aid to match the targeted values, the hearing aid is evaluated. Again, the audiologist can choose from several hearing aid evaluation procedures. These alternatives have a common goal: evaluation of the benefit provided by the hearing aid when it is worn by the patient with hearing loss. Because the primary benefit to be derived from use of the hearing aid is improved understanding of speech, the hearing aid evaluation usually involves measurement of the patient's speech recognition performance with and without the hearing aid. This is done using loudspeakers with the patient positioned in the sound field. Standardized tape-recorded speech materials are preferred for testing (see Chapter 4). The patient is typically presented with a sample of continuous speech or speech-shaped noise at a level approximating conversational levels (65 or 70 dB SPL). While listening to this stimulus, the patient adjusts the volume control on the hearing aid (if any) to a comfortable setting. Next, speech recognition testing is conducted, with the materials presented at the same overall level (65 to 70 dB SPL). Speech recognition testing is often performed in a background of noise or multiple-talker babble to permit evaluation of the benefit provided by the hearing aid for conditions representative of those in which the hearing aid is to be worn. With this in mind, a speech-to-noise or speech-to-babble ratio of +6 to 8 dB is recommended for use. This range of values represents "typical" noisy conditions encountered by most patients. The speech recognition measure is also often obtained from the patient under identical stimulus conditions without the hearing aid. The difference in performance between the aided

In recent years, verification of the fitting from sound level measurements in the patient's ear canal has become more popular. Rather than prescribing target amounts of gain based on some underlying theoretical objective and then verifying that gain in the patient's ear canal (Vignette 7.5), this approach seeks to verify the objectives directly without using gain. Consider, for example, the following theoretical objective for a fitting approach: the full amplitude range of speech, about a 30-dB range at each frequency, should be made audible but not uncomfortably loud at 200 to 6000 Hz.

The graph illustrates an approach to direct verification of this theoretical objective. Thresholds representing the limit to audibility and LDLs representing the maximum tolerable sound levels appear on this graph. Both are expressed in *ear canal* sound pressure level. Both threshold and LDL could be measured in the sound field while a probe tube microphone was positioned in the ear canal to measure the sound level in decibels SPL, but typically this is not the case. Instead, thresholds and LDLs obtained with an insert earphone are converted to ear canal sound pressure levels with the help of some software (and some additional probe tube microphone measurements from the patient). Once these lower (threshold) and upper (LDL) boundaries have been established, speech or speechlike sounds can be presented from the loudspeaker while the sound levels are measured in the patient's ear canal. In the graph, these acoustical measurements have verified that the lower speech amplitudes are above threshold over the whole frequency range and that the higher speech amplitudes never exceed LDL. Thus, the theoretical objectives of this fitting rationale have been verified directly in the wearer's ear canal. Of course, this same approach can be used to verify a number of theoretical objectives aside from the one described here. However, the one described here is one of the frequently used approaches.

Although the graph reveals a good match of the hearing aid fit to the targeted theoretical objectives, this is not always the case, especially in the initial fit. Frequently, insufficient gain is provided in the high frequencies for the low speech amplitudes or too much output is provided at other frequencies. In these circumstances, the audiologist uses a personal computer to change the gain, compression, or output-limiting parameters at specific frequencies and then redoes the acoustical measurements with the speechlike sounds measured in the ear canal. This process of measurement and adjustment continues until the targeted objectives of the fitting approach have been accomplished, as shown in the graph.

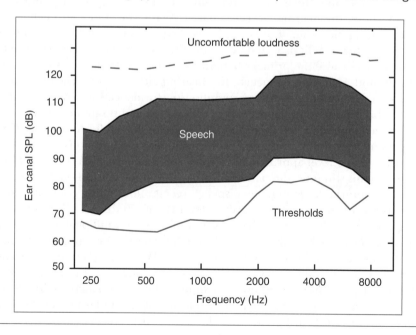

and unaided measures provides a general indication of the benefit provided by the hearing aid under typical listening conditions. These direct measures of the effects of the hearing aid on speech recognition have sometimes been referred to as *objective* measures of benefit (see Vignette 7.7).

VIGNETTE 7.7   Effects of a hearing aid on speech understanding in quiet and in noise

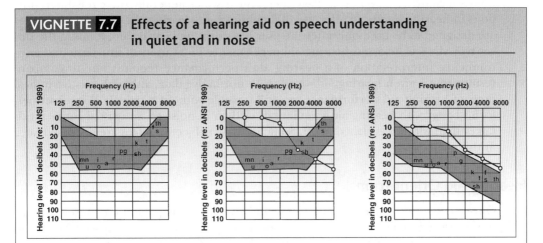

The *left-hand panel* in the figure shows the distribution of various speech sounds at conversational levels on the coordinates of the audiogram. We will refer to this type of plot in this chapter as the speech audiogram. The full range of speech sounds is audible to an individual with normal hearing in quiet conditions. Also, several speech sounds, such as /f, s, and t/, are low in intensity and high in frequency.

In the *middle panel*, a high-frequency sensorineural hearing loss similar to that found in many elderly individuals has been superimposed on the speech audiogram. Many of the high-frequency, low-intensity consonants are no longer heard by the individual with this hearing loss, although many low- and mid-frequency speech sounds (such as vowels and nasal sounds) remain audible. A frequent complaint of individuals with this very common type of hearing loss is that they can hear speech but they can't understand it. When presented with the word set *wife, white, wide, wipe, wise,* for example, the individual may hear only the word "why" repeated several times. The high-frequency consonant at the end of each word is not heard, and the words are misperceived.

In the *right-hand panel*, the speech sounds have been amplified by a well-fitted hearing aid. In this case, a well-fitted hearing aid amplifies the high frequencies to make those consonants audible to the patient while not amplifying the low frequencies, where hearing is essentially normal. With the audibility of all of the speech sounds in conversational speech restored by the hearing aid, the hearing aid wearer will regain the ability to understand speech as well as a normal-hearing listener. Depending in part on how long the person has been accustomed to hearing speech through the hearing loss, the time required to perform normally will vary from patient to patient.

In noise, however, the microphone of the hearing aid amplifies the noise as much as the speech; thus, the speech-to-noise ratio is not improved by the conventional hearing aid. If the conversational speech of the person in front of the listener is 6 dB greater at the input to the hearing aid (microphone) than the background of babble produced by the other attendees at a cocktail party, this 6-dB speech-to-noise ratio will remain at the output from the hearing aid. The speech will be made audible by the hearing aid, but so will the noise. Consequently, conventional hearing aids are generally not considered to work as well in noise as in quiet.

In addition to these objective measures of hearing aid benefit, the hearing aid evaluation should include some subjective measures of performance and benefit. Most commonly, self-assessment surveys or inventories of hearing handicap and hearing aid performance have been used. The self-assessment scale, generally consisting of approximately 25 items, is administered before delivery of the hearing aid and sometime afterward (e.g., 30 or 45 days later). Such scales generally show reliable reductions in hearing handicap after use of amplification. Hearing aid performance scales are designed to be used only after the user has worn the hearing aid. Items in the survey typically seek to assess hearing aid performance in a variety of situations and environments. Interpretation of a hearing aid's performance requires one to compare results from a given hearing aid wearer with normative data, although relative indications of hearing aid performance are still possible without norms (e.g., patient performs better with hearing aid in quiet rather than in noise or with visual contact with talker than without visual contact). Some of these subjective scales are discussed later in this chapter.

Hearing Aid Orientation

Once the hearing aid has been selected and evaluated, the patient is counseled about the measured benefits, the limitations of hearing aids, the cost, and so forth. If the patient decides to purchase the hearing aid, the audiologist may either dispense it or refer the patient to another party who sells it. Another common model is to have the patient purchase the aid or aids before selection and evaluation (after the audiological evaluation), with a refund provided if dissatisfied with the result. The particular dispensing model followed varies from clinic to clinic and can vary with the type or style of instrument. For example, a one-size-fits-all open-fit BTE can be selected and evaluated without delay, as long as identical units are available for use in the audiologist's office. In this case, it would be feasible to do a selection and evaluation prior to purchase. On the other hand, custom ITE devices require ear impressions that are sent to the manufacturer prior to product delivery. In this case, the patient is more likely to make at least a partial payment toward the purchase of the aid or aids prior to selection and evaluation.

Hearing aids are typically sold on a 30-day trial basis in the United States; dissatisfied patients are given a refund at the end of that trial period. During the trial period, the patient is encouraged to visit the audiologist two or three times for orientation. During the orientations, the patient is instructed in the use and care of the hearing aid, counseled about its limitations, given strategies to maximize its benefit, and given an opportunity to voice any complaints about its function. Frequently, modification of the earmold or the earpiece (shell) of the aid is needed to make it fit more comfortably in the patient's ear. The hearing aid may require some electronic adjustments as well. After the trial period, the user is encouraged to return for further evaluation in a year, or sooner if he or she has difficulty.

Alternative Rehabilitative Devices

Assistive Listening Devices

As mentioned previously, full-time use of a hearing aid is not necessary or beneficial for many individuals with hearing loss. A number of people with mild hearing loss require only part-time use of a hearing aid or alternative device. For many of these individuals, a practical alternative is a class of devices known as assistive listening devices. These devices are typically electroacoustic devices designed for a much more limited purpose than that of the conventional hearing aid. Two of the most common uses of these devices are use of the telephone and listening to the television. Several telephone handsets have been developed to amplify the telephone signal by 15 to 30 dB. These devices are effective for people with mild hearing loss who have difficulty communicating over the telephone.

Many of the assistive listening devices physically separate the microphone from the rest of the device so that the microphone can be placed closer to the source of the desired sound. Recall that the microphone converts an acoustic signal into an electrical one so that it can be amplified by the device. If the microphone on the assistive listening device is separated by a great distance from the rest of the device, the electrical signal from the microphone must somehow be sent to the amplifier. This is accomplished in various ways, with some devices simply running a wire several feet long directly from the microphone to the amplifier. Other devices convert the electrical signal from the microphone into radio waves (FM) or invisible light waves (infrared) and send the signal to a receiver adjacent to the amplifier and worn by the individual. The receiver converts the FM or infrared signal back to an electrical signal and sends it to the amplifier.

The FM and infrared systems are frequently referred to as wireless systems because they eliminate the long wire running directly from the microphone to the amplifier. The wireless feature of these assistive listening devices makes them more versatile and easier to use, but it also makes them more expensive. These assistive listening devices overcome the primary disadvantage of the conventional hearing aid; they improve the speech-to-noise ratio. Separating the microphone from the rest of the device and positioning it closer to the sound source (e.g., the talker's mouth or the loudspeaker of the television set) amplifies the primary signal of interest more than the surrounding background noise. On a conventional hearing aid, the ear-level microphone amplifies both the speech and the surrounding noise equally well; therefore, the speech-to-noise ratio is not improved, and all sound at the position of the microphone is simply made louder by the conventional hearing aid (Vignette 7.8).

Separating the microphone from the rest of the device has its drawbacks. It is only a reasonable alternative when the sound source is fairly stable over time. If the microphone is positioned near the loudspeaker of the television, for example, the voice of a talker seated next to the impaired person will not be amplified. The impaired individual is forced to listen to the sound source closest to the microphone. For assistive listening devices, this is not a serious drawback because they have a limited purpose.

Selection and evaluation of assistive listening devices is not as formalized as it is for hearing aids. Most clinics today have a room designated as the assistive listening device area. This room or area is set up to simulate the conditions under which the devices are to be used. Typically, the room takes on the atmosphere of a living room or family room, with television, stereo, and telephones available. After the patient's needs have been assessed through a written or oral questionnaire, the patient tries several assistive devices under controlled conditions in the simulated environment. If the patient finds the device beneficial, it is dispensed by the audiologist, or the patient is referred to an appropriate source for its purchase.

Assistive devices of various types also benefit the severely or profoundly impaired. In addition to the devices mentioned earlier, some nonauditory devices have been developed. Some flash lights in response to various acoustic signals in the home, such

---

VIGNETTE 7.8   Improving the speech-to-noise ratio with an assistive listening device or classroom system

In this vignette, we make use of the speech audiogram concept used in Vignette 7.7. The *left-hand panel* shows the speech audiogram for conversational speech with background noise (several other people talking) as it has been amplified by a hearing aid. This is the same as the *right-hand panel* of Vignette 7.7 with the addition of background noise. The level of the noise is indicated by the *heavy dashed line*. The speech and noise levels shown here represent those measured through the hearing aid with the listener in the middle of a living room or classroom full of people at about 1 m from the desired talker.

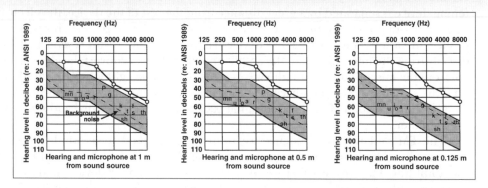

In the *middle panel*, the microphone has been detached from the hearing aid and is positioned about half a meter from the primary talker. (The hearing aid's microphone can't actually be detached. We're just pretending to illustrate the concept behind assistive listening devices.) According to the inverse-square law (see Chapter 2), as the distance to the sound source is halved (from 1 m to 0.5 m), the sound level increases by 6 dB. The speech is now 6 dB higher than it was in the *left-hand panel*, whereas the diffuse background noise (*dashed line*) coming from a variety of sources, including reflections from walls and the ceiling, remains unchanged. Thus, the speech-to-noise ratio has improved 6 dB.

In the *right-hand panel*, we have positioned the microphone still closer to the sound source, approximately 0.125 m (4–5 inches) from the primary talker's mouth. As a result, the speech level from the talker has increased another 12 dB (two more halvings of the distance), and the speech-to-noise ratio has been improved a total of 18 dB compared with that in the *left-hand panel*.

As noted in Vignette 7.7, the conventional hearing aid does not improve the signal-to-noise ratio but simply amplifies the acoustic signals, speech and noise alike, that arrive at the microphone (*left panel*). Moving the microphone closer to the desired sound source (*middle* and *right panels*), whether a talker or a loudspeaker, increases the speech signal level without affecting the background noise. The result is an improved speech-to-noise ratio and better communication. This is the primary operational principle behind many assistive listening devices and similar classroom amplification systems.

---

as the ringing of the doorbell or the telephone. Other special telephone devices enable text to be sent over phone lines (in printed form) so that a profoundly impaired person can carry on a telephone conversation by sending and receiving text messages. Special keyboard-like devices are needed at both ends of the phone line to enable such communication. A summary of assistive devices along with their advantages and disadvantages is listed in Table 7.1.

TABLE 7.1 Summary of Accessory Amplification Devices

Input	Device	Description	Advantages	Disadvantages
Telephone	Internal telephone amplifier	Volume control installed by phone company in telephone receiver	Volume control easily adjusted; good range in gain; clear signal	Telephone usage restricted to modified phone; monthly fee; not available on all styles of phones
	External telephone amplifier	Hearing aid telecoil	A personal hearing aid can be used if aid equipped with circuit; adjustable volume control (can also be used with induction-loop systems)	Strength not always dependable; does not work on all phone styles
		Small device attaches to phone earpiece (used without hearing aid induction coil)	Portable; adjustable volume control; inexpensive; one-time expense	Battery operated; alignment problems
		Amplifier snaps on to earpiece (operates in conjunction with hearing aid induction coil)	Portable; adjustable gain control; provides extra power when used with hearing aid telecoil; versatile (some models can also be used as a television and radio amplifier)	Battery operated; alignment problems; relatively expensive
		Loudspeaker	Option for persons who have trouble manipulating T-switch or holding the receiver to aid for any length of time (provides extra gain without feedback problems when used in addition to one's personal hearing aid)	Limits phone usage to the modified phone
Television	Amplifier without a direct connection to source	Induction loop TV/radio kit: Kit includes materials for setting up an induction loop system in home or office (components can also be purchased separately from local TV/radio stores)	Mobility around room; improved signal/noise ratio	Trouble and expense of setting up; must have aid with T-switch; unable to hear environmental sound
Radio	Same options as TV	Radio with TV band	Good quality; can be used as radio	Fairly expensive
Tape recorder	Same options as TV			
Signaling devices	Telephone signal amplifier	Suction cup, attaches to surface of phone or doorbell, produces a loud tone	Allows individual to hear phone signal at some distance	Battery operated
	High-intensity doorbell	Large doorbell which provides much greater intensity than standard bells or chimes	Alerts person from some distance away	Installation

From Ricketts TA, Bess FH, DeChicchis AR: Hearing aids and assistive listening devices. In Bailey BJ, ed. Head and Neck Surgery-Otolaryngology. 3rd Ed. Philadelphia: Lippincott Williams & Wilkins, 2001.

Classroom Amplification

A discussion of hearing aids would not be complete without a review of the special amplification systems designed for education. *Classroom amplification* is a term used to describe a device that provides amplified sound to a group of children. Classroom amplification gained added importance with the advent of IDEA, a federal mandate regarding the education of all handicapped children. The law requires that schools provide children with hearing loss with adequate services and funding. This includes habilitative or rehabilitative services, such as selection and evaluation of personal hearing aids and group systems, auditory training, speech training, speech reading, and any other services deemed necessary for the child's educational development.

Why should a child need a special educational amplification system? A primary concern is the acoustic environment of the classroom. Children are continually bombarded with excessively high noise levels that interfere with their ability to understand the teacher. These noise levels originate from sources outside the school building (aircraft or car traffic), within the school building (adjacent classrooms and hallways, activity areas, heating and cooling systems), and within the classroom itself (students talking, feet shuffling, noise from moving furniture). These various sources contribute to noise levels ranging from 40 to 67 dBA.[1] Such high noise levels result in an unfavorable signal-to-noise ratio (SNR) or speech-to-noise ratio reaching the child's ear. Recall that the SNR represents the difference in decibels between speech (from the teacher) and the overall ambient noise in the classroom. For example, an SNR of +10 dB means that the teacher's speech is 10 dB more intense than the noise in the classroom. Ideally, an SNR of +20 dB is necessary if a child with hearing loss is to understand speech maximally. Noise surveys in classrooms have shown that SNRs typically range from −6 to +6 dB, a listening environment that precludes maximal understanding even for normal-hearing children.

Classroom noise is not the only variable that contributes to a difficult listening environment. Reverberation time, or the amount of time it takes for sound to decrease by 60 dB after the termination of a signal, also contributes to an adverse acoustic environment. When a teacher talks to the child, some of the speech signal reaches the child's amplification system within just a few milliseconds. The remainder of the signal strikes surrounding areas in the form of reflections after the initial sound reaches the child's ear. The strength and duration of these reflections are affected by the absorption quality of the surrounding surfaces and the size (volume) of the classroom. If an area has hard walls, ceilings, and floors, the room will have a long reverberation time. In contrast, an acoustically treated room with carpeting, drapes, and an acoustic tile ceiling will have a shorter reverberation time. Generally, as reverberation time increases, the proportion of reflected speech sound reaching the listener increases and speech recognition decreases. In addition, the smaller the room, the greater the reverberation. Many classrooms for those with hearing loss have reverberation times ranging from a very mild value of 0.2 second to more severe reverberation, with times greater than 1 second.

---

[1]As note previously sound level meters have three weighting networks (A, B, C) that are designed to respond differently to noise frequencies. The A network weighs (filters) the low frequencies and approximates the response characteristics of the human ear. The B network also filters the low frequencies but not as much as the A network. The C scale provides a fairly flat response. The federal government recommends the A network for measuring noise levels.

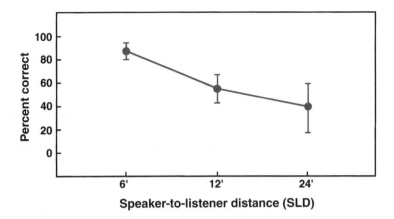

FIGURE 7.8 Typical speech recognition scores for normal-hearing children at different speaker-to-listener distances. At 6 feet, the signal-to-noise ratio is +6 dB and the reverberation time is 0.46s.

These factors, noise and reverberation, adversely affect speech recognition. As the noise levels and reverberation times increase, the SNR becomes less favorable and there is a significant breakdown in speech understanding. Further, as the distance between the talker and listener increases, the SNR worsens. Figure 7.8 illustrates this phenomenon by showing the speech recognition scores for sentence materials in a group of normal-hearing children who listened to speech with noise levels and reverberation times similar to those in a classroom. The reverberation time is 0.46 seconds, and the SNR at 6 feet is +6 dB. Speech recognition deteriorates with increasing distance. At 6 feet, speech recognition is seen to average approximately 90%, whereas at 24 feet, it averages 40%. Table 7.2 shows how noise and reverberation can produce a hardship for young children with hearing loss. These data represent the unaided speech recognition scores of children with hearing loss in a quiet environment and under different SNRs and reverberation times. As the noise levels increase, speech recognition decreases. Further, as reverberation increases, speech recognition decreases. At an SNR of +6 dB (a common listening condition in the classroom) with a reverberation time of 0.4 second, the mean recognition score is 52%; when reverberation time is 1.2 seconds, recognition is only 27%. It is not surprising that a child with hearing loss will find it difficult to learn under such adverse conditions.

TABLE 7.2 Mean Word Recognition Scores for Children Wearing Hearing Aids Under Various Noise and Reverberant Conditions

Reverberation Time (s)	SNR (dB)			
	Quiet	+12	+6	0
0.0 (nonreverberant)	83	70	60	39
0.4	74	60	52	28
1.2	45	41	27	11

Adapted from Finitzo-Hieber T, Tillman TW. Room acoustic effects on monosyllabic word discrimination ability for normal children and children with hearing loss. J Speech Hear Res 21:440–448, 1978.

Children with hearing loss not only have difficulty understanding speech in difficult listening situations, but they also expend a great deal of effort in attending to the spoken message. Not only does the presence of noise increase learning effort; it even reduces the energy available for performing other cognitive functions. Even young school-age children with very mild forms of hearing loss have reported less energy or were tired more frequently than children with normal hearing.

These findings may well be a result of these children's difficulties with listening under adverse listening conditions. One can speculate that toward the end of a school day, children with hearing loss will be physically and mentally spent as a result of focusing intently on the teacher's speech and on the conversations of other children. This expenditure of effort will no doubt compromise a child's ability to learn in the classroom.

Several types of special educational amplification systems have been designed to overcome the adverse effects of the classroom environment by offering a better SNR. These system types include hardwire systems, FM wireless systems, infrared systems, and a system that combines the FM wireless system with a personal hearing aid. More recently, sound field amplification systems have been developed as yet another option for use in the classroom and one that may benefit *all* students in the classroom, not just those with hearing loss. The concept behind these systems is similar to that described for the assistive listening devices. The microphone is moved closer to the desired sound source, the teacher. A brief description of each of these systems follows.

Hardwire System

In this system, a microphone worn by the teacher is wired to an amplifier. Each student wears headphones or insert receivers that are connected to the amplifier by wires so that the teacher and the students are in effect tethered together (Fig. 7.9, *top*). The primary advantage of a hardwire system is the high fidelity and high level of output available through earphones. These systems are inexpensive, simple, and easy to operate. The obvious disadvantage is the restricted mobility of both the teacher and students. Hardwire systems are not commonplace in classrooms today.

FM Wireless Systems

Most classrooms for those with hearing loss use either FM devices or a combination of an FM system and a personal hearing aid. A microphone transmitter is worn around the teacher's neck, and a signal is broadcast to an FM receiver worn by the child (Fig. 7.9, *bottom*). Most FM receivers have an environmental microphone so that the child can monitor his or her own voice, the voices of his or her peers, and other environmental sounds. When the environmental microphone is used, the SNR is compromised because of the distance between the talker and the microphone. The advantage to this system is the mobility it allows. The teacher and the students are free to move around the room, and the students will continue to receive amplification.

Infrared Systems

Infrared group amplification is seldom used in classrooms but is used widely as an assistive device in theaters, churches, and other public facilities. As mentioned earlier, the system uses an infrared emitter that transmits the speech signal from the input microphone to individually worn infrared receiver–audio amplifier units. It is similar

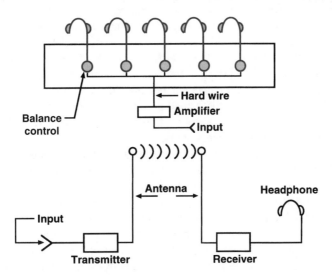

FIGURE 7.9 Two classroom amplification systems. *Top*, Hard wire. *Bottom*, FM. The personal hearing aid could replace the headphones shown at bottom to produce a dovetailed system.

in design to the FM system shown in Figure 7.9 (*bottom*), except that infrared light waves are used to send the signal from the transmitter to the receiver rather than FM radio waves. Infrared systems are somewhat limited in power output.

Coupling the FM Wireless System to the Child's Ear

With personal FM systems, the teacher wears a microphone-transmitter that broadcasts carrier waves to a receiver worn by the child. A number of options are available for coupling the FM system to the child's ear. A summary of the coupling options that can be used with FM systems is shown in Vignette 7.9.

Sound-Field Amplification

A more recent development in this area has been to broadcast the signal from the teacher's transmitter via FM transmission to an amplifier connected to a series of loudspeakers placed strategically around the classroom (Fig. 7.10). Often the loudspeakers are suspended from the ceiling, with at least two in the front and two at the rear of the classroom. The basic idea is that because the teacher's voice comes from loudspeakers dispersed throughout the classroom, no student is too far from the primary signal (the teacher's voice), and a favorable SNR is maintained throughout the classroom. Thus, the amplified signal is delivered uniformly to *all* students, rather than just those with hearing loss. This can benefit not just other students with special needs but normal-hearing children as well. As noted previously, the acoustics in many classrooms are poor, and even normal-hearing children may find listening a challenge at times.

Similar to other amplification devices, the sound-field system has limitations—the amount of amplification is limited (8 to 10 dB), and the system amplifies only the teacher's voice, not the voices of other children. Of course, the child with hearing loss can receive additional benefit from the use of a personal hearing aid in a classroom

Several options exist for coupling the FM system to the ear. One option is to combine the FM device with the personal hearing aid. This approach, commonly called dovetailing, is done to take advantage of the benefits of both systems: the improved speech-to-noise ratio offered by the FM system and the custom fitting of the personal hearing aid. One approach for combining the FM system with the personal hearing aid is the incorporation of an FM receiver into an audio boot. When the boot is slipped on to an appropriate hearing aid, FM reception is possible. Some boots use an electrical connection from the receiver to the hearing aid; some manufacturers have developed wireless boots.

Another approach to coupling a personal hearing aid to the FM system is via inductive coupling. With this device, the FM signal, which is sometimes mixed with an environmental signal in the student receiver, is converted to an electromagnetic field via a wire loop encircling the child's neck. The personal hearing aid is worn in the telecoil position, thereby inductively coupling a hearing aid to the FM receiver–miniloop combination. A third approach is the use of a BTE FM receiver, a development brought about through advances in microminiature FM technology. The BTE houses, at ear level, both the FM receiver and the hearing aid circuitry, which eliminates the need for cords, neck loops, and body-worn receivers. The BTE FM system device looks like a conventional BTE hearing aid. Other techniques for coupling the FM receiver to the child's ear include an FM system receiver with Sony Walkman–type ear bud headphones or simply a self-contained FM receiver with a button or BTE transducer.

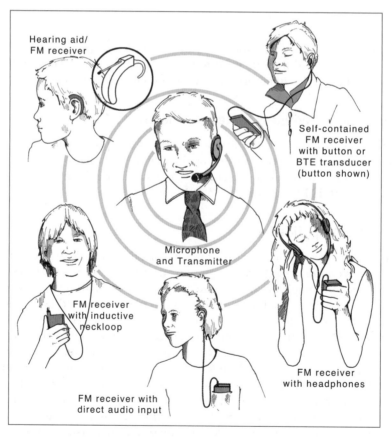

Hearing aid/
FM receiver

Self-contained
FM receiver
with button or
BTE transducer
(button shown)

Microphone
and Transmitter

FM receiver
with inductive
neckloop

FM receiver
with headphones

FM receiver with
direct audio input

Figure adapted from Lewis DE. Classroom amplification. In Bess FH, ed. Children With Hearing Impairment: Contemporary Trends. Nashville: Bill Wilkerson Center, 1998.

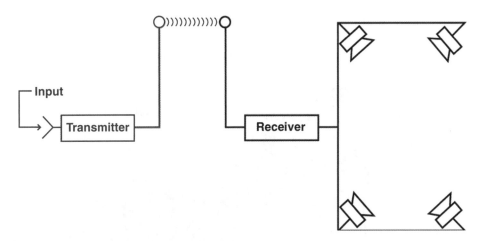

FIGURE 7.10 Sound-field amplification system.

equipped with sound-field amplification. The low cost of the system and its potential benefit to many students in the classroom, though, make it an attractive option for many schools.

A number of other populations known to have difficulty in classroom-type noise conditions may also receive benefit from sound-field amplification. These populations include children under age 15 years, children with phonological disorders, children with language disorders, children who are learning disabled, non–native English speakers, children with central auditory processing deficits, and children with a history of middle ear disease with effusion.

Bone-Anchored Hearing Aid

Some patients with hearing loss are unable to use conventional air conduction hearing aids because of pinna abnormalities (see Fig. 5.3), atresia (absence of ear canal), or chronic ear disease. Under such circumstances, bone conduction hearing aids can be a viable option. Traditional bone conduction hearing aids are devices that deliver amplified sound to the cochlea through a bone vibrator placed on the mastoid behind the ear. Traditionally, such devices have been used with body aids or with eyeglass hearing aids. With body instruments, the bone oscillator is mounted on one side of a headband and spring tension holds the vibrator firmly against the skull. With eyeglass hearing aids, the bone vibrator is fastened to the stem piece of the glasses. Bone conduction hearing aids typically have a number of drawbacks, including discomfort because of constant pressure from the steel spring, poor sound quality because the skin attenuates sound at higher frequencies, poor aesthetics, and insecure positioning of the vibrator. In recent years, there has been development of the bone-anchored hearing aid (BAHA), which appears to avoid many of the disadvantages of a conventional bone conduction hearing aid. BAHAs provide mechanical vibration that is transmitted to the skull by way of a titanium screw embedded in the mastoid. A small titanium implant in the skull behind the ear osseointegrates (bonds) with the living bone. An abutment is attached to the implant and a sound processor is clipped on— the sound processor can be worn or taken off at any time (Fig. 7.11).

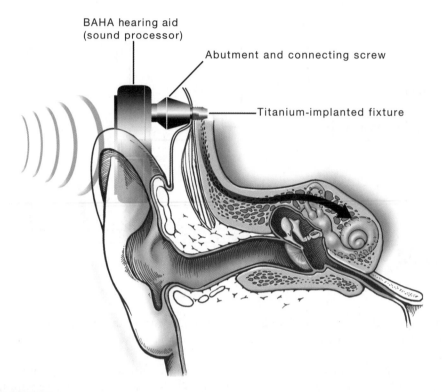

BAHA hearing aid
(sound processor)

Abutment and connecting screw

Titanium-implanted fixture

FIGURE 7.11 The BAHA (bone-anchored hearing aid). Note the amplified sound waves traveling to the inner ear. Adapted from http://www.cochlearamericas.com/products/2127.asp.

Candidates for this device are individuals with bone conduction thresholds better than or equal to 45 dB HL (0.5, 1, 2, 3 kHz). In addition to conductive and mixed hearing losses, BAHAs have been advocated for single-sided deafness due to trauma or surgery. For young children who can benefit from bone conduction hearing aids, implants are typically delayed until age 5—a time when the skull is thicker and stronger. Prior to the age of 5 years, children can wear an elastic band to hold the processor firmly in place.

Cochlear Implants

In the 1980s, the cochlear implant emerged as a viable alternative to conventional amplification for individuals with profound hearing loss. Several types of cochlear implants are available commercially today. They all share a common conceptual framework but differ in its implementation. The cochlear implant is a device that is surgically implanted, with its stimulating electrode array (wire) inserted directly into the cochlea. The implant contains 1 to 22 channels. Although some individuals still have the earlier single-channel cochlear implants, all contemporary devices make use of multiple electrode arrays. The electrode is used to stimulate the auditory nerve directly with electric current, bypassing the damaged cochlear structures. As in the conventional hearing aid, a microphone is used to convert the acoustic signal into an electrical one. The electrical signal is amplified and processed in various ways in a separate body-worn component, the stimulator. The stimulator is about the size of a body-worn hearing aid or a package of cigarettes. Recently, however, the stimulator and microphone have been combined into one ear-level unit, very similar to a BTE hearing aid. The output of the stimulator is sent to an external receiver worn behind the ear. This external receiver activates a similar internal receiver implanted surgically just under the skin and behind the ear. The implanted internal receiver converts the received signal into an electrical one and directs it to the electrode array penetrating the cochlea. This electrical signal, when routed to the electrode array, stimulates the remaining healthy auditory nerve fibers of the damaged inner ear. Figure 7.12 illustrates a typical arrangement for a cochlear implant and compares this device with a conventional hearing aid. As can be seen, these two devices share many features.

As previously noted, contemporary cochlear implants are multiple-channel devices. The channels essentially are adjacent bands in the frequency domain analogous to a series of band-pass filters. The sound picked up by the microphone is analyzed and sorted into several frequency-specific packets, or channels, of information by the processor. The output of each channel is routed to a corresponding electrode in the array, which is positioned in a specific location along the length of the cochlea. Thus, low-frequency channels are connected to electrodes in the more apical region of the cochlea, whereas high-frequency channels are connected to electrodes in more basal locations. This system is an attempt to restore tonotopic mapping (see Chapter 3) to the damaged cochlea.

For older children and adults, the *ideal* candidates for cochlear implants are those who acquired profound bilateral sensorineural hearing loss after acquiring language. Cochlear implants, however, appear to hold even greater promise for profoundly impaired children under 2 or 3 years of age, although research regarding the comparative benefits of rehabilitative devices in this population is still in progress. Although the results of clinical trials with these devices have varied markedly between patients, the best performance has been achieved with the multiple-channel devices. There are examples of so-called star patients who perform remarkably well with the device without any visual cues and do so almost immediately. At a minimum, just about every recipient benefits from the device as an aid to speech reading. Its primary usefulness as an aid to speech reading seems to lie in making gross cues of timing and voicing available to the patient. Great strides continue to be made in the devices and in the training programs after implantation, such that implants are probably the rehabilitative device of choice for the profoundly impaired, especially if implanted before acquisition of language for pre-lingual deafness.

Vibrotactile Devices

Many persons with profound hearing loss can receive little or no meaningful information through the ear. This is true whether the ear is stimulated with an acoustic signal in the case of the conventional hearing aid or an electrical one in the case of the cochlear implant. Often, this results in the use of alternative means of communication using normally functioning senses. Manual communication, or sign language, takes advantage of the normal sight of most of the population with hearing loss, including those with profound impairments. Adoption of manual communication as a primary means of communicating, however, restricts one to communicating with the small percentage of the population able to converse in sign language.

Other senses have also been explored for use as alternative means of encoding the acoustic signal. Various vibrotactile devices use tactual (touch) stimulation as an alternative to auditory stimulation. A microphone converts the acoustic signal to an electrical

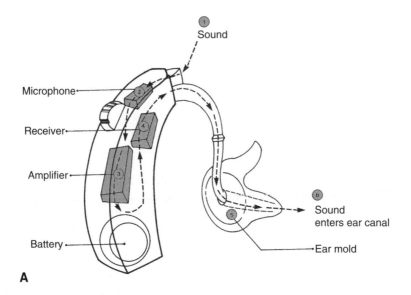

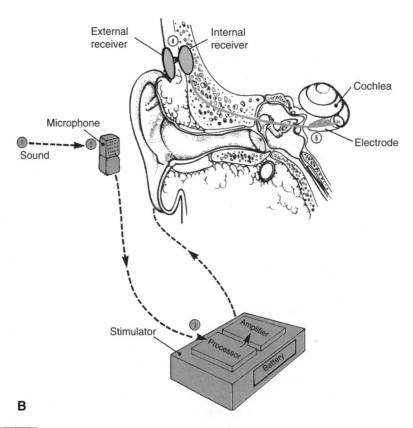

FIGURE 7.12 Similarities between conventional behind-the-ear hearing aid **(A)** and cochlear implant device **(B)**. The components of the systems are numbered identically to highlight the similarities.

one, as in the hearing aid and cochlear implant. The vibrotactile device uses this electrical signal to activate a series of vibrators. The vibrators, when activated by the electrical signal, make contact with the skin and stimulate the patient's sense of touch. The most common clinical vibrotactile devices are single-channel instruments. They stimulate the skin at a constant rate or frequency and increase the amplitude of vibration as the intensity of the acoustic signal increases. The vibrators for most clinical devices are worn on the hand, wrist, arm, or thigh. Multichannel devices, which attempt to mimic the auditory system's tonotopic organization (see Chapter 3) by routing sounds of different frequencies to vibrators at separate locations on the skin (along the length of the wrist or the length of the waist, for example) have been developed and are undergoing clinical evaluation. Generally, however, vibrotactile devices are primarily used as aids to speech reading and are much less common than either hearing aids or cochlear implants.

Device Management

The prosthetic device, whether a hearing aid, FM classroom device, cochlear implant, or vibrotactile aid, is one of the most important aspects of rehabilitation for most individuals with hearing loss. It is essential that every precaution be taken to ensure that the device is always in good working order.

For most individuals with hearing loss, the conventional electroacoustic hearing aid is the prosthetic device of choice. Care must be taken to avoid dropping the instrument or exposing the aid to severe environmental conditions, such as excessive moisture or heat. If dampness reaches the microphone or receiver, it can render the unit inoperable. It is also important to check the earmold or canal portion of the device periodically for blockage by cerumen and signs of wear from extended use, such as a cracked earmold or tubing. Perhaps the most common problem that interferes with adequate hearing aid performance is the battery or battery compartment area. Old batteries that have lost their charge, inappropriate battery size, inadequate battery contact, and improper battery placement are all problems that can contribute to a nonfunctional hearing aid.

Consistent amplification for the young child with hearing loss is essential, yet numerous school surveys have revealed that approximately half of children's hearing aids do not perform satisfactorily. The most common problems among children with hearing loss are weak batteries, inadequate earmolds, broken cords, bad receivers (sometimes the wrong receiver), and high distortion levels. Even the FM wireless systems are susceptible to faulty performance. Approximately 30 to 50% of these systems have been reported to perform unsatisfactorily in the classroom. The solution to inconsistent and inadequate amplification is implementation of a daily hearing aid check using a form like the one shown in Figure 7.13. In addition, the school audiologist must conduct a periodic electroacoustic analysis of every child's hearing aid.

REHABILITATION OF THE CHILD WITH HEARING LOSS

Management of the child with hearing loss is a monumental challenge to the clinical audiologist. In learning to understand the spoken language of others and to speak it, there is no adequate substitute for an intact auditory system. Without normal or near-normal hearing, it is extremely difficult to acquire an adequate oral communication system. Because so much language learning occurs in the first few years of life, there has been considerable emphasis on early identification and intervention for young children with hearing loss. The various approaches to early identification were outlined in Chapter 6 and are not restated here. For the most part, however, the earlier

```
Student _____
Teacher _____ Aid make/model _____
School _____ Serial no. _____
Classroom _____
Electroacoustic check _____ Y _____ N
Date of inspection _____
Overall condition: ____ Satisfactory _____ Marginal ____ Unsatisfactory ____ Missing
Recommendations _____
_____
_____

Examiner _____
```

Problem Checklist			

| | Inspected? | | |
Item	Yes	No	Comments
Battery	___	___	_____
Battery compartment	___	___	_____
Microphone	___	___	_____
Power switch	___	___	_____
Gain control	___	___	_____
Telephone switch	___	___	_____
Tone control	___	___	_____
Amplifier	___	___	_____
Cord	___	___	_____
Receiver	___	___	_____
Earmold	___	___	_____
Clip/case	___	___	_____
Harness	___	___	_____
Other	___	___	_____

```
As-worn setting:
  Volume control    _____
  Tone control      _____
  Receiver type     _____
```

FIGURE 7.13 Sample monitoring form for a personal hearing aid worn by a child.

one can identify the hearing loss, preferably during the first year of life, the sooner intervention can begin and the better the chances for a favorable outcome. Generally speaking, children with hearing loss who exhibit the best spoken language and show the most satisfactory progress in school are those who have had the benefit of early identification and intervention. The intervention must include adequate parent-infant management, wearable amplification, speech and language training, and development of perceptual and cognitive skills.

Choosing the Appropriate Communication Mode

An important issue facing audiologists, teachers, and school officials is determining which educational approach is most appropriate for a given child with hearing loss. Presently, two primary modes of instruction are recommended in the educational system: auditory-oral communication and total communication. The auditory-oral approach places emphasis entirely on the auditory system for developing receptive and expressive forms of communication, whereas total communication emphasizes a combination of audition, vision, finger spelling, and signs for achieving the same goal. These approaches are discussed in greater detail in Chapter 8. Although most would agree that oral language maximizes the options available to the child, the reality is that not all children are able to learn spoken English. Even in total communication programs, decisions are sometimes made about whether to emphasize oral language or manual communication. How, then, does one determine which mode of communication is most beneficial?

Two approaches have been proposed for audiologists who must determine whether a child with hearing loss would be better off in an auditory-oral or a total-communication program of instruction. One is the Deafness Management Quotient (DMQ). The DMQ uses a weighted point system (total of 100 points) to quantify a number of factors about the child and the child's environment. These factors include the amount of residual hearing (30 points), central auditory system intactness (30 points), intellectual factors (20 points), family constellation (10 points), and socioeconomic issues (10 points). A child scoring more than 80 points is recommended for an auditory-oral program. Unfortunately, it is very difficult to quantify objectively the recommended factors, and more important, the DMQ has not been adequately validated. An alternative index, known as the Spoken Language Predictor (SLP), was proposed and validated. Similar to the DMQ, the SLP incorporates five factors considered important to a child's success in an auditory-oral program. The factors are weighted, and a point score (total of 100 points) is derived. The factors include hearing capacity (30 points), language competence (25 points), nonverbal intelligence (20 points), family support (15 points), and speech communication attitude (10 points). Children with scores of 80 to 100 are judged to have excellent potential for developing spoken language. Not only can the SLP be of use in deciding on placement, but it can also verify the appropriateness of placement for an older child already enrolled in a program.

Let us now review some of the appropriate management strategies for children with hearing loss. The approaches to be discussed can accommodate either an auditory-oral or a total communication emphasis.

Parent-Infant Management

The first 3 years of life are critical to a child's general development, especially with respect to communication, and the parents of young handicapped children often lack the skills necessary to optimize family-infant interactions, which could facilitate the child's communication development. Awareness of this situation has led to parent-infant intervention programs. In addition to espousing early identification and intervention, most parent-oriented programs include family support for parents and members of the child's extended family. Information exchange, demonstration teaching (in which the family explores a variety of strategies to assist the child in achieving communication), and educational advocacy for the parents are also frequently included. The latter entails helping the parents to become effective consumers of services and knowledgeable child advocates.

An important component of a parent-infant curriculum is audiologic management and amplification. Here the emphasis is on helping the child to develop his or her auditory potential. Emphasis is placed on further clarification of the nature of the hearing loss, selection of amplification, and the development of full-time hearing aid use.

Teaching parents the importance of care and maintenance of hearing aids is also an important dimension. Another element of effective parent-infant management is auditory training, an organized sequential approach to the development of listening skills. Here, the emphasis is on developing a program of auditory training experiences that will guide the parents through a developmental sequence for their child that parallels the development of auditory perceptual skills in the normal-hearing infant. The hierarchy of skills can be divided into the following levels:

1. Auditory perception of both environmental sounds and the human voice
2. Awareness of environmental sounds and the human voice as conveyors of information and association of sounds with their physical sources
3. Development of an auditory-vocal feedback mechanism in which the child monitors his or her own speech
4. Comprehension of meaning in syllables, words, phrases, and sentences
5. Increasing verbal comprehension and the emergence of auditory memory and sequencing skills

Another important component of parent-infant management is vocal play strategies for speech habilitation. The initiation and maintenance of vocal behavior is a major area of the early-intervention program that is critical to young children. Full-time use of amplification is important so that the child with hearing loss can hear his or her own speech as well as the speech of others. The use of an auditory program to enhance the use of the auditory feedback mechanism is also important. Further, parents are taught to use vocal play interaction techniques that are necessary for the development of prelinguistic speech skills. Parents must also learn to develop strategies that facilitate social and communicative turn taking.

Finally, there are the verbal interaction techniques of language programming. At this point, the focus is on teaching the parent communicative interaction styles, particularly verbal interaction patterns, which enhance the child's acquisition of language. Linguistic development is maximized by training parents to incorporate the principles of adult-child interaction patterns that are reported to occur during the language acquisition of normal children.

Amplification

The importance of amplification to the child with hearing loss cannot be overemphasized. The personal hearing aid and other amplification devices are the primary link many of these children have to an auditory society. If these children are to develop speech and language in a manner somewhat similar to that of the normal-hearing child, everything possible must be done to capitalize on whatever residual hearing exists. Toward this end, the child receives amplification (usually binaural) soon after identification. The audiologist then offers periodic hearing evaluations and modifies the hearing aid as more is learned about the child's hearing sensitivity.

Language: Characteristics, Assessment, and Training

Language may be defined as a systematic code used to represent the concepts that designate experience and to facilitate social interaction. Oral language is the primary means by which humans communicate with one another. Although a comprehensive review of language is beyond the scope of this book, a general knowledge of the dimensions of language is important to the understanding of management issues.

Most would agree that there are three components of language: form, content, and use. Form pertains to the elements of language and the rules for combining those elements. The three aspects of form include phonology (the sounds or phonemes of the language), syntax (word order rules), and morphology (the internal structure of words). In learning phonology, children acquire the rules for how sounds can be sequenced to formulate words. For example, in English, the/mp/sequence of phonemes can appear at the end of a word (e.g., jump) but not at the beginning of a word. In learning syntax, children acquire the rules for how words are combined to form grammatical sentences. For example, in a question, a subject noun and an auxiliary can be inverted (e.g., Is he eating cookies?) but a subject noun and main verb cannot be inverted (e.g., Eats he cookies?). In learning morphology, children acquire the rules for how inflections are added to words (e.g., the plural of *cookie* is *cookies*). To learn language, children must process language input (e.g., the talk of their caregiver) and hypothesize the rules to formulate grammatical sentences.

The second component of language is content, also referred to as semantics. Children must learn the meaning of individual words and of particular phrases (e.g., raining cats and dogs). The final component of language is pragmatics, or the ability to use language to communicate effectively, such as how to engage in conversation and how to use language to meet a variety of goals (e.g., seek information, answer questions). The development of language is an extremely complex process involving the acquisition of skill in each component of language.

Therefore, it is not surprising to learn that children with hearing loss have great difficulty in learning language through speech. This difficulty increases with increasing hearing loss. Most research dealing with the language characteristics of children with hearing loss has focused on the form component because errors in form (phonemes, morphemes, and syntax) are relatively easy to quantify. In addition, the acquisition of form may be more challenging than the acquisition of content and use. Nevertheless, it is important to realize that researchers have documented language learning difficulties in all aspects of language—form, content, and use—for children with hearing loss.

Many commercially available instruments are designed to assist the clinician in the ongoing evaluation of a child's language development. Although formal language tests explore a wide range of language skills, for the most part they do not adequately evaluate a child's ability to use language in day-to-day situations. Hence, clinicians always have to explore informal nonstandardized tasks to obtain information in areas not covered by the standard diagnostic tools. Language sampling can be an invaluable tool in determining the extent to which hearing loss is affecting the development and the interaction of content, form, and use in the child's language system as the child engages in authentic communication.

A number of approaches have been used in language intervention, most of which have focused on the syntactic forms of language. These approaches can be classified as either analytic or natural methods for teaching language. Analytic methods have concentrated on the form of a child's language, and most techniques categorize the various parts of speech grammatically. These approaches are also characterized by extensive drills and exercises. An example of the analytical method is the Fitzgerald key, which emphasizes the analysis of relationships among discrete units through the visual aid of written language. Students classify words from a sentence as to whether they belong in a *who*, *what*, or *where* category. The natural approach, sometimes called the experiential method, holds that language is learned through experiences, not systematic drills and exercises. This content/unit approach emphasizes identifying areas of interest for the child that serve as the basis for teaching vocabulary and sentence structure in meaningful contexts and practicing spoken and later written language.

More recently, language intervention approaches have begun to consider modern language theory and to develop strategies that attempt to integrate syntactic, pragmatic, and semantic levels. The reader interested in learning more should consult the suggested readings at the end of this chapter.

Speech Production: Characteristics, Assessment, and Training

We noted earlier that significant hearing losses make it difficult not only to understand speech but also to produce it. Nevertheless, it is the consensus that many children with hearing loss, even those with profound losses, can develop speech skills. Children with hearing loss manifest a variety of speech production errors categorized as either segmental (i.e., phonemic and phonetic) or suprasegmental (i.e., related to intonation and prosody). The most common segmental errors include the omission of word-final sounds and substitution errors for both consonants and vowels. Suprasegmental errors include inadequate timing, which results in very slow, labored speech, and poor control of the fundamental frequency, causing abnormal pitch and distorted intonation. Predictably, as the frequency of errors increases, overall intelligibility decreases.

Assessment of speech production is not as easy as one might predict, because many of the tools were designed for normal-hearing children. The evaluation of segmental errors is usually conducted with commonly available picture identification tests. Because most of these tests do not consider the unavoidable problems of testing the child with hearing loss, it is fairly common for the clinician to develop informal tests that will focus on specific segmental errors frequently seen in this population. Assessment of overall intelligibility of conversational speech is also important for the planning of an intervention program. Some clinicians record spontaneous speech samples, which are judged by a group of listeners to evaluate a child's intelligibility.

Perhaps the most popular method for teaching speech to the child with hearing loss is an approach advocated by Daniel Ling. Very briefly, this method focuses on using the child's residual hearing to monitor speech production and to understand the speech of others. The attempt is to duplicate the experience of normal-hearing children. The teaching of speech is carried out primarily at the phonetic and phonologic levels, with emphasis on the phonetic domain. At the phonetic level, there is emphasis on nonsense syllable drills (i.e., /ta, ta, ta/, or /ti, ta, to/). Several stages are proposed in which target behaviors are established using criterion-referenced skills. A child must complete each phase satisfactorily before moving on to the next level. These stages include undifferentiated vocalizations; suprasegmental voice patterns; a range of distinctly different vowel sounds; consonants contrasted in manner of production; consonants contrasted in manner and place of production; consonants contrasted in manner, place, and voicing; and consonant blends. The following additional strategies have been suggested to supplement the Ling approach:

1. Production by imitation: the child produces the target sound using auditory clues only
2. Production on demand: the child produces the target sound from visual cues
3. Discrimination: the child selects the speech pattern from a closed set of alternative speech patterns produced by the clinician or model
4. Self-evaluation: the child evaluates his or her own speech production

REHABILITATION OF THE ADULT WITH HEARING LOSS

The rehabilitation techniques used with the adult with hearing loss are quite different from the approaches used with children. There are similarities, however. The individual must receive a careful assessment to determine the nature and extent of the problem; amplification plays a major role in the rehabilitation; and the techniques and strategies used in rehabilitation are determined by the information elicited in the assessment phase.

Assessment Issues

In the introduction to this chapter, we talked about the importance of the assessment phase and how it is used to establish a rehabilitative program. The assessment or identification phase typically consists of a comprehensive case history, pure-tone audiometry, immittance measurements, speech recognition tests, a communication-specific self-assessment questionnaire, and occasionally a measure of speech-reading ability. Because we have already reviewed in some detail the basic assessment battery (case history, pure-tone audiometry, immittance measurements, and speech recognition), we focus here on questionnaires and speech-reading skills in the planning of rehabilitation programs.

Assessment With Communication Scales

Communication scales must be a part of every assessment approach. These scales usually assess how the hearing loss affects everyday living, that is, the way in which the hearing deficit affects psychosocial, emotional, or vocational performance. Such information can be valuable in determining the need for and probable success of amplification, irrespective of the degree of hearing loss and the specific areas in which the rehabilitation should occur. Most scales focus on communication-specific skills. Examples of questions that could be included in such a scale: *Do you have difficulty hearing when someone speaks in a whisper? Does a hearing problem cause you difficulty when listening to TV or radio?*

The answers to such questions illuminate listening problems. Once the areas of difficulty have been identified, possible solutions can be considered. For example, if the individual reports difficulty only when listening to a television or radio, an assistive listening device might be considered. If a patient reports difficulty in a variety of listening situations and notes a tendency to withdraw from social activities because of the hearing loss, the individual is a good candidate for a personal hearing aid. Counseling for this patient and the patient's relatives might also be indicated. Furthermore, the audiologist may wish to develop techniques for improving speech reading and auditory training skills in situations that present listening difficulty. Numerous communication scales are available to the audiologist, and it is not possible to review all of them in an introductory book. Four commonly used scales are the HHIE-S, the Abbreviated Profile of Hearing Aid Benefit (APHAB), the Client Oriented Scale of Improvement (COSI), and the Hearing Performance Inventory (HPI). The HHIE-S is described in some detail in Chapter 6. Briefly, the HHIE-S is a self-administered 10-item questionnaire designed to detect emotional and social problems associated with hearing loss. Subjects respond to questions about circumstances related to hearing by stating whether the situation presents a problem. The questions for the HHIE-S appear in Table 6.7. The APHAB is a 24-item questionnaire—half of the questions are used to assess unaided ability; the other half are used to assess aided ability. The APHAB was designed to survey communication abilities and the sound quality of hearing aids. The APHAB is scored separately for its subscales—ease of communication (EC), reverberation (RV), background noise (BN), and the aversiveness of sounds (AV). Patients respond to the different questions on a rating scale from always to never. Examples of questions include the following: *When I am in a grocery store, talking with a cashier, can I follow the conversation? Are unexpected sounds, like a smoke detector or alarm bell, uncomfortable. Are traffic noises too loud.* The examiner administers the unaided part of the scale first—this portion of the scale offers valuable information about the types of difficulties the patient has in everyday listening situations. Several weeks after the patient receives the hearing aids, the aided portion of the APHAB can be administered. The difference in the aided versus the unaided performance yields a percentage of aided benefit. With the COSI, at the initial interview the audiologist identifies important listening situations in which the patient would like to hear more clearly. Typically, five listening situations are sufficient to provide a focus for the rehabilitation program. Once the listening situations have been identified, it is possible to determine the patients' expectations of hearing aids. The situations identified in the initial interview can be used post hearing aid fitting and rehabilitation to determine the benefits provided.

Finally, the HPI is a more comprehensive scale than the HHS. It probes hearing-impaired patients across several dimensions rather than only one. These dimensions include speech comprehension, signal intensity, response to auditory failure, social effects of hearing loss, personal effects of hearing loss, and occupational difficulties. Examples of items on the HPI are as follows: *"You are home reading in a quiet room. Do you hear the telephone ring when it is in another room?"* "At the beginning of a conversation, do you let a stranger know that you have a hearing problem?" In this inventory, the patient is queried about a specific listening environment and responds to each item with practically always, frequently, about half the time, occasionally, or almost never. The original version of the HPI was quite long, taking approximately 60 minutes to administer and score. A shortened version (approximately 35 minutes) is also available. The HPI affords valuable information regarding the impact of hearing loss on communication and identifies the general listening situations in which the patient has trouble. It is also useful as a formal performance measure that can be used at the initial assessment and to track progress during rehabilitation.

Assessment of Speech Reading Skills

The ability to use vision as an aid to understanding spoken English is another important area of assessment. Several tests are available for assessing a patient's speech reading or lipreading skills. One such test is the Denver Quick Test of Lipreading Ability, a group of 20 short, simple statements (Table 7.3). The test is scored in terms of percentage correct, with each test item representing 5%. The test can be used to assess speech reading abilities in a vision-only mode or in a combination of vision and hearing. Performance in the vision-only mode can offer valuable diagnostic information. A low score on the Denver Test suggests that the patient needs speech reading instruction, that is, instruction in paying attention to visual cues to complement auditory input. The use of both modes offers insight into how the patient will perform under realistic conditions and should also be helpful in determining how well the individual will perform with amplification.

TABLE 7.3	Items on the Denver Quick Test of Lipreading Ability

1. Good morning.	11. May I help you?
2. How old are you?	12. I feel fine.
3. I live in [state of residence].	13. It is time for dinner.
4. I only have one dollar.	14. Turn right at the corner.
5. There is somebody at the door.	15. Are you ready to order?
6. Is that all?	16. Is this charge or cash?
7. Where are you going?	17. What time is it?
8. Let's have a coffee break.	18. I have a headache.
9. Park your car in the lot.	19. How about going out tonight?
10. What is your address?	20. Please lend me 50 cents.

Reprinted from Alpiner JG, Schow RL. Rehabilitative evaluation of hearing-impaired adult. In Alpiner JG, McCarthy PA, eds. Rehabilitative Audiology: Children and Adults. 2nd ed. Baltimore: Williams & Wilkins, 1993.

Management Strategies For the Adult With Hearing Loss

Importance of Counseling

Counseling should be a central focus of any management strategy for the adult with hearing loss. In fact, the adult with hearing loss should receive counseling both before and after receiving a hearing aid. Counseling is a vital part of the assessment phase because it elicits information about the patient's communication problems. The first component of counseling is to explain to the patient, in lay terms, the nature and extent of the hearing loss. If the audiologist believes that the patient can benefit from amplification, counseling is needed to discuss with the patient the value of a hearing aid and what can be expected from it. Modification of the patient's motivation and attitudes may also be appropriate at this juncture. The audiologist will have information from the assessment data on the patient's feelings about wearing a hearing aid. Often the patient has no real interest in a hearing aid but is simply responding to the will of a spouse or significant other. Some receive misleading information about hearing aids from friends or from advertisements. In fact, the Internet has resulted in a large increase in the amount of hearing aid information and misinformation being distributed. Unsubstantiated and substantiated claims and direct-to-consumer marketing have greatly influenced patients' expectations. Some patients are concerned about whether the hearing aid will show because of the stigma commonly associated with deafness or aging in the United States (Vignette 7.10). Under such circumstances, the objective of the audiologist is to help the individual with hearing loss realize that many of the fears or concerns about hearing loss or hearing aids are unwarranted. The individual should be counseled about how the use of amplification can help in a variety of listening situations.

Counseling is also sometimes appropriate for relatives and friends who have developed erroneous impressions about hearing loss and amplification. For example, a patient with a high-frequency sensorineural hearing loss typically has difficulty in understanding speech. Relatives and friends sometimes interpret this difficulty as a sign of senility, inattention, or even stupidity. It is helpful for the audiologist to counsel relatives and friends about the nature and extent of hearing loss and the psychosocial complications associated with a hearing deficit. Reviewing such information

VIGNETTE 7.10   The hearing aid effect

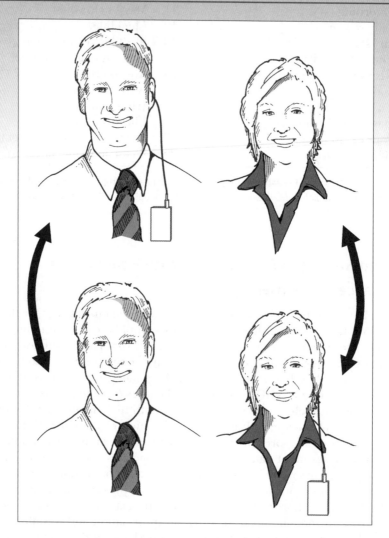

Examine the two top pictures. How would you rate the person on the left on a continuum from bright to dull or from smart to dumb or from pretty to ugly? How about the person on the right at the top?

Now, examine the two pictures at the bottom. How would you rate these two individuals on the same continua?

The two people pictured in the top are the same as the two in the bottom, but the one wearing the hearing aid has changed. Researchers have had large groups of subjects rate their impressions of real photographs similar to these drawings along similar continua. The researchers counterbalanced the design so that each person is pictured wearing a hearing aid by the conclusion of the testing. The results indicate that the presence of a hearing aid on the individual in the photo leads to lower ratings on many continua. This negative image associated with the wearing of a hearing aid is called the hearing aid effect. It has been documented in adults and children alike and is part of the stigma hearing aid wearers must overcome.

with loved ones helps them to understand better and to be more tolerant of the listening difficulties caused by a significant hearing loss. The audiologist may also choose to offer suggestions for enhancing communication. The significant other can be counseled in the use of deliberate, unhurried speech, good illumination of the speaker's face, and care to ensure that the lips are clearly visible.

Once the hearing aid has been purchased or just before a purchase, the patient is counseled about the use and care of a hearing aid. The audiologist reviews the manipulation of the various controls, the function of the battery compartment, troubleshooting techniques in cases of malfunction, the proper care of the earmold or shell, and the warranty of the hearing aid. A potential difficulty is that patients often have unrealistic expectations for a hearing aid, especially in the initial stages of use. The audiologist must take care to advise the patient with hearing loss about the limitations of amplification and to help the individual adjust to very difficult listening situations, such as competing speech and competing background noise. Finally, some patients need special help in the manipulation of hearing aid controls. This common problem among the elderly is discussed in more detail later in this chapter.

Throughout the rehabilitation cycle, counseling is a continuing process. The audiologist spends time listening, advising, and responding to the needs and concerns of the individual with hearing loss.

Instruction for Speech Reading and Auditory Training

The two primary training aspects of aural rehabilitation for the adult are speech reading and auditory training. Speech reading refers to the ability of a person, any person, to use vision as a supplement to audition when communicating. All persons, regardless of the degree of impairment, can benefit from visual cues. At one time, speech reading was referred to as simply as *lipreading*. The change in label to *speech reading* has come about in recognition of the fact that more than just the talker's lips provide important visual cues to understanding speech.

Speech reading should be viewed not as a replacement for auditory coding of speech but as an important supplement. With visual information alone, approximately 50 to 60% of a spoken message typically can be understood by the average person. However, individuals vary widely in this ability.

Acquisition of speech reading skills can take hours of training. There are two basic approaches to speech reading training: analytic and synthetic. Analytic methods begin with training on individual speech sounds and progress to words, phrases, sentences, and continuous discourse, in sequence. The synthetic approach begins training at the phrase or sentence level. The synthetic approach seems to be more widely used by audiologists. Training usually begins with simple, commonly encountered questions such as *What is your name?* or *What time is it?* It then progresses to less frequently encountered statements and continuous discourse.

Auditory training refers to training the individual with hearing loss to use his or her hearing as well as possible. The approaches vary with the onset of the hearing loss. Typically, a hierarchy of skills is developed at the phoneme and word level, beginning with detection of the sound or word. (Can the patient hear anything when the sound is spoken?) The next goal is discrimination of the targeted sound or word. (Is it the same or different from some other sounds or words?) This is followed by development of skills in identification of the sound or word. (Which one of several words or sounds was it?) The final goal is often to develop proficiency in the open-set recognition of the speech sound or word. (What sound or word was it?) Auditory training is encouraged for all individuals wearing a hearing aid for the first time. It takes time and training to learn to understand speech with a hearing aid. Many individuals with hearing loss have never heard speech or have heard it through the distortion of the hearing loss—in many cases, for several years—before seeking assistance. Fitting the hearing aid or other rehabilitative device will not bring about an instant restoration of normal function. Recent research indicates that at least 3 to 6 months may be required for many hearing aid wearers to attain maximum levels of speech communication with their hearing aids. In fact, many patients will probably never perform *completely* as well as a normal-hearing person does, especially in the adverse listening conditions all too commonly encountered in everyday communication. With continued training, however, they can come much closer to achieving this objective. Auditory training is designed to maximize the use of residual hearing, whereas speech reading is meant to supplement the reduced information received through the auditory system. Extensive training in both areas can result in very effective use of the rehabilitative device chosen for the patient.

Listening Training, Speech Conservation, and Speech Tracking

Another role of the audiologist is to help the patient with hearing loss develop or maintain good listening skills and to assist the patient in maintaining good speech production skills. Listening training refers to helping the patient to attend better to the spoken message. Some people simply have poor listening skills, and this problem is exacerbated in the presence of a hearing loss. The emphasis in listening training is on teaching the impaired listener to be alert, attentive, and ready to receive the spoken message. Training should focus on eliminating or avoiding distractions, learning to focus on the speaker's main points, attending to nonverbal information, keeping visual contact with the speaker, and mentally preparing oneself to listen to the speaker.

As hearing loss increases, it becomes more difficult for an individual to monitor his or her own speech production. This inability results in faulty speech characterized by poor vocal quality, nasality, segmental errors, and suprasegmental errors. Under such conditions, learning the effective use of kinesthetic (sensation of movement) cues is essential for awareness of the segmental elements of speech. The patient must become physically aware of the kinesthetic qualities of each phonetic element in speech. Auditory training and speech reading can also help in preserving the perception of subtle nuances in the speech message. Those with hearing loss need techniques for developing an awareness of the rhythm, quality, intonation, and loudness of one's own speech. Finally, the importance of listening is critical to this population, and the enhancement of listening skills should be part of any speech conservation program.

Speech tracking is a procedure in which a reader presents connected speech and a listener repeats the message, word for word or syllable for syllable. Both the speaker and the listener participate in the procedure, with the impaired listener attempting to immediately imitate the speaker. The technique has great face validity because the material approximates normal communication more closely than single words do. Tracking ability is measured in terms of the number of words tracked per minute. Rate of speech tracking improves with rehabilitative training (speech reading and/or auditory training) and with the use of amplification or alternative rehabilitation devices. Speech tracking can be used as a tool in aural rehabilitation, especially for measuring the effects of rehabilitation or training.

Special Considerations for the Elderly With Hearing Loss

We have noted on several occasions throughout this text that a large number of elderly people exhibit significant hearing losses. Typically, the hearing loss in the aged is a mild to moderate bilateral high-frequency sensorineural hearing loss with associated difficulty in understanding conversational speech (see Chapter 5). The loss usually begins around 50 years of age and progresses. In addition, speech understanding difficulties become greater when the listening task is made more difficult. Such hearing loss adversely affects both the functional health status and the psychosocial well-being of the impaired individual. It is generally thought that hearing loss can produce withdrawal, poor self-concept, depression, frustration, irritability, senility, isolation, and loneliness.

Despite the high prevalence of hearing loss among the elderly and the accepted psychosocial complications, the elderly with hearing loss are not usually referred for audiologic intervention. Frequently, they are not considered candidates for amplification until they reach advanced old age. The reasons for this are not clear. Some elderly persons believe that their deafness is simply another unavoidable aspect of aging. This feeling lessens the person's felt need to seek rehabilitation or the ability to justify it. This belief, combined with an inadequate knowledge and low expectations of rehabilitative measures, seems to discourage these individuals from seeking assistance. Even those who do seek assistance often fail to use their hearing aids to the fullest. In fact, some stop using their amplification systems soon after purchase.

The special problems of the elderly with hearing loss require that the audiologist educate physicians and lay persons about the benefits of hearing aids. Audiologists must also recognize the special needs of this population. For example, during the assessment phase, one must determine whether there are any limitations in upper body movement or any arthritis. These conditions can interfere with an individual's ability to reach, grasp, or manipulate a hearing aid. Such information is most helpful in deciding on the type of hearing aid to be recommended. For example, a small ITC hearing aid with tiny controls is inappropriate for an individual who has arthritis affecting the hands and arms (Vignette 7.11). Another important consideration in the assessment phase is the visual acuity of the patient. Like hearing, vision declines with increasing age. Because visual acuity is important for receiving auditory-visual information, it is prudent for the audiologist to assess the visual abilities of an elderly patient. This can be done simply by posing questions about visual status to the person with hearing loss. Examples of such questions include these:

1. Do you have problems with your vision? If so, what kind?
2. Do you wear eyeglasses? Do they help you to see?
3. Are you able to see my mouth clearly?

Some audiologists actually test for far visual acuity using the well-known Snellen eye chart.

A check of mental status is also appropriate for the elderly population. Many elderly individuals exhibit declines in cognitive function that would reduce the likelihood of successful use of a hearing aid. Formal tests are available to assess mental status. In lieu of these, however, the audiologist can simply pose questions about the patient's cognitive functioning (i.e., memory, general knowledge, orientation). If there are problems with mental status, the audiologist will need to work closely with a significant other to ensure appropriate use and care of the hearing aid.

VIGNETTE 7.11   Remote controls for hearing aids

One way to overcome manual dexterity and vision difficulties of many elderly persons while using hearing aids is to use a remote control. The hearing aid remote control is a handheld device not unlike the remote controls used with many televisions, DVD players, and stereo systems. The remote control communicates with the hearing aid and adjusts its settings via infrared transmission. An example of one type of remote control is shown in the drawing. The large size makes it easier both to manipulate and to see than the corresponding controls on a BTE or ITE hearing aid. The remote controls can include on-off switches, volume controls for one or two hearing aids, and for multiple-program digital hearing aids, a program selector (much like the channel selector on a TV remote control), which lets the wearer choose the set of hearing aid settings he or she wishes to use in specific situations.

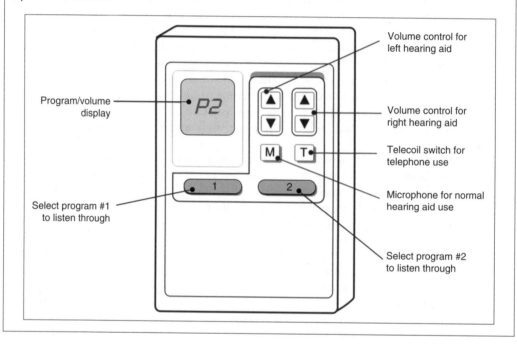

Program/volume display

P2

Volume control for left hearing aid

Volume control for right hearing aid

Telecoil switch for telephone use

Microphone for normal hearing aid use

Select program #1 to listen through

Select program #2 to listen through

Other factors to be considered before amplification is recommended to an elderly person include motivation, family support, financial resources, and lifestyle. Special attention is also important for the elderly during the hearing aid orientation program. Greater care is required to explain the various components of a hearing aid. Furthermore, the audiologist should schedule elderly patients for periodic follow-up visits to monitor the patients' progress and to review questions and concerns that they may have about their amplification devices. When considering amplification for this group, one must recognize that they could benefit from many of the assistive listening devices described earlier in this chapter. Many of the problems exhibited by this group center on using the telephone, watching television, and understanding speech in group situations, such as church or public auditoriums.

To summarize, the elderly with hearing loss have unique problems and concerns that require the special consideration of the audiologist throughout the rehabilitation process. If the audiologist attends to these needs and concerns, there is a far greater probability that use of a hearing aid will be successful.

SUMMARY

This chapter reviews and discusses the pertinent aspects of amplification and rehabilitation of children and adults with hearing loss. The hearing aid is the most important rehabilitative tool available for management of those with hearing loss. Numerous types of amplification systems, including personal hearing aids, assistive listening devices, and classroom systems, are available for the habilitation or rehabilitation of individuals with hearing loss. Further, this chapter addresses some of the varied rehabilitative approaches used for children and adults with hearing loss.

References and Suggested Readings

Bess FH, Gravel JS, Tharpe AM. Amplification for Children With Auditory Deficits. Nashville: Bill Wilkerson Center, 1996.

Bloom L, Lahey M. Language Development and Language Disorders. New York: Wiley, 1978.

Byrne D. Theoretical prescriptive approaches to selecting the gain and frequency response of a hearing aid. Monogr Contemp Audiol 4:1–40, 1983.

Clark JG, Martin FN. Effective Counseling in Audiology: Perspectives and Practice. Englewood Cliffs, NJ: Prentice Hall, 1994.

Dillon H. Hearing Aids. New York: Thieme, 2001.

Fitzgerald MT, Bess FH. Parent/infant training for hearing-impaired children. Monogr Contemp Audiol 3:1–24, 1982.

Geers AE, Moog JS. Predicting spoken language acquisition of profoundly hearing impaired children. J Speech Hear Dis 52:84–94, 1987.

Hawkins D, Yacullo W. The signal-to-noise ratio advantage of binaural hearing aids and directional microphones under different levels of reverberation. J Speech Hearing Dis 49:278–286, 1984.

Katz J. Handbook of Clinical Audiology. 5th ed. Baltimore: Lippincott Williams & Wilkins, in 2001.

Kretschmer RR, Kretschmer LW. Communication/language assessment of the hearing-impaired child. In Bess FH, ed. Hearing Impairment in Children. Parkton, MD: York, 1988.

Ling D. Speech and the Hearing-Impaired Child: Theory and Practice. Washington: Alexander Graham Bell Association for the Deaf, 1976.

Moeller MP, Brunt MA. Management of preschool hearing-impaired children: A cognitive-linguistic approach. In Bess FH, ed. Hearing Impairment in Children. Parkton, MD: York, 1988.

Moeller MP, Carney AE. Assessment and intervention with preschool hearing-impaired children. In Alpiner JG, McCarthy PA, eds. Rehabilitative Audiology: Children and Adults. 2nd ed. Baltimore: Williams & Wilkins, 1993.

Mueller HG, Johnson EE, Carter AS. Hearing aids and assistive devices. In Schow RL, Nerbonne MA, eds. Introduction to Audiologic Rehabilitation. 5th ed. Boston: Allyn & Bacon, 2007.

Mueller HG, Hawkins DB, Northern JL. Probe Microphone Measurements: Hearing Aid Selection and Assessment. San Diego: Singular, 1992.

Norlin PF, Van Tassell DJ. Linguistic skills of hearing-impaired children. Monogr Contemp Audiol 2:1–32, 1980.

Northern JL, Downs MP. Hearing in Children. 5th ed. Baltimore: Lippincott Williams & Wilkins, 2002.

Pascoe DP. Hearing Aids. Who Needs Them? St. Louis: Big Bend, 1991.

Ricketts TA, Tharpe AM, DeChicchis AR, Bess FH. Amplification selection for children with hearing impairment. In Bluestone CD, Alper CM, Arjmand EM, et al., eds. Pediatric Otolaryngology. 4th ed. Philadelphia: Harcourt Health Sciences, 2001.

Sanders DA. Management of Hearing Handicap: Infants to Elderly. 4th ed. Englewood Cliffs, NJ: Prentice Hall, 1999.

Seewald RC, ed. A Sound Foundation Through Early Amplification. Chicago: Phonak, 2000.

Seewald RC, Gravel JS, eds. A Sound Foundation Through Early Amplification, 2001. Chicago: Phonak, 2002.

Schow RL, Nerbonne MA, eds. Introduction to Audiologic Rehabilitation. 5th ed. Boston: Pearson Education, 2007.

Skinner MW. Hearing Aid Evaluation. Englewood Cliffs, NJ: Prentice-Hall, 1988.

Studebaker GA, Bess FH, eds. Vanderbilt Hearing Aid Report. Monogr Contemp Audiol, 1982.

Studebaker GA, Bess FH, Beck LB, eds. Vanderbilt Hearing Aid Report II. Parkton, MD: York, 1991.

Pediatric Work Group of the Conference on Amplification for Children With Auditory Deficits: Amplification for infants and children with hearing loss. Am J Audiol 5:53–68, 1996.

CHAPTER 8

Audiology and the Education of Individuals With Hearing Loss

After completion of this chapter the reader should be able to:

- List and describe the legislative provisions for children with hearing loss and their families.
- Describe the educational programs and settings available for children with hearing loss.
- Describe the educational achievements exhibited by today's children with hearing loss.
- Understand the impact of varying degrees of hearing loss on educational performance.
- Develop an appreciation for the role of audiology in the educational setting.

Previous chapters referred to the importance of the auditory system for acquiring information about the world. Significant hearing loss can result in serious developmental complications, such as delays in development of language, speech production and understanding, and cognition. Also, in the absence of hearing, the symbol system we traditionally use for developing and verbally expressing thoughts and ideas is not automatically perceived and learned. Given this background, it should come as no surprise to learn that children with hearing loss often exhibit significant lags in educational achievement.

Education is a process of imparting to individuals information that will prepare them for life and enable them to use their native abilities in a meaningful and constructive manner. When one considers the method by which information is imparted, it becomes apparent that auditory input from teacher to student and from student to student is critical to acquiring an education in the typical manner. Vision also plays a vital role but is secondary to hearing. One need only watch a television program without the sound to gain some realization of what children with hearing loss experience in the classroom. Communication through hearing, so natural and automatic that it is taken for granted by most people, is reduced dramatically between a teacher and a child with hearing loss. Many students enrolled in an introductory audiology class are likely to be faced with the responsibility of working with a child with hearing loss later in their career. This chapter, therefore, focuses on educational programming and the educational difficulties of children with hearing loss.

LEGISLATIVE PROVISIONS FOR HANDICAPPED CHILDREN

In 1975, part B of the Education of the Handicapped Act (known as the Education for All Handicapped Children Act—Public Law 94-142) was passed by Congress and signed into law. Public Law (PL) 94-142 focuses on the rights and protection of handicapped children and their parents. Briefly, the law has four major functions. First, it guarantees the availability of a special education program to all handicapped children and youth who require it. This is true without regard for factors, such as geographic residence, that contributed to many inequities of opportunity in the past. Second, the law assures fair and appropriate decision making in providing special education to handicapped children and youth. Third, PL 94-142 established, at every level of government, clear management, auditing requirements, and procedures for special education. Fourth, the law assists the special education efforts of state and local governments through the use of federal funds.

Importantly, the law does not mandate special education for every handicapped child but only for those who by reason of one or more disabilities require it. Many children with disabilities can and should enroll in regular classes without program modification. The law further implies that special education is "special" and includes only instruction aimed at meeting the unique needs of a handicapped child. The law also makes it clear that handicapped children may require related services that may not be available from the school system itself. These services are to be provided through contractual relations with other agencies, either public or private, and with outside specialists. The act demonstrates a clear and logical progression: the child is handicapped and needs special education and/or related services; special education is the specially designed instruction program to meet the child's unique needs; and related services are those necessary to enable the child to benefit from special education instruction.

An important milestone was the passage of PL 99-457, the Education of the Handicapped Amendment (EHA) of 1986. The amendment reauthorized PL 94-142 and authorized the extension of EHA to infants and toddlers 0 to 2 years of age. Known as part H of the EHA, this legislation was designed to assist states in the development and implementation of comprehensive, coordinated, interdisciplinary programs of early intervention for handicapped infants, toddlers, and their families. Children with delays in language and speech development are among those covered by part H of the EHA. Early intervention is defined as "developmental services which include. . . speech pathology and audiology . . . and are provided by qualified personnel, including speech and language pathologists and audiologists" (United States House of Representatives, 99th Congress, Report 99-860, 1986). Other services covered in the law include early identification, screening, and assessment; psychological services; medical services for diagnostic or evaluation purposes only; and any other services deemed appropriate for helping infants and toddlers benefit from early intervention. In addition, the bill strengthens portions of the original act by developing better incentives for states to serve the 3- to 5-year-old population (part B). Finally, not only does the bill help to expand the services to young infants and toddlers, but it also helps to ensure that states use appropriately trained personnel.

In considering this bill, Congress recognized these needs:

- To enhance the development of handicapped infants and toddlers and to minimize their potential for developmental delay;
- To reduce the educational costs to society, including schools, by minimizing the need for special education and related services after handicapped infants and toddlers reach school age;
- To minimize the likelihood of institutionalization of handicapped individuals and maximize the potential for their independent living in society; and
- To enhance the capacity of families to meet the special needs of their infants and toddlers with handicaps.

Implementation of this law entails a multidisciplinary evaluation to determine eligibility and to develop an individualized educational plan (IEP) for the child. The IEP is discussed in more detail later in this chapter. Other components of the law include nondiscriminatory evaluation, rights of the parents to be involved in the decisions affecting the child, and education in the least restrictive environment.

As noted in Chapter 1, PL 94-142 and 99-457 became known as the Individuals With Disabilities Education Act (IDEA) in 1990; the law was reauthorized, updated, and expanded in 1997. Signed into law by President Clinton, it is PL-105-17, the Individuals With Disabilities Education Act Amendments of 1997 (IDEA 1997). In 2004, President Bush signed a new law, PL 108-446. This law is commonly called the Individuals With Disabilities Education Improvement Act (IDEIA 2004). IDEIA 2004 continues to expand the services to very young children with disabilities and their families. Although IDEIA 2004 retains many of the provisions offered in previous versions of the law, differences do exist between IDEA 1997 and IDEIA 2004. Some of the major differences between the two bills are detailed in Table 8.1.

Another important legislative initiative for individuals with disabilities is the Rehabilitation Act of 1973 (Title V, Section 504, Subpart D: Preschool, Elementary, and Secondary Education). This law, amended in 1978, was developed to protect disabled individuals from discriminatory action; in effect, a person with a handicap should have the same rights and benefits (e.g., accessibility to public facilities) as one who does not have a handicap. Hence, the bill, sometimes referred to as the bill of rights for individuals with handicaps, offers special provisions beyond instructional services. For example, these services might include availability of special devices such as fire alarms, public announcement systems, and telephone services for children with hearing loss.

Finally, in 1990, the Americans With Disabilities Act (ADA) was passed in an effort to prevent discrimination against individuals with handicapping conditions, particularly in employment. To this end, President Reagan's National Council on Disability wrote the ADA, designed to afford the handicapped equal opportunities in employment, public accommodations, transportation, and state and local services in telecommunications.

All of this legislation has significantly improved the life quality of individuals with hearing loss. It has created an environment in which individuals with hearing loss can compete effectively in all aspects of our society.

TABLE 8.1   The Major Differences Between IDEA 1997 and IDEIA 2004

Topic	IDEA 1997	IDEIA 2004
"Highly qualified" special education teachers	States set qualifications for educating children with disabilities	Requires certification in special education. Teachers must meet NCLB "highly qualified" standard.
IEP	Must meet annually to write IEP. Entire team must be present to change IEP.	Parents and school districts can agree to change IEP without a formal meeting. 15 states can write up an IEP for up to 3 y.
Early childhood	School districts can fund special services for at-risk special needs students. Part C program for children with disabilities, birth to age 2 y.	States can elect to extend part C to kindergarten.
Parental choice for private schools	Children in private schools have no rights to receive special education and related services in the public system.	School districts may use IDEIA funds for services chosen by parents in schools identified as needing improvement under NCLB.
Definition of assistive technology device	Makes no reference to medically implanted devices.	Medically implanted devices and replacement excluded.
Overidentification, overreferral	Not mentioned.	States required to reduce overidentification of minority students; eliminate IQ discrepancy model; child must have a disability as defined by law *and* have educational needs; disability alone will not qualify a child for services.
Funding	Federal goal has always been to fund IDEA by 40%; however, federal funding covers only about 17% of the national average cost per student.	6-y plan to reach 40% goal. For FY 2005, federal government cut special education budget.

NCLB, No Child Left Behind; IEP, individual education plan; FY, fiscal year.
From Bradham T. Personal communication, 2007.

THE CULTURE OF DEAFNESS

Historically, hearing health care professionals have treated deafness as a pathologic medical condition. The audiologist's general goal has been to mainstream the deaf child into a normal-hearing world, to provide the child with speech (English) or some other means of communication, and to help the child and the child's family to make educational and social decisions. In the past 25 years, however, there has been a strong movement toward considering the deaf as not just a group of people with a medical condition but a cultural and linguistic minority. There is a move to acknowledge the cultural values of the deaf population and to view the differences between deaf and normal-hearing people as cultural differences, not as deviations from the norm. Deaf people now promote the deaf culture to get hearing people to understand deaf people as they understand themselves. The book *Deaf in America: Voices from a Culture* made the following statement:

> The traditional way of writing about Deaf people is to focus on the fact of their condition— that they do not hear—and to interpret all other aspects of their lives as consequences of this fact. . . . In contrast to the long history of writings that treat them as medical cases, or as people with "disabilities" who compensate for their deafness by using sign language, we want to portray the lives they live, their art and performances, their everyday talk, their shared myths, and the lessons they teach one another. We have always felt that the attention given to the physical condition of not hearing has obscured far more interesting facets of Deaf people's lives (Padden and Humphries, 1988).

This statement offers some valuable insight into the differences between hearing and deaf views of deafness. For hearing health care professionals, the emphasis seems to be placed on the handicap, the audiologic data, or the mode of communication, whereas deaf people are more concerned with social, linguistic, and cultural aspects of the deaf experience. Hence, it is important for all hearing health care professionals to recognize and understand the attitudes and feelings of deaf people. Audiologists must be cognizant of and sensitive to the characteristics and problems of deaf people and not just view the deaf as persons affected by a pathologic condition but rather as a group of people with specific language and behavior patterns and a proud history.

The contrasting views of the deaf community and hearing health professionals can best be illustrated with the debate on cochlear implants for children. As one might expect, audiologists, otolaryngologists, and some deaf educators are strong advocates of cochlear implants for prelingually deaf children. Implants allow an individual with significant hearing loss to receive auditory signals—to maximize their potential for listening, speaking, and learning (see Chapter 7). In contrast, some members of the deaf community question the value of implant efficacy and suggest that the long-term burdens associated with a surgical implant and the subsequent rehabilitation are significant for deaf children and their families. Moreover, some members of the deaf community believe that implants are looked upon as a panacea, or cure-all, for deafness, which in turn perpetuates negative attitudes toward deafness and deaf people. It is believed that if a family decides not to pursue cochlear implantation and instead opts to use sign language as the principal means for communication, the child will be well received into the deaf community—a community which contains a rich history, a valued language, and a value system of its very own. Stated otherwise, the family that allows a child to remain deaf and to develop language through sign will become an active member of a vibrant cultural and linguistic minority group. Those among the deaf community maintain that this association with the deaf population will lead to better psychosocial development, a better quality of life, and subsequently, personal happiness. Hence, the emphasis is on simply letting the deaf be deaf.

Children as young as 4 months of age have received cochlear implants. The debate about the appropriateness of cochlear implants in children has intensified as the age of implantation became younger and younger. Central to this debate is the question of whether deafness is a medical problem to be remedied or a central feature of an individual's identity and culture that should be left unchanged. The questions raised in the debate about cochlear implants in children are likely to intensify as work on the human genome progresses and genetic "cures" for deafness emerge. Although these questions can often become philosophical and abstract for most of us, for the parents of a deaf child, most of whom are normal hearing themselves (see Chapter 5), the decision regarding the best course of action for their child poses an immediate dilemma for them. Often, their decision is based on the preferred communication mode for their child, both educationally and socially.

COMMUNICATION MODES USED IN EDUCATIONAL INSTRUCTION

Chapter 7 briefly discusses the various modes of communication used for educational instruction: auditory-oral and total communication. It is not our intent here to suggest that one mode of communication is better than another. Unquestionably, the two most common approaches used in education are the auditory-oral and total communication methods. Recall that the auditory-oral method, sometimes referred to as the oral-aural approach, emphasizes use of the child's existing residual hearing to develop oral communication. The method is referred to as the auditory-verbal approach if only listening is advocated with no emphasis on vision for receiving information. Others emphasize vision over hearing or stress the combined use of hearing and vision. Whatever modification is used, this approach does not permit the use of signs or finger spelling. The only means of expression allowed is speech.

The other popular approach to educational instruction is the method known as total communication. Total communication combines the auditory-oral method with signs and finger spelling. The emphasis is on receiving information by all possible means, including amplification, vision, signs, and finger spelling. Similarly, expression can occur by speech or through signs and/or finger spelling. Like advocates of the auditory-oral approach, proponents of total communication believe that the method should be introduced in early infancy, if possible, and that parents should be intensively involved. The difference, of course, is that with total communication, the parents assist the child in the development of language using all means available.

At this point, a brief discussion of manual communication is warranted because it is an important component of the total approach. Variations of the auditory method will also be presented to help the reader contrast the different instructional approaches used in children with hearing loss. Language development in children depends on the nature of the language presented to the child (English or American Sign Language) and the type of communication system used (manual versus oral). As shown in Figure 8.1, language is coded into three basic forms, American Sign Language (ASL), Manually Coded English (MCE), and Oral English (OE). Each of

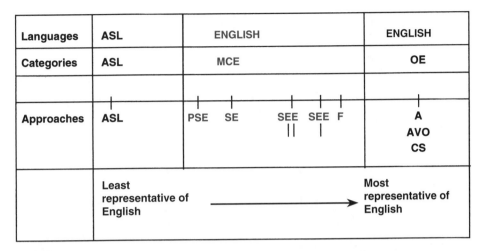

Languages	ASL	ENGLISH	ENGLISH
Categories	ASL	MCE	OE
Approaches	ASL	PSE SE SEE SEE F	A AVO CS
	Least representative of English	⟶	Most representative of English

FIGURE 8.1   Summary of the approaches used to teach communication and language skills to children with hearing loss. The approaches fall on a continuum according to how closely they resemble the English language. ASL, American Sign Language; MCE, Manually Coded English; OE, Oral English; PSE, Pidgin Sign English; SE, Signed English; SEE II, Signed Exact English; SEE I, Seeing Essential English; F, finger spelling; A, auditory; AVO, auditory-visual-oral; CS, cued speech. (From Quigley SP, Paul PV. Language and Deafness. San Diego: College-Hill, 1984.)

these forms varies according to how closely it resembles the structure of the English language. For MCE and OE, several additional subdivisions further complicate the classification scheme.

One means by which a word or idea can be presented manually is through a sign. There are four basic features common to all signs. These include general position, configuration, orientation (direction of the palms), and movement of the hands. These four features are combined in various ways to formulate signs of different meanings. Figure 8.2 shows examples of signs. Although the different signs in this figure all use the same hand shape (index and middle fingers extended), the movement, position, and palm orientation alter the meaning. The manual communicator has the flexibility to use finger spelling only, sign only, or a combination of the two. The sign language used in the United States is generally called ASL to differentiate it from some of the more recent modifications devised to make signs conform more closely to the syntax of the English language. ASL is a rich and complex visual-gestural language system—it has its own vocabulary and grammatic structure. In fact, many believe that ASL should be taught as the primary language to all children with hearing loss and that English should be taught as a second language. ASL users do not typically speak while signing, and hence, sound is not used as an information source. ASL is the primary language used by the adult deaf community. The community comprises individuals who share common experiences, values, interests, and language. Within the deaf community, there is a clear sense of cohesion and pride, particularly in regard to the use of ASL.

MCE uses gestures, signs, finger spelling, or some combination of these to approximate English. Varying forms of MCE that attempt to bring ASL closer to English include Pidgin Sign English (PSE), Signed English (SE), Signing Exact English (SEE II), Seeing Essential English (SEE I), and finger spelling. With the exception of finger spelling, each of these systems is based on ASL but uses the word order of English.

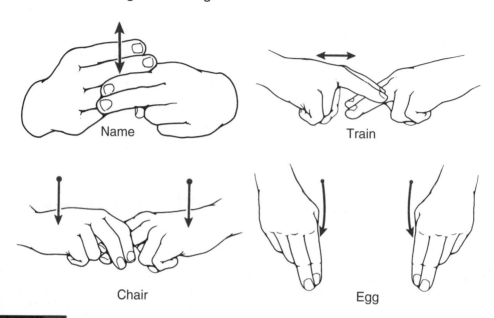

FIGURE 8.2   A group of signs. Although each sign has a similar hand shape, there are differences in movement, placement, and orientation of the hands. (From Schleper D. Communicating with Deaf People: An Introduction. Washington: National Information Center on Deafness, Gallaudet University, 1987.)

PSE, sometimes referred to as a contact sign, is used by deaf adults to approximate English using sign and finger spelling. The term *pidgin* means simplified speech used for communicating between two people with different languages. Hence, PSE is often used between hearing persons, most of whom are not familiar with ASL, and deaf persons. SE, originally designed for preschool children, consists of both signs and finger spelling. Each of the approximately 3500 signed words in the SE system parallels the meaning of a separate word entry in a standard English dictionary. Morphologic sign markers are used to represent the regular and irregular plurals, and thus, SE more closely approximates English than does PSE. SEE II is one of the more widely contrived systems that adds morphemes such as prefixes and suffixes that are not included in the basic signs. Examples include the morphemes *-ed* as in *talked* and *-ly* as in *friendly*. A common way to accomplish this is through finger spelling. SEE I was developed before SEE II and in fact was one of the first attempts to use signs in a structure that replicated English. SEE I has a vocabulary of about 5000 words, and signs are used to represent word forms and even word parts such as roots, prefixes, and suffixes. Compound words were made by putting two words together. For example, the sign for *understand* was made by joining the signs of *under* and *stand*. SEE I and SEE II differ in that they use different rules for establishing sign boundaries. SE, SEE II, and SEE I have some common characteristics: (*a*) They borrow from the ASL vocabulary. (*b*) They were developed for use by hearing parents of deaf children and teachers. (*c*) They attempt to use signs for such elements of speech as pronouns, affixes, and verb tenses.

Finger spelling simply is spelling a word letter by letter, representing each letter by a specific sign that corresponds to a letter in the English alphabet. As noted earlier, finger spelling is often used in combination with sign. The hand is held at about chest level, and different finger configurations are formed. The presentation rate is somewhat

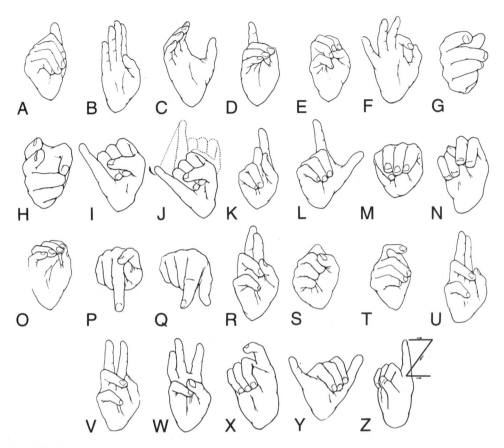

FIGURE 8.3 The American Manual Alphabet (shown as signs appear to person reading them). (Reprinted from Schleper D. Communicating with Deaf People: An Introduction. Washington: National Information Center on Deafness, Gallaudet University, 1987.)

similar to that of speech. Figure 8.3 shows the manual alphabet used in the United States, with 26 hand shapes representing the letters in the English alphabet. Those who desire a more detailed coverage of manual communication are referred to the suggested readings at the end of this chapter.

Figure 8.1 shows that the approach that most closely approximates English is OE. This approach emphasizes the key role of acoustic input as a means of developing skill in both understanding and producing connected speech as the primary mode of communication. Major characteristics of this approach include maximum emphasis on hearing, comprehensive intervention well beyond the traditional setting, and emphasis on connected speech. The use of sign or finger spelling is not typically allowed. Early full-time use of a rehabilitative device, such as a hearing aid or implant, with periodic reexamination of hearing to monitor the child's auditory capacities with and without the device, is crucial to this method. In general, the assumption is that language is best learned by hearing it, just as it is with normal-hearing persons. Approaches that focus on residual hearing (*A*) are referred to as auditory, auditory-oral, auditory-verbal, or acoupedics, whereas techniques that use vision (lipreading) as part of training are referred to as auditory-visual-oral (AVO).

Another approach classified as oral is cued speech (CS). CS is a system that incorporates eight hand configurations and four hand positions near the lips to aid hearing and speech reading. The premise is that the hand cues can supplement speech reading and audition by signaling differences between sounds. For example, the words *bee* and *me* look alike to the speech reader. A hand cue made simultaneously at the lips signals the difference between the two look-alike words.

The auditory-oral method was easily the most widely used method of instruction until the mid-1970s; then the combination of sign and speech (total communication) became the more popular method used in educational programs in the United States, regardless of grade level. This approach gained widespread acceptance after research showed that deaf children exposed to manual communication by deaf parents exhibited better educational performance than deaf children of hearing parents. At the same time, the two groups of children showed essentially no differences in their speech. Today, auditory-oral and auditory-verbal programs in the United States are increasing, probably because of the emphasis on early identification (newborn screening), the growing number of children receiving cochlear implants, and the growing number of mild hearing losses seen in the schools (discussed later). A recent summary of the primary methods used in teaching children with hearing loss is shown in Table 8.2.

Given so many choices, how does one decide which is the best method? Chapter 7 discusses the approaches used to determine whether a child with hearing loss would benefit most from an auditory-oral or a total communication program of instruction. Many believe that the best method for a given child is the one that the family selects based on unbiased information. It is important that families be well informed of the various options available—this means that the families must carefully investigate each option and be able to answer the following basic questions: Do you know what your options are for communication? Do you understand these options? Have you examined them in person? Do you understand all test results? How much time do you have to devote to learning the system? Once families are able to answer these questions, they must carefully examine what options are available in their community. It would not make good sense, for example, to opt for an auditory-verbal approach if the closest program was many miles away. Moreover, a child with a profound sensorineural hearing loss who was identified late (3–4 years of age) will probably not be the ideal candidate for an auditory-oral approach. All methods require a good deal of work on the part of the family, and no method is easy.

TABLE 8.2   Methods Used to Teach Young Children With Hearing Loss (N = 42,361)

Methods of Teaching	%
Speech only	46.1
Sign and speech	44.9
Sign only	7.6
Cued speech	0.4
Other	0.9

Data taken from Regional and National Summary Report of Data from the 2001–2002 Annual Survey of Deaf and Hard of Hearing Children and Youth. Washington: GRI, Gallaudet University.

EDUCATIONAL SETTINGS

What are the settings used to educate children with hearing loss? There are numerous types of programs, both public and private, designed to serve children with hearing loss of all ages. One of the best-recognized educational programs is the residential school. Residential programs maintain facilities for room and board as well as instruction and recreation. Most residential schools are operated by state governments. There are, however, some well-known private residential programs in the United States. Today, many children commute as day students to residential facilities, especially if the school is in a metropolitan area.

Also found in large metropolitan areas are private and public day schools for those with hearing loss. In these schools, the children with hearing loss commute as normal-hearing children do. Day classes are another type of instructional format for children with hearing loss. Here, classes for those with hearing loss are conducted in public schools at which most of the children have normal hearing. Instruction may take place entirely in classrooms containing only students with hearing loss, or the children may be integrated into a regular classroom, a situation commonly referred to as *inclusion*. Inclusion may occur on a full-time or part-time basis. Special classes (resource rooms) are arranged for areas in which the child needs individual tutorial assistance, but most of the student's time is spent in regular classrooms. Finally, there are itinerant programs, in which a child with hearing loss attends regular classrooms full time but receives support services from an itinerant teacher. Itinerant programs are typically used as a supplement or an alternative to resource rooms. Typically, the itinerant teacher moves from one school to another throughout the week, offering support services to children with special needs. Table 8.3 lists the percentage of children with hearing loss attending various instructional settings.

It is interesting how these placement options have changed over the past several decades. First, there are many more children with hearing loss in public day classes today than there were in the 1980s and even in the 1990s. Paralleling the increase in public day classes was a decrease in public schools for the hearing impaired. Also noteworthy is the decrease in all types of private schools throughout the United States. Between 1974 and 1986, the percentage of deaf children attending private residential and day schools dropped from 6% to 1.5%. Since approximately 1974, there has been a trend toward an increase in the role of the public schools in educating students with

TABLE 8.3 **Instructional Settings Attended by Children With Hearing Loss (N = 43,361)**

Instructional Settings	%
Special school or center	26.6
Self-contained classroom	32.9
Resource room	13.5
Regular education	45.2
Home	2.7
Other	5.1

Data taken from Regional and National Summary Report of Data from the 2001–2002 Annual Survey of Deaf and Hard of Hearing Children and Youth. Washington: GRI, Gallaudet University.

hearing loss, mostly through day school programs (public day classes). This trend is no doubt a result of the mandate of IDEA 1997 and IDEIA 2004.

A number of postsecondary educational opportunities are available for the deaf and hard-of-hearing population in the United States. Foremost is Gallaudet University, which was for many years the only higher educational program in the world developed specifically for people with hearing loss. The establishment of the university was spearheaded by the efforts of Edward Minor Gallaudet and Amos Kendall, two resourceful professionals who were committed to serving the population with hearing loss. The university was named after Edward Gallaudet's father, Thomas Gallaudet, a pioneer in deaf education (Vignette 8.1). Today, Gallaudet serves as a major source of leadership to individuals with hearing loss in the United States. In addition to offering liberal arts

---

VIGNETTE 8.1 **Pioneers in deaf education**

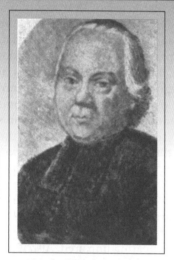

CHARLES-MICHEL DE L'ÉPÉE

One of the most prominent names in the history of deaf education worldwide is that of Abbé de l'Épée, the person credited with making education of the hearing impaired a matter of public concern. He was also interested in making education available to the indigent population. Charles-Michel de l'Épée was born in Versailles, France, in 1712. He was well educated and chose the priesthood as his profession. His interest in deafness stemmed from his knowledge of twin sisters who were severely to profoundly hearing impaired. Because of his concern for these sisters, he agreed to instruct them, and soon his success gained him widespread recognition. From this time on he devoted his life to working with the hearing impaired. He established a school, and educators from all over the world came to study his technique. Also, de l'Épée helped develop and expand sign language for the hearing impaired and served as an advocate for manual communication.

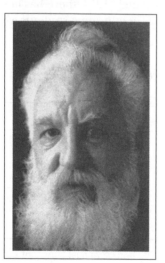

ALEXANDER GRAHAM BELL

Alexander Graham Bell is recognized as one of the great teachers of the deaf in the United States. He was born March 3, 1847, in Edinburgh, Scotland. At 24 years of age, he came to the United States to visit a school for deaf children. He was most impressed with how children with hearing loss used lipreading and speech. This initial experience motivated Bell to become more involved with the hearing impaired. Bell spearheaded the development of the auditory-oral method for teaching the deaf in the United States.

In 1872, Bell opened a training school for teachers of the deaf in Boston. His plan to develop an auditory-oral training school was greatly opposed by advocates of the manual approach. His desire to develop a mechanical means of making speech visible to the hearing impaired led Bell to experiment with the electrical transmission of sound.

VIGNETTE 8.1   **Pioneers in deaf education (Continued)**

He hoped to develop a means of amplification for the hearing impaired. These experiments resulted in the development of the telephone. Bell later married Mabel Hubbard, a deaf woman who helped start the auditory-oral approach in the United States. Throughout his later years, Bell maintained his interest in the education of the hearing impaired and served as an advocate for the population with hearing loss.

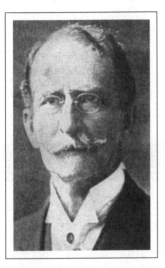

EDWARD MINOR GALLAUDET

Edward Minor Gallaudet was the son of Thomas Hopkins Gallaudet, a pioneering teacher of the hearing impaired in the United States and the man for whom Gallaudet University in Washington, D.C., was named. Edward Minor Gallaudet studied under his father and served as the first president of Candle School, a private school for the hearing impaired. The school was later renamed Gallaudet College in honor of his father. Candle School became the preparatory department at this college. Edward Minor Gallaudet studied both oral and manual techniques; he supported the combined method but was convinced that manual communication was the most appropriate and natural approach for the educational instruction of children with hearing loss.

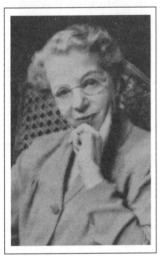

IRENE R. EWING

Irene R. Ewing is one of the modern pioneers in the education and audiologic management of children with hearing loss. During the war years between 1939 and 1945, nurseries, clinics, and hospitals in Great Britain kept a steady and careful watch over the general development of their young infants and children. Children with abnormal responses or behavior were quickly noted and referred to appropriate clinics. Children who exhibited abnormal responses to sound were typically referred to Ewing's clinic for deaf children at Manchester University. The worldwide reputation of this program for children with hearing loss came about primarily because of Ewing's persistent and undaunted efforts as a teacher and as one who had a unique ability to impart knowledge to others. She demonstrated worldwide the benefits of early identification and intervention, the importance of parent-home training for the development of speech, and the techniques for testing young children with hearing loss. From her clinic's opening in 1919 until her retirement in 1949, she encouraged and aided successive groups of students with her own enthusiasm and conveyed to them something of her steadfast principles on educating children with hearing loss. She also encouraged others to pursue a professional career in deaf education. Her efforts won worldwide renown, and her advice and consultation were sought throughout the United Kingdom and the world.

and graduate education for the hearing impaired, Gallaudet also trains professionals, such as school administrators, audiologists, speech-language pathologists, teachers, and researchers, to serve the population with hearing loss. There is no comparable postsecondary program for individuals with hearing loss in the United States.

Technical schools for those with hearing loss also exist in this country. Perhaps the best known is the National Technical Institute for the Deaf (NTID), a technical school of higher education that serves deaf students in association with the Rochester Institute of Technology in Rochester, New York. The educational programs can lead to certificate programs, associate degrees, or bachelor's degrees. The NTID is also involved in carrying out research concerned with the deaf and hard-of-hearing populations.

Finally, a number of state universities and community colleges throughout the United States have federally funded programs providing vocational or liberal arts training to those with hearing loss. In fact, some of these programs serve as feeder programs for the NTID and Gallaudet University.

EDUCATIONAL ACHIEVEMENT OF CHILDREN WITH HEARING LOSS

One need only contrast the manner in which a normal-hearing child develops oral speech and language with the situation of the child with hearing loss to appreciate the learning difficulties of children with auditory deficits. The typical normal-hearing child comes to kindergarten or first grade with a wide array of auditory experiences and a well-developed language symbol system. The child with hearing loss has had limited auditory experiences and was most likely not even identified as having hearing loss until 1 to 2 years of age. (With the recent advent of newborn hearing screening, age of identification is improving; see Chapter 6.) Therefore, the child with hearing loss has been wearing hearing aids for only a few years. The child with a significant hearing loss has far fewer learning readiness experiences before entering first grade. Thus, we find that children with hearing loss lag behind normal-hearing children in educational achievement.

The educational opportunities for deaf students are many, and the number of deaf individuals enrolling in postsecondary programs has more than doubled over the past few decades. Nevertheless, many deaf students do not take advantage of the opportunities. Close to half of the deaf students in high school drop out before completion or simply receive a certificate of attendance. Moreover, of those who graduate from high school and go on to a postsecondary education, many will drop out.

Indeed, the influences of both education and communication are reflected in the incomes earned by the deaf population. Deaf persons with the most education generally earn the highest incomes. Those using only manual communication or gestures report the lowest median earnings. Of deaf individuals in the upper half of the income range, most use speech to communicate at work, with about half of these persons using speech combined with one or more other modes of communication and half using speech exclusively.

Although employment opportunities have improved substantially over the past 2 decades, unemployment rates among the deaf continue to be higher on the average than in the hearing population; underemployment, however, is a much more serious problem, especially for the female deaf population. For example, few are employed in professional, technical, or managerial positions, and fewer than 1% are employed in sales. A large percentage of the deaf are engaged in clerical, craft, or machine opera-tor positions—the latter being one of the largest occupations. No doubt, underem-ployment of the deaf is in part because of employers' lack of understanding about deafness and their failure to recognize that deaf individuals are as intellectually capa-ble as hearing individuals—they are stellar and dependable employees. Certainly, the ADA should result in improvement in job opportunities for workers with hearing loss. The ADA prohibits discrimination against qualified individuals because of any type of impairment, including hearing loss. Other reasons for underemployment will become apparent as we review the educational difficulties of children with varying degrees of hearing loss. The case illustrations of seven school-age children with hearing loss pre-sented in Vignettes 8.2 through 8.8 also provide some insight into the problem.

VIGNETTE 8.2   A child with profound bilateral sensorineural hearing loss receiving excellent benefit from a cochlear implant

This 4.5-year-old girl was identified at 18 months of age as having a bilateral profound sensorineural hearing loss. She received amplification binaurally within 2 months and implants at age 2 years. As shown in the accompanying figure, when the child wore amplification, sound-field thresholds (A-A) improved significantly compared with unaided thresholds; sound-field threshold data for the implant (CI-CI) provided even more improvement than the hearing aids. She initially wore a processor on her body but has recently switched to a behind-the-ear processor.

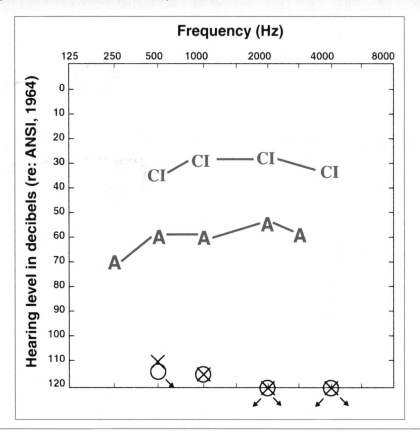

(continued)

VIGNETTE 8.2   **A child with profound bilateral sensorineural hearing loss receiving excellent benefit from a cochlear implant (Continued)**

The child was enrolled in an auditory-verbal program soon after she received amplification. At the time she received the implants, she exhibited no receptive skills other than a few words based on pattern perception, such as no, and a few everyday phrases that she understood in structured therapy settings. She had no verbal skills and communicated mainly through some vocalization combined with pointing.

After implantation, she continued in the auditory-verbal program in weekly sessions. By 10 months after the implant, she could understand sentences with two key words; basic what, where, and when questions; and early descriptors, and she could follow single-step directions without any contextual cues. All of these tasks were performed with no visual cues while she was not looking at the speaker. She had some trouble with lip rounding for a few vowels and diphthongs, but all age-appropriate consonants were established. She used three-word utterances to communicate, which were approximately 75% intelligible to unfamiliar listeners. Longer utterances were usually intelligible to her family. At 1 year after implant, her understanding of concepts was at or above age level in all areas except time and sequence concepts.

By 2 years after implant, the child's auditory skills had developed to the point that she could listen and sequence three events of a story and listen to a paragraph with informational content and recall two details. Her receptive language was a year above her chronologic age. She used narratives and a variety of idioms. Her understanding of language enabled her to say, "I shouldn't eat sweets because I get wound up like a spring." Her speech was 90% intelligible to strangers.

Since age 3, this child has attended a regular preschool. She was discharged from the auditory-verbal program at 4.3 years of age and returns only for monitoring and consultation. She subsequently entered a public school kindergarten.

VIGNETTE 8.3   **A child with profound bilateral sensorineural hearing loss receiving marginal benefit from a cochlear implant**

This 5.2-year-old boy was hospitalized soon after birth because of oxygen deprivation. He was identified as having a bilateral profound hearing loss soon thereafter and was fitted with binaural amplification; at 2.2 years of age, the child received an implant. The accompanying figure shows the unaided audiogram and the improvement in sound-field thresholds the child received with amplification (A-A) and with the implant (CI-CI). Clearly, both devices resulted in improved thresholds compared with the unaided data; the implant provided the most improvement in threshold sensitivity. At 12 months of age, he was diagnosed with cerebral palsy and severe food allergies.

The parents initially chose a total communication approach for the child but opted for an auditory approach when he was 13 months old. After approximately 12 months of auditory-verbal training, he was detecting all vowels, understanding patterns, associating animal and vehicle sounds with their objects, and vocalizing intentionally to communicate. His motor skills were poor, he needed propping up to sit, and his arm movements were random. He was able to hold up his head. Developmentally, he was very difficult to assess. However, he did demonstrate object permanence, means-end, and cause-effect skills. In addition to the

VIGNETTE 8.3 A child with profound bilateral sensorineural hearing loss receiving marginal benefit from a cochlear implant *(Continued)*

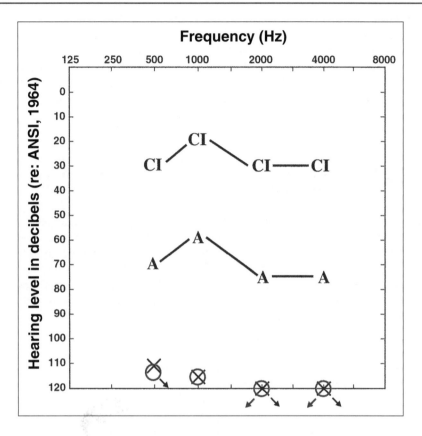

auditory-verbal program, he began intensive oral-motor exercises and received physical and occupational therapy on a weekly basis.

For the first 3 months after the implant, he showed no signs of detecting any sounds and stopped vocalizing. By 1 year after implant, he had begun to detect sounds consistently without prompting. He could understand a variety of words and phrases using audition alone. On a standardized test, his receptive skills were a year delayed when compared with his chronologic age. He had made a 15-month gain in the 1 year after his implant in his receptive skills. He continued to use pointing with intentional vocalization. With a special seat he was able to sit independently for short periods,. In the interim, he was hospitalized several times with severe viral infections.

By 2 years after implant, at age 4.2 years, he had begun to walk with support. His receptive skills began to develop rapidly; however, he used only a few key words. At this point, a very structured approach, the Association Method, which pairs audition, written symbols, and visual cues, was begun for his consonant and vowel production. At the same time, consultation for an augmentative communication device was recommended because communication with his parents was breaking down.

After 6 months of the Association Method, he was using two- and three-word utterances that were intelligible to strangers, his receptive skills had soared and were only a few months delayed, and he was walking independently. His parents had never used any augmentative communication device during this period.

(continued)

VIGNETTE 8.3 A child with profound bilateral sensorineural hearing loss receiving marginal benefit from a cochlear implant *(Continued)*

His receptive skills when compared with those of children with normal hearing are at the low end of normal but within one standard deviation. He uses three- to five-word sentences that are intelligible to strangers and has all age-appropriate vowels and consonants in his spontaneous speech. He receives physical therapy and occupational therapy through his school system and continues in the auditory-verbal program. His social skills are poor, and although he attends a regular preschool, he does not use much communicative language there. His parents are looking into a variety of options for kindergarten.

VIGNETTE 8.4 A child with bilateral moderately severe to profound sensorineural hearing loss

---

This 10-year-old boy was identified at age 17 months as having a moderately severe to profound bilateral sensorineural hearing loss. Binaural amplification was introduced within a month; the accompanying figure shows an audiogram obtained after 2 months of amplification *(left panel)*. Thresholds obtained in a sound field (S-S) reveal a severe to profound hearing loss. When the child wears a hearing aid, the sound-field thresholds (A-A) improve markedly compared with unaided thresholds. A more recent pure-tone audiogram is shown in the *right panel*. Data for aided thresholds are also presented.

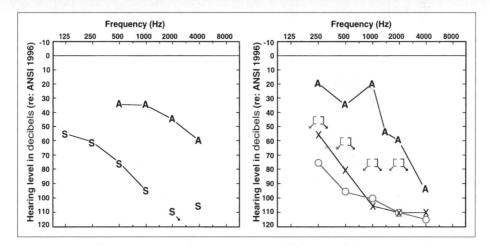

The child was enrolled in an auditory-oral parent-infant training program as soon as amplification was introduced. His parents were taught speech, language, and auditory stimulation techniques and were excellent in carrying out auditory training at home. The child progressed rapidly and was making single-word approximations accompanied by jargon at 1 year after amplification.

At 3 years of age, he was enrolled in a half-day oral-acoustic nursery for children with hearing loss. He wore an FM wireless system during school hours. By 5 years of age, he was using simple sentences to communicate orally, and he was mainstreamed into a private prekindergarten classroom with support services from the local school. The support services consisted of individual speech and language therapy and assistance in reading, math, science, and social studies.

VIGNETTE 8.4 **A child with bilateral moderately severe to profound sensorineural hearing loss (Continued)**

The child continues to be mainstreamed in a private school, with supportive speech and language therapy. He is in the third grade and functioning at grade level in reading comprehension and math. He is functioning below age level in vocabulary development and language associated with logical thinking skills (i.e., sequencing events, predicting outcomes, verbal analogies, and multiple meanings).

Intelligibility of speech production is good, with approximately 90% of his speech understood by peers, teachers, and family members. The child orally presents essays and other assignments on a par with other children in his class.

He probably will require speech and language therapy throughout his school years along with special assistance with academic subjects. However, this is a case in which appropriate early identification combined with proper educational management and parental determination has led to a life in the mainstream.

VIGNETTE 8.5 **A child with bilateral moderate to severe sensorineural hearing loss**

This 11-year-old girl was identified as having a bilateral moderate to severe sensorineural hearing loss at age 5 years and was referred to a hearing clinic. The etiology of the hearing loss is unknown. Her audiogram at age 5 is shown in the accompanying figure (*left panel*). The most recent audiogram indicated a moderate to severe sensorineural hearing loss in the right ear and a moderate to profound sensorineural hearing loss in the left ear (*right panel*).

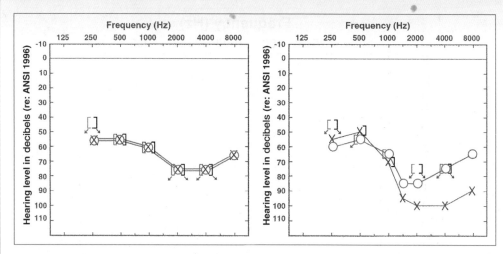

The child was enrolled in both a self-contained kindergarten classroom in a local school system and in a parent-infant training program. Her communicative skills were fair, and she responded well to amplification. Her speech was judged to be partially intelligible, and her language skills were similar to those of a 3- to 4-year-old. She has continued in a

(continued)

VIGNETTE 8.5 **A child with bilateral moderate to severe sensorineural hearing loss** *(Continued)*

---

self-contained classroom with additional individual speech and language therapy. She is in a second-grade self-contained classroom. Her reading skills are at age level, and she is functioning at grade level in math and social sciences. When compared with normal-hearing children, expressive language skills are at the 7-year-old level.

Mainstreaming has been considered but has not been implemented because of concerns regarding her ability to work independently and because of a lack of qualified personnel to provide the necessary support services. It is probable that she will be mainstreamed, at least partially, when she is older and more able to work independently.

VIGNETTE 8.6 **A child with unilateral severe to profound sensorineural hearing loss**

This 6-year-old boy has a severe to profound sensorineural hearing loss in the left ear and normal hearing in the right ear. Pertinent medical history includes maternal diabetes and syphilis, meningitis at 1 year of age, and head trauma at 5 years of age. He is attending first grade and receives preferential seating (seated to the right side of the teacher so that the good ear is fully exposed to the teacher). The teacher indicated that the child would be retained in the first grade for the next year. She reported that he is a "slow learner," although he is more capable than he demonstrates. He also attends a reading resource class and receives articulation therapy.

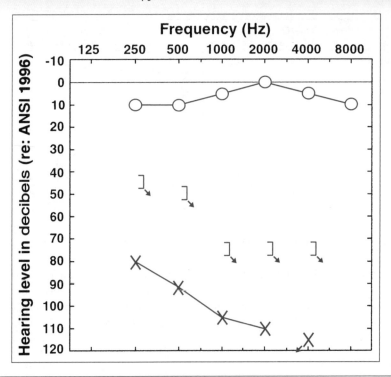

VIGNETTE 8.6 A child with unilateral severe to profound sensorineural hearing loss *(Continued)*

Before a 2-week trial with an FM system, the teacher rated his ability to understand and/or follow directions as fair in small groups and as very poor in large groups. The teacher also rated his ability to concentrate on tasks as poor.

Use of an FM wireless system reportedly resulted in a marked improvement in his performance. His ability to understand and follow directions in small and large groups and to concentrate on tasks while using the FM wireless system was now rated by the teacher as good. In addition, the teacher felt that peer acceptance of the FM wireless system was excellent. According to the teacher, the FM wireless system was especially useful in classroom learning situations.

Both the teachers and the parents were counseled about the dangers that children with unilateral hearing loss can encounter in such routine activities as crossing busy streets and bike riding in heavy traffic. In addition, the teachers and the parents were counseled about the need for practicing good hearing health care. Monitoring the child for possible conductive hearing loss resulting from effusion in either ear and progressive sensorineural hearing loss was emphasized. Furthermore, the practice of using ear protection in any high-noise environment was recommended as a conservation measure.

VIGNETTE 8.7 A child with bilateral minimal hearing loss

This 6-year-old boy has a long history of middle ear disease with effusion. He has had persistent otitis media for several years and a history of myringotomy with insertion tubes beginning at age 6 months. The child had seven or eight sets of tubes during the first 6 years

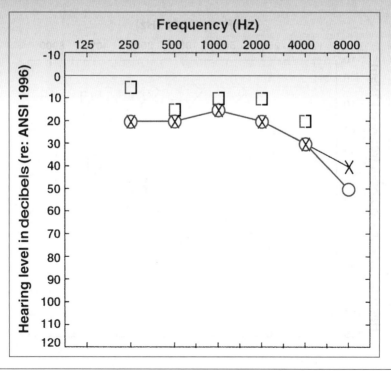

(continued)

VIGNETTE 8.7 **A child with bilateral minimal hearing loss** *(Continued)*

---

of life. He was hospitalized 22 times for refractory (unmanageable) otitis media, and he underwent mastoidectomy and tympanoplasty on the right side.

The audiogram shows that the child has a very mild bilateral hearing loss through the speech frequency range and a somewhat precipitous drop in the high frequencies. The child had considerable difficulty understanding speech in a background of noise. When tested in a sound-field situation in the presence of background noise (16 dB SNR), the child was able to understand only 76% of the material.

He is enrolled in kindergarten, where he is having considerable difficulty. There is serious question as to whether he will progress to the first grade. He is reportedly immature and hyperactive. Language skills, especially vocabulary, are delayed by 1 to 2 years.

Based on these results, a number of recommendations were made: (*a*) He should continue with otologic management for middle ear disease with effusion. (*b*) He should receive support in the form of an FM system for use in the academic setting (this system was recommended to improve the SNR in the noisy classroom environment). (*c*) The board of education should be notified of the child's circumstance so that his audiologic and academic needs can be monitored. (*d*) The child should be seen by the audiologist every 6 months to monitor progress.

VIGNETTE 8.8 **A child with unilateral conductive hearing loss**

This 5-year-old girl has a history of early otitis media. The child underwent myringotomy with tubes inserted at 1 year of age, a second set at 2 years of age, and a third set at 2.5 years of age. When this audiogram was taken, the child did not have tubes. At 5 years, she presented with a perforation in the left ear and underwent tympanoplasty to repair the eardrum. An ear

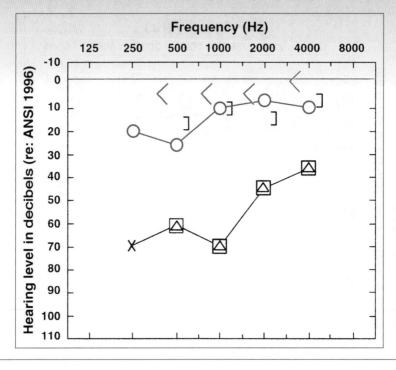

VIGNETTE 8.8	A child with unilateral conductive hearing loss *(Continued)*

infection shortly after the tympanoplasty compounded the child's conductive problem. The child is enrolled in a Head Start program, where she is having difficulty understanding speech and is delayed in speech and language by approximately 1 year.

  Based on these results, the following recommendations were made: (*a*) The child should receive a comprehensive speech and language evaluation and evaluations every 6 to 8 months. (*b*) The child should be evaluated for the use of an FM system to help her in the classroom. (*c*) The child should be placed in a special education class in the fall. (*d*) The child should receive classroom seating preference.

Children With Severe to Profound Hearing Loss

In general terms, there seems to be an association between the severity of hearing loss and the degree of educational delay. The milder the hearing loss, however, the more difficult it is to predict the educational potential of the child. Since the 1920s, it has been acknowledged that deafness causes an educational lag of 4 to 5 years. This lowered achievement is thought to result from the difficulty of acquiring language and communication skills. Delayed speech and language in the important preschool years cannot help but be reflected when a child learns to read, because reading achievement is an important indicator of linguistic competence. Reading is a basic learning tool that directly influences the mastery of all other academic content. For years, educators of deaf children have been concerned with the apparent plateau effect that begins at approximately 9 to 10 years of age and persists through the teens. This effect is reflected in very minimal gains in reading level over several years of instruction. The average gain in reading level between 10 and 16 years of age among deaf students is less than a year. One can expect most children with profound hearing loss to be delayed 7 to 8 years in reading vocabulary by age 18 years. There are, however, many exceptions.

  There have been a number of national surveys of the population with hearing loss. In general, for deaf individuals who could not hear and understand speech and who had lost that ability by 19 years of age (or never had it), approximately half had not completed high school, and close to one-third had not completed the ninth grade. Although such information should be interpreted with caution because the census reports years of school completed and not achievement level, it does offer insight into some of the educational difficulties of the deaf population. Figure 8.4 shows the results from the most recent nationwide norms on the Stanford Achievement Test (SAT) for reading comprehension and mathematics for children with hearing loss as a function of age. The two charts show the scaled scores for the subtest on the left ordinate; the right ordinate provides the corresponding grade equivalents for hearing students. For reading comprehension (*left panel*), the average 18-year-old student with hearing loss is reading at only the fourth grade level. Moreover, the average child with hearing loss increased reading ability only about two grade equivalents between 9 and 18 years of age. Finally, whereas children at 8 years of age are delayed approximately 2 years in grade level compared with normal-hearing children, the children at 15 years of age have fallen even further behind and are delayed more than 7 years. In contrast, mathematics procedure scores (*right panel*)

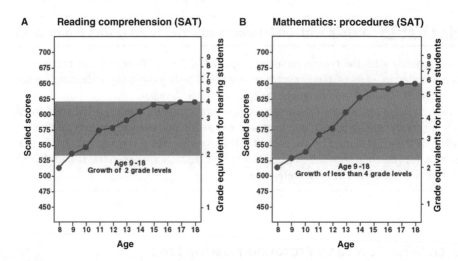

FIGURE 8.4 Stanford Achievement Test (SAT) scores for students with hearing loss (1996 data). Scaled scores for the subtest appear on the left ordinate; the right ordinate shows the corresponding grade equivalents for hearing students. **A.** Reading comprehension levels as a function of age in years for children with hearing loss. **B.** The scores of children with hearing loss for mathematics procedures. (Data courtesy of Gallaudet Research Institute, Gallaudet University, Washington, 1996.)

are less affected by hearing loss, approaching the sixth-grade level at age 17 years. These data clearly illustrate the educational lag that is common to deaf and partially hearing children enrolled in special programs.

Children With Mild to Moderate Hearing Loss

Thus far, our discussion has focused on the impact of severe to profound hearing loss on education. What about children with the milder forms of hearing loss, sometimes called the hard-of-hearing or the population with partial hearing loss? Once again, we find that even those with milder hearing losses can have difficulty in school. In 1968, researchers examined the educational potential of 116 children with hearing loss using subtests of the SAT. Table 8.4 summarizes the results from this study and shows the differences between expected performance (computed from the birth dates of the children) and actual performance for children with varying degrees of hearing loss on the subtests of word meaning, paragraph meaning, and language. Several important points are evident. First, there is a slight trend toward decreasing IQ with increasing hearing loss. Second, all groups of children with hearing loss, even those with losses as mild as 15 to 26 dB, lagged in educational performance. This is indicated by the appearance of negative numbers in the table. Third, one can see by looking at the subtest averages that the discrepancy between expected performance and actual performance increases with increasing hearing loss. The average difference between expected performance and actual performance for all groups was −1.25 grades. These data, although not universally acknowledged as valid, demonstrate that some children with slight hearing loss are not realizing their educational potential.

TABLE 8.4   Differences Between Expected and Actual Performance of Children on the Stanford Achievement Test

Average Hearing Threshold Subtest (Better Ear) (dB)	No. of Children	IQ	Word Meaning[a]	Paragraph Meaning[a]	Language[a]	Subtest Average[a]
<15	59	105.14	−1.04	−0.47	−0.78	−0.73
15–26	37	100.81	−1.40	−0.86	−1.16	−1.11
27–40	6	103.50	−3.48	−1.78	−1.95	−2.31
41–55	9	97.89	−3.84	−2.54	−2.93	−3.08
56–70	5	92.40	−2.78	−2.20	−3.52	−2.87

[a]Negative values indicate a deficit in measured grade level compared to normal-hearing children.
(Adapted from Quigley SP. Some Effects of Hearing Loss Upon School Performance. Springfield, IL: Division of Special Education Services, Department of Special Education Development and Education, 1968.)

The data in Table 8.4 prompted other investigators to explore the impact of milder hearing losses on educational achievement. Foremost in this effort has been the work of Davis and coworkers published in 1981 and in 1986. Davis and coworkers conducted two comprehensive studies on the educational abilities of children with hearing loss in the schools. In the first study, data were taken from the school files of more than 1000 children with mild to moderately severe hearing loss. The findings of this retrospective study revealed that the children with mild to moderate degrees of hearing loss (three-frequency pure-tone average of ≤50 dB) did not show significant educational problems. Those with average hearing losses of more than 50 dB, however, exhibited significant deficits in academic achievement, and these problems increased over time. In contrast, most of the children with hearing loss, even those with mild losses, demonstrated difficulties with language.

In a follow-up investigation, a prospective study was performed on a group of 40 children with mild to moderately severe hearing loss. Rather than rely on test scores from the school files, as before, the researchers administered the same battery of educational achievement tests to all subjects in the sample. Importantly, and in contrast to the previous study, it was not possible to predict educational performance solely on the basis of hearing level; it was possible for a child with minimal hearing loss to exhibit as much (or even more) difficulty with a given task as a child with a mild to moderate hearing loss. The difficulties experienced by these children could be lumped into three general areas: verbal skills, academic skills, and social development. Verbal skills seemed to be affected most, and this area was also reported to be the most closely associated with hearing loss. These researchers emphasized the heterogeneity of the population with hearing loss and concluded that children with any degree of hearing loss can be at risk for delayed verbal skills and reduced educational progress.

Another important finding of this study was that many of these children exhibited behavioral problems. Many were also concerned about peer acceptance. One of the children from the study related the following: "I don't have very many friends. Oh, people say, 'Hi, Kris, hi, Kris,' but only 'Hi, Kris,' never anything—you know—go out for lunch or go out on dates or anything like that. The only friends I almost have are my teachers and my counselors" (Davis, Elfenbein, Schum, and Bentler, 1986).

Children With Moderate to Severe Unilateral Sensorineural Hearing Loss

Not only are children with mild hearing loss at risk, but it seems that children with moderate to severe unilateral sensorineural hearing loss also have difficulty in the schools. The auditory, linguistic, and psychoeducational skills of a group of school-age children with unilateral sensorineural hearing loss have been examined extensively. In a survey of 60 children with unilateral hearing loss, 35% were found to have failed at least one grade, and an additional 13% needed special assistance. Moreover, children with unilateral sensorineural hearing loss exhibited greater difficulty than children with normal hearing in understanding speech in the presence of competing background noise and localizing sound in the horizontal plane. Children with severe to profound unilateral hearing loss exhibited lower IQs than did children with milder unilateral loss; and those who failed a grade in elementary school exhibited verbal IQs that were significantly lower than those of children with unilateral hearing loss who had not failed a grade. Perhaps the most interesting finding from this study was that children with right-ear impairments were at greater risk for academic failure than children with left-ear impairments. Finally, teachers rated children with unilateral losses as having greater difficulty in peer relations, less social confidence, greater likelihood of acting out or withdrawn behavior in the classroom, greater frustration and dependence on the teacher, and more frequent distractibility.

Before this research, the prevailing belief was that children with unilateral hearing loss do not have any problems in school. It had always been assumed that one good ear is sufficient to enable a child to achieve satisfactorily in school.

Children With Minimal Conductive and Sensorineural Hearing Losses

Conductive Hearing Loss

For almost 4 decades, there has been a growing awareness of the potential psychoeducational complications associated with recurrent otitis media (ROM) during the early developmental years. Although many of the research studies conducted in this area have flaws in design, most imply a link between a history of ROM, associated hearing loss, and some area of child development. Otitis proneness in children has been linked to learning disabilities, academic problems, lower intelligence levels, behavior and attention problems, difficulties in understanding speech in a background of noise, and delayed language development.

How is it that the mild, fluctuating hearing loss associated with otitis media can interfere with the development of auditory, linguistic, and psychoeducational skills? Recall from Chapter 5 that children with otitis media have hearing loss averaging about 30 dB through the speech-frequency range. During the early developmental period for speech and language, the otitis-prone child is likely to have an inconsistent and perhaps a somewhat distorted auditory signal. In fact, many of the speech sounds that have low energy, such as /f/, /s/, /u/, /k/, /p/, /h/, /z/, and /v/, may well be missed altogether in the presence of a mild 30-dB hearing loss. Similarly, important acoustic information, such as morphologic markers (i.e., plural -s, past tense -ed) and inflections may be especially difficult to identify.

The loss of acoustic energy partly explains trouble in the developmental years. Once the otitis-prone years have passed, can the child make up for the lost input?

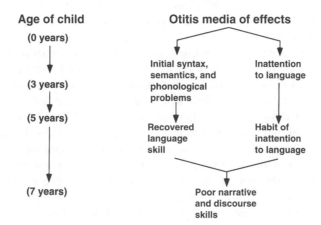

Effects of Otitis Media

FIGURE 8.5   Hypothetical model to explain how later language functioning might be affected by early persistent otitis media. (Reprinted from Feagans L. Otitis media: A model for long term effects with implications for intervention. In Kavanagh JF, ed. Otitis Media and Child Development. Parkton, MD: York, 1986.)

Unfortunately, some evidence suggests that some children do not. Otitis media can produce both delays in language and an inattention to language. Once the otitis media resolves or the episodes become less frequent, the child can recover basic language skills, but the habit of not attending to language may persist. Some of the more basic language components, such as syntax and semantics, may not be as seriously affected as discourse and narrative skills. The latter require some amount of attention to language. Figure 8.5 summarizes the possible sequence of events that could occur from repeated bouts of early otitis media.

Sensorineural Hearing Loss

Since the mid-1980s audiologists have discussed the potential educational and psychosocial problems associated with minimal sensorineural hearing loss (MSHL). MSHL typically refers to three different types of hearing loss: unilateral sensorineural hearing loss, bilateral sensorineural hearing loss, and high-frequency sensorineural hearing loss. Unilateral sensorineural hearing loss is defined as an average air conduction threshold of 20 dB HL or greater in the impaired ear—unilateral losses that are milder than discussed earlier. Bilateral sensorineural hearing loss in this context is defined as an average pure-tone threshold between 20 and 40 dB bilaterally with average air-bone gaps no greater than 10 dB at frequencies 1, 2, and 4 kHz. High-frequency sensorineural hearing loss is defined as air conduction thresholds greater than 25 dB HL at two or more frequencies above the 2 kHz (i.e., 3, 4, 6, 8 kHz) in one or both ears.

When using such definitions, the prevalence of MSHL in the schools (grades 3, 6, and 9) is 5.4%. That is, 1 in 20, or close to 2.5 million children, exhibit very mild sensorineural hearing loss. Unilateral sensorineural hearing loss is the most prevalent form, followed by high-frequency and bilateral sensorineural hearing loss. Interestingly, MSHL is more prevalent in the schools than conductive hearing loss. Finally, when all forms of hearing loss are considered, the prevalence of hearing loss among school-aged children is 11.3%, approximately twice the 5 to 6% prevalence rate often reported in the schools.

The general cause of sensorineural hearing loss is not known. However, recreational noise, chronic otitis media, and survival rate of premature at-risk infants have all been mentioned as possible factors. It seems that children with MSHL can have a variety of educational and psychosocial problems. Recently, a group at Vanderbilt University conducted a study designed to assess the relationship of MSHL to educational performance and functional health status. More than 1000 children in grades 3, 6, and 9 served as the study sample. Third-grade children identified with minimal loss were found to exhibit significantly lower scores on many subtests of an academic achievement test than did a matched group of normal-hearing children. Moreover, children with minimal loss were found to be at greater risk for academic failure than their normal-hearing counterparts, as determined by a screening tool administered to the teachers of the children with hearing loss. The subtest on communication from the screening tool showed the greatest discrepancy between children with minimal loss and children with normal hearing. The communication subtest focuses on the students' understanding ability, vocabulary and word usage skills, and story-telling abilities; all very important skills for learning.

In support of the teacher's survey, 37% of children with MSHL failed at least one grade, compared with the district norm failure rate of 3%. A breakdown of the failure rate for children with minimal losses as compared to normal hearing children across grades 3, 6, and 9 is shown in Figure 8.6. Retention rates increase with increasing grade; almost half the children in the 9th grade with MSHL had failed at least one grade. The Vanderbilt study also demonstrated that children with MSHL exhibit greater psychosocial

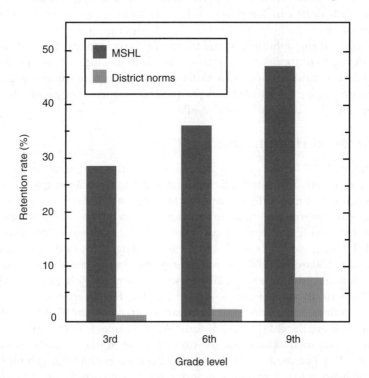

FIGURE 8.6 School retention rates for children with MSHL at each grade level (3, 6, 9). School district norm retention rates are included for comparison. (Reprinted from Bess FH, Dodd JD, Parker RA. Children with minimal sensorineural hearing loss: Prevalence, educational performance and functional health status. Ear Hear 19:339–354, 1998.)

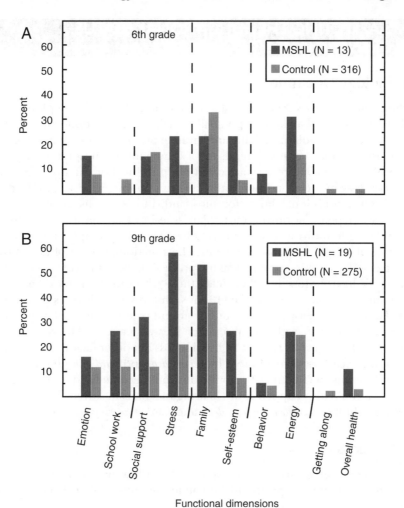

FIGURE 8.7 Percentage of children with MSHL and normal-hearing counterparts in grades 6 **(A)** and 9 **(B)** who exhibited scores of 4 or 5 (greater dysfunction) on a measure of functional health status. (Adapted from Bess FH, Dodd JD, Parker RA. Children with minimal sensorineural hearing loss: Prevalence, educational performance and functional health status. Ear Hear 19:339–354, 1998.)

dysfunction than normal-hearing children. These data are shown in Figure 8.7. This figure shows the percentage of children with MSHL in grades 6 and 9 who exhibited high scores (greater dysfunction) on a measure of functional health status. The children with MSHL tended to perform worse than normal-hearing children on many of the social and emotional domains, especially self-esteem, energy, stress, and social support. Social skills are known to play an important role in an individual's receipt of social, academic, and emotional rewards. Problems in social and emotional behavior are linked to peer status, school maladjustment, dropping out of school, and juvenile delinquency. Indeed, the results from this study suggest the need for audiologists, speech-language pathologists, and educators to examine carefully our identification and management approaches with this population. Better efforts to manage these children could result in meaningful improvement in their educational progress and their psychosocial well-being.

FACTORS AFFECTING THE EDUCATIONAL STATUS OF CHILDREN WITH HEARING LOSS

The Terminology Dilemma

Leading commentators over the past 2 decades have frequently deplored the growing tendency for issues of all kinds—political, social, religious, ethnic, minority, and many others—to become polarized. This unfortunate predilection seldom benefits either of the opposing groups because it tends to lock them into such rigidly exclusive positions that flexibility and compromise are often not possible. For example, the terms *liberal* and *conservative* in social and political affairs can no longer be accurately described or defined along traditional lines, for most individuals are likely to cross over these boundaries, depending on the particular issue involved. So it is with the use of the terms relating to individuals with hearing loss. Despite attempts to emphasize the various interrelating factors that determine the functioning level of an individual with hearing loss, lay people, as well as many professionals, continue to dichotomize individuals with hearing loss as either deaf (those who cannot hear) or hard of hearing (those who can hear, at least partially). Thus, children with degrees of hearing loss designated as mild, moderate, severe, and profound could in fact spend their lives in one or the other category with its subsequent lifestyle pattern. The determinant would then be not the degree or severity of hearing loss but other factors, most of which were present in the earliest years of life. The terms *deaf* and *hard of hearing* are not mutually exclusive, because a child may begin life deaf but become hard of hearing. Of course, the reverse could also happen if the hearing mechanism suffers further damage. The following definitions of *hearing loss, deaf,* and *hard of hearing* may be useful.

Hearing Loss

Hearing loss or *hearing impaired* is a generic term indicating disability that may range in severity from very mild to profound; it includes the subsets of deaf and hard of hearing.

Deaf

Deaf describes one whose disability precluded successful processing of linguistic information through audition with or without a hearing aid.

Hard of Hearing

Hard of hearing describes one who generally, with the use of a hearing aid or cochlear implant, has residual hearing sufficient to enable successful processing of linguistic information by way of audition. The term *partially hearing* is sometimes used synonymously with *hard of hearing*.

Although these definitions are likely to be inappropriately used and interpreted, they present a thoughtful and reasonable approach to a very complex issue. There is a need to recognize that *hearing loss* includes all gradients of severity of hearing loss. The term has too often been used redundantly in the phrase *the deaf and the hearing impaired*. To be deaf is to be impaired in hearing, but *hearing impaired* is often used as if it were synonymous with *hard of hearing* or *partially hearing*. Such definitions suffer the same fault that has been inherent in most other definitions; most children with hearing loss cannot be classified either as deaf or hard of hearing early in life. Nor will the label necessarily remain appropriate from that time forth. The distinction made in the definitions relates to the present auditory capabilities. Many individual variables determine the borderline between the residuum of hearing for which aural linguistic processing is not possible and that for which it is possible. It is not unusual, for example, for a child with only a moderate hearing loss to function more like a deaf child whose hearing loss is in the profound range. Thus, although some levels of hearing loss do preclude linguistic processing by audition, for many severely impaired persons, the more important factor is the age at which auditory experience through individual amplification or implantation is initiated and how successfully it is monitored and maintained.

Degree of Hearing Loss

In general, the more severe the hearing loss is, the greater the likelihood that a child will be enrolled in a special education program. In fact, approximately 80% of children enrolled in special programs have losses greater than 55 dB HL in the better ear.

The serious nature of the educational handicap of hearing loss requires that parents and professionals diligently seek every possible advantage needed by children with hearing loss. However, although many will enthusiastically endorse this established principle, it is not always put into practice. For example, although early detection, intervention, and use of appropriate rehabilitative technology are pretty much universally endorsed regardless of the particular method supported, most children enrolled in special education programs have not had such opportunities.

Age of Intervention

The rubella epidemic that swept across the United States during 1964 and 1965 sharply increased awareness of childhood deafness and its challenges to educators. During the late 1960s, several well-known programs were developed for parents and their deaf babies aged birth to 3 years. These programs emphasized parent counseling and training instead of focusing the training efforts on the child. The theory was that formal procedures were not yet suitable for such young children. By demonstration and example, parents were tutored in principles of communicating with their children. They were shown the importance of amplification and adaptation to use of hearing as a primary source of language input in the first years of life, which for all children is the most natural time for language acquisition. Although several highly successful programs were organized and conducted, such facilities were not always within the reach of children with hearing loss and their parents. Most children with hearing loss are affected at birth or before age 3 years. Congenital and other forms of prelingual hearing loss are the most handicapping educationally, as evidenced by the need for special education facilities. If the impairment had occurred after language acquisition, many of these children might have been enrolled in regular education.

The advent of universal newborn hearing screening has resulted in a systematic decrease in the age of identification for hearing loss and intervention. Importantly, universal newborn screening was advocated because it was generally believed that the critical period for language development occurred within the first 2 years of life and that auditory deprivation in that first year results in deprivation of language learning—hence, the importance of early intervention. The value of early intervention is discussed further in Vignette 8.9.

VIGNETTE 8.9   Early versus late intervention

Are the outcomes for children with congenital hearing loss more favorable if treatment is begun early in infancy rather than later in childhood (i.e., 6 months versus 18 months)? Much theoretical understanding, intuitive belief, and clinical experience argue in favor of early intervention. Advocates point to the animal research demonstrating that early acoustic deprivation results in morphologic changes in the central neural pathways. Extrapolating such findings to humans, however, would indeed be speculative. Moreover, at least until recently, behavioral data to support the proposition that early intervention leads to more favorable outcomes has been limited. A research team from the University of Colorado shed some light on the benefits of early versus late identification of children with hearing loss. Very briefly, the Colorado group compared the language skills of children identified by 6 months of age with the language skills of children identified after 6 months. Their study showed that children who were identified before 6 months of age exhibited significantly better receptive and expressive language skills than did children whose hearing losses were identified after 6 months of age. The Colorado group concluded that when their data were considered with other investigations, the first year of life, especially the first 6 months of life, is a critical period of intervention for children with hearing loss.

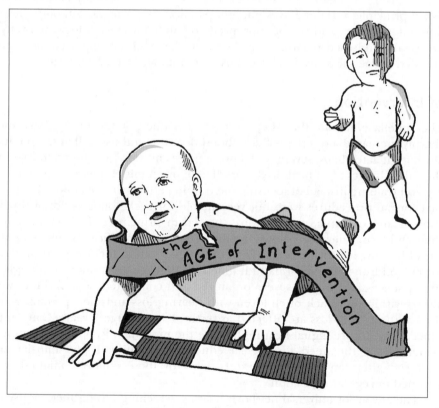

A more recent study from Boys Town National Research Hospital offered additional support for the findings obtained by the Colorado team. The Boys Town study systematically investigated this question: is there a relationship between age of intervention and language skills at age 5? The study included 112 children with hearing loss. The children were evaluated

---

VIGNETTE 8.9 **Early versus late intervention *(Continued)***

---

for language and verbal reasoning as a function of age of intervention. Early intervention was found to result in improved outcomes for the children at 5 years of age. The later the children received intervention, the poorer the outcomes. Moreover, family involvement was a key variable to positive outcomes.

The table below pointedly illustrates the value of early intervention and the importance of family involvement. The children (n = 80) were categorized into three groups based on their verbal reasoning test scores (i.e., high performers, average performers, and low performers). Clearly, the best performers benefited from early intervention, had the most family involvement (a rating of 5 indicated the greatest involvement, whereas a rating of 1 indicated the least involvement) and the mildest impairment.

Hence, based on the research of these investigators and several other pilot studies, it is the general belief among most hearing health care professionals that infants with hearing loss who are identified by 6 months of age and receive early intervention will no doubt come closer to realizing their maximum potential.

Characteristics of Children Scoring at Various Levels on a Test of Verbal Reasoning[a]

Performance Category	Age of Enrollment (y)	Family Involvement Rating	Better-Ear Pure-Tone Average (dB)
Highest performers (at or above 25th percentile)	1.2	4.4	71
Average performers (10th to 25th percentile)	1.8	3.6	75
Low performers	2.3	2.6	80

[a]Data represent mean scores.
Reprinted from Moeller MP. Intervention and outcomes for young children who are deaf and hard of hearing and their families. In Kurtzer-White E, Luterman D, eds. Early Childhood Deafness. Baltimore: York, 2001.

Communication Patterns

In general, speech, either oral English alone or in combination with other modes, is the communication pattern most frequently used by parents and students with hearing loss in their interaction. The children use signs somewhat more than their parents do, and they use speech a bit less. Approximately 69% of family members do not sign regularly, whereas regular signing in the home is used by 26% of family members. Speech alone and speech supplemented with gestures account for approximately 50% of the parent-to-student communication and 40% of student-to-parent communication. In general, the communication patterns of children with hearing loss yield the following conclusions: (*a*) Children who have hearing loss vary widely in their communication patterns. (*b*) Combinations of methods rather than a single method are the rule in the classroom but far less so at home. (*c*) Speech alone is the single most common pattern at home, whereas a combination of speech signs, finger spelling, writing, and gestures is the single most common pattern at school. (*d*) There is relatively little consistency between patterns of communication used at home and in school.

In the view of most educators, there should be consistency in the communication patterns used by parents and teachers, regardless of the particular educational philosophy held. Much improvement could be made through more intensive efforts for parent participation in the education process for children with hearing loss.

Ethnic Background

In general, whites score higher on reading comprehension tests than either African-American or Hispanic students, a fact thought to be a consequence of socioeconomic and cultural elements and possibly differences among these populations in access to medical, education, and other remedial services. For Hispanic students, the problem is compounded by the fact that Spanish is the primary language spoken in the home and English is the primary language spoken in the schools. Very few programs for children with hearing loss in this country can adequately deal with the problems raised by bilingual spoken language acquisition, not to mention the issues of signing and written language. No doubt, as the numbers of minorities increase among children with hearing impairment, this issue of ethnicity will become increasingly important.

Presence of an Additional Handicapping Condition

It is generally estimated that about one-third of children with hearing loss have at least one additional handicapping condition that affects education. Close to 10% have at least two additional handicaps in combination. These conditions include visual impairment, brain damage or injury, mental retardation, epilepsy, learning disabilities, cerebral palsy, orthopedic problems, and emotional and behavioral problems. These children are likely to be placed in special education settings only. Clearly, such handicapping conditions adversely affect the child's ability to learn in the schools.

Understandably, children with multiple disabilities represent a challenge to the audiologist. Major differences among these children are considerable; they function at different levels, and they learn in different ways. Moreover, these children are typically identified somewhat later than deaf children. Finally, many of these children are managed as if they do have a hearing loss; it is sometimes several years before the additional handicaps are recognized.

To summarize to this point, hearing loss in childhood is a serious barrier to the normal educational process. However, this problem is related not just to one or two but to many interacting variables. When this cluster of variables is for the most part favorable, even severely and profoundly impaired children can achieve remarkably well in comparison to hearing children.

AUDIOLOGY IN THE SCHOOLS

We have just seen that children with varying degrees of hearing loss undergo considerable hardship in school and typically lag behind their normal-hearing peers in terms of academic achievement. The audiologist can play an important role in the management of these children in the schools. The following discussion focuses on the role of the audiologist in the educational setting.

Models for Delivering Audiologic Services to the Schools

The delivery of audiologic services within the educational environment varies considerably from one local educational agency (LEA) to the next. Educational systems offer programs ranging from comprehensive audiologic management to only minimal services. Although models for the provision of audiologic management to the schools are numerous, there are three commonly used approaches. These models are the *parent referral* approach, the *cooperative interagency* approach, and the *audiology approach within the schools.*

Parent Referral Model

The parent referral model is the most traditional approach to the delivery of audiologic services in the schools. The LEA provides identification and intervention services; the more comprehensive assessment and evaluation services are supplied by agencies or parties outside of the LEA. The success of this model depends highly on the parents, who become responsible for the management and follow-up of their child. Once the school has notified the parents that their child is in need of further testing, they must make arrangements on their own for an audiologic or medical evaluation. The results of these evaluations are given directly to the parent, with feedback supplied to the LEA. The advantages to this model are that services are provided at a minimal cost to the LEA and that the school system uses resources that already exist within the community, avoiding unnecessary duplication of services. Unfortunately, there are more disadvantages than advantages to the parent referral model. The LEA has no control over the management of a child and must rely on the cooperation of the parent, the hearing and speech center, and the physician to supply the necessary information and recommendations. Because the LEA does not monitor referred children, many complications can arise. For example, there is no mechanism for ensuring that diagnostic reports will be sent to the school within a reasonable period or that they will be sent at all. In addition, the received reports may be incomplete or perhaps inappropriate in that the information provided may not assist the school or teacher in helping the child educationally. Seldom does the report supply sufficient information relative to the child's educational placement and/or management. Even if such information is available, the model provides no assurance that the child will receive appropriate follow-up. Finally, the parent referral model is conducive only to an annual evaluation and not to continuous audiologic management.

Cooperative Interagency Model

An alternative to the provision of audiologic services in the schools is a contractual arrangement between the LEA and a community hearing and speech center, a hospital, or a private practice. Once the child is identified, the school notifies the parents and the contracting agency. Although dependent on the contracted services, the agency ordinarily provides audiologic management of the child and maintains constant feedback to an LEA designate, usually the coordinator of the program for those with hearing loss. In some instances, an audiologist coordinates the referral and management. The parent initiates a referral to the physician, if necessary, at the recommendation of the school. The physician in turn provides feedback to the parent, school, and contract agency.

The success of this model depends on the types of services contracted. The more knowledgeable the administrator, the more comprehensive the contract and the more successful the program. The agreement works best when an audiologist from the agency is solely responsible for coordinating the audiologic services. The contact person at the LEA and the teachers must have one person to whom they can refer questions or problems. This model offers several advantages and eliminates some of the disadvantages associated with the parent referral model. It is particularly useful for educational systems with small numbers of children with hearing loss (such as schools in rural areas). Duplication of services is avoided, and as with the parent referral model, the LEA need not be concerned with the high cost of equipment and facilities. At a time when funding is a primary concern in education, this must be considered a distinct advantage. This model also has several limitations. Unless responsibilities and lines of authority are clearly defined and monitored on a continuing basis, communication can break down. Because the LEA is paying for the audiologic services, there is a tendency for the educational administration to dictate the type and extent of services to be provided. Open lines of communication, willingness to cooperate with the LEA staff, and general agreement on services to be delivered are essential. Another potential difficulty is the LEA's loss of control over expenditures, although this problem can be eliminated by carefully defining in the contract how funds will be expended.

School Audiology Model

The final model is development of a comprehensive audiologic program within the LEA. In this model, services are provided by a coordinating audiologist and associated staff. This model provides the LEA with complete central control of audiologic services. Identification, assessment, and management are all under the jurisdiction of the coordinating school audiologist. The advantage to such a model is that the audiologist is where the children are—in the schools. IEPs for the students with hearing loss can be developed and implemented in the schools. Effective input to these plans would be difficult for professionals outside the system. Other advantages of this model include immediate access to diagnostic information, development of evaluation data tailored to the educational setting, greater control over follow-up, good communication between the LEA staff and the school audiologist, and better potential for ongoing in-service education. The limitations of the model are the high costs of equipping a complete audiologic facility and employing the needed personnel and the problems that arise from duplicating services that are available within the community. Now that we have reviewed three of the models used for delivering services to the schools, let us briefly examine some of the responsibilities of the school audiologist.

Responsibilities of Audiologists in the Schools

The duties of the audiologist in the school setting are numerous and require highly specialized skills and knowledge. The American Speech-Language-Hearing Association developed a comprehensive list of suggested responsibilities for audiologists in education. This information is summarized in Table 8.5. Some of the basic responsibilities discussed here include identification, assessment, audiologic management including amplification, educational admission and placement, in-service training, and provision of rehabilitative services.

TABLE 8.5   **Suggested Responsibilities of Audiologists Employed in the Schools**

- Provide community leadership to ensure that all infants, toddlers, and youth with impaired hearing are promptly identified, evaluated, and provided with appropriate intervention services.
- Collaborate with community resources to develop a high-risk registry and follow-up.
- Develop and supervise a hearing screening program for preschool and school-age children.
- Train audiometric technicians or other appropriate personnel to screen for hearing loss.
- Perform follow-up comprehensive audiologic evaluations.
- Assess central auditory function.
- Make appropriate referrals for further audiologic, communication, educational, psychosocial, or medical assessment.
- Interpret audiologic assessment results to other school personnel.
- Serve on the educational team in evaluation, planning, and placement. Make recommendations regarding placement, service needs, communication needs, and modification of classroom for students with auditory problems.
- Provide in-service training on hearing and hearing loss and their implications to school personnel, children, and parents.
- Educate parents, children, and school personnel about prevention of hearing loss.
- Make recommendations about use of hearing aids, cochlear implants, group and classroom amplification, and assistive listening devices.
- Ensure proper fit and function of hearing aids, cochlear implants, group and classroom amplification, and assistive listening devices.
- Analyze classroom noise and acoustics and make recommendations for improving the listening environment.
- Manage the use and calibration of audiometric equipment.
- Collaborate with school, parents, teachers, special support personnel, and relevant community agencies and professionals to ensure delivery of appropriate services.
- Make recommendations for assistive devices (radio, television, telephone, alerting, and convenience) for students with hearing loss.
- Provide services, including some programming if appropriate, in speech reading, listening, communication strategies, use and care of amplification, including cochlear implants, and self-management of hearing needs.

Reprinted from Guidelines for audiology services in the schools by the American Speech-Language-Hearing Association. ASHA Desk Reference for Audiology and Speech-Language Pathology, II. 1995, p 71; DeConde Johnson C, Benson PV, Seaton JB. Roles and responsibilities of the educational audiologist. In Educational Audiology Handbook. San Diego: Singular, 1997, 17–25.

Identification

Ideally, the educational audiologist should have primary responsibility for the identification of preschool and school-age children with hearing loss or middle ear disease. Even if identification services are not offered directly by the school program, the educational audiologist should coordinate the screening program. Techniques for setting up screening programs are discussed in Chapter 6.

Assessment

A major responsibility of the educational audiologist is to assess the communicative efficiency of children with hearing loss in the schools. The assessment battery should include traditional measurements of auditory function (pure-tone audiometry, speech audiometry, and immittance measures) as well as the evaluation of auditory processing and communication skills. Assessment protocols are addressed in Chapter 4.

Audiologic Management, Including Amplification

The school audiologist plays an important role in the audiologic management of the child with hearing loss. The associated responsibilities might include selection and evaluation of amplification and assistive listening devices, maintenance of amplification devices, monitoring classroom noise, coordination of habilitation or rehabilitation activities, and parent counseling.

The selection and evaluation of amplification is a fundamental concern to the audiologist in education and warrants additional comment at this point. After the hearing aid is selected, periodic reevaluations of the child's performance with amplification are essential. Occasionally it is necessary to make minor modifications in the electroacoustic parameters of the hearing aid as more is learned about the child's hearing or as hearing sensitivity changes. The educational audiologist is responsible not only for the selection and evaluation of the personal hearing aid but also for the classroom amplification system. The audiologist spends considerable time and effort in the selection and evaluation of a personal hearing aid for a child with hearing loss; however, this is not always true regarding the selection and evaluation of classroom systems. Whatever is appropriate in the selection and evaluation of the child's personal aid should also be important in the selection and evaluation of the child's classroom system. The educational audiologist should make sure that the characteristics of both the personal and classroom hearing aids of a child are comparable and provide consistency in auditory input.

Far too often, hearing aids in the school do not function properly. To help eliminate these problems, a well-organized amplification maintenance program should be implemented in the schools. A maintenance program should contain the following essential elements: (*a*) education of parents and teachers on the use and care of a hearing aid, (*b*) a daily visual and listening examination, (*c*) monthly electroacoustic checks, and (*d*) comprehensive physical inspections of the hearing aid. At the outset, both the parents and the teachers should be taught how to troubleshoot a hearing aid and should be given a kit that permits simple inspection of a hearing aid. A traditional troubleshooting kit would include a drying agent for removing moisture, pipe cleaners, a battery tester, a hearing aid stethoscope, spare batteries, and an extra receiver. The parent should be instructed to examine the child's hearing aid each day before school, and the teacher or an assistant should recheck the instrument once each morning. It is important for teachers to have a supply of batteries in the classroom. A good maintenance program should also include an adequate stock of loaner aids (aids used as substitutes for personal hearing aids that are in need of repair).

Although the focus in the preceding paragraphs is on the provision and monitoring of hearing aids, because they still represent the rehabilitative device most commonly encountered by the audiologist, the same principles apply to other devices, such as cochlear implants. Every effort should be made to monitor the performance of the implant periodically to ensure that it is programmed appropriately and functioning properly.

Educational Admission and Placement

The audiologist should be an active member of the staff that reviews a child's school status to decide placement or admission. The audiologist's input should be evident in the IEP of PL 94-142 or the individual family service plan (IFSP) of PL 99-457 as it relates to amplification needs, the amount and type of language and speech intervention required, the classroom acoustic environment, parent and child counseling, and support systems for the classroom teacher. IEPs are written statements that detail the educational management of a given child and meet the unique needs of the family. These statements are generated because the child's condition precludes the use of a standard school curriculum. The IEP details special educational needs and special services the child will need on a daily basis. Hence, the IEP provides the child with an individualized and appropriate education in the least restrictive environment possible. It is critical that the child's audiologic needs be built into the IEP; otherwise, the local LEA will have no obligation to include such services in the child's educational management plan. Hence, the audiologist must become an advocate for the child and his or her parents from an audiologic standpoint.

In general, the IEP should include the following components:

- Statement of the child's educational performance;
- Statement of goals, including short-term and instructional objectives;
- Statement of the specific special education and related services to be provided to the child to enable him or her to participate in regular educational programs;
- Projected date for initiation and anticipated duration of such services; and
- Appropriate objective criteria and evaluation procedures and schedules for determining (at least annually) whether short-term instructional objectives are being achieved and whether placement is appropriate.

The following information should be included in the IFSP:

- Child's current status and present levels of development as determined by objective criteria;
- Family information needed for facilitating the development of the child;
- Expected outcomes of the early intervention program;
- Details of the specific plan for the delivery, location, and method of payment for early intervention;
- Other services not required by law but needed by the child (e.g., medical services)
- Duration and dates of the specific early intervention services;
- Designation of the case manager to ensure proper implementation of the IFSP; and
- Plans for transition into the school system. Unfortunately, the audiologist is generally not included in the development of the IEP/IFSP unless specifically requested by the parent or teacher.

An example of a portion of an IEP is shown in Table 8.6.

In-Service Education

An important responsibility of the audiologist in the schools is the development of in-service education programs for school personnel who come in frequent contact with children with hearing loss. In addition to providing in-service training to speech-language pathologists and teachers of those with hearing loss, more general in-service

TABLE 8.6   Segment of an Individual Education Program

Domain	Status	Annual Goal	Short-Term Objective
Audiologic	Can discriminate two utterances that differ in syllable length and intonation, such as *hello* from *how are you?*	Achieve closed-set identification of monosyllabic everyday words	Correctly identify a spoken word presented in the context of four, then six alternatives with 80% accuracy
Language	Does not use bound morphemes, such as -ed, -ing	Establish consistent use of word endings in expressive and written communication	Demonstrate use of past tense endings in 80% of written samples and 70% of spontaneous spoken language samples
Speech	Neutralizes vowels and omits final word consonant	Improve speech intelligibility	Distinguish between /i/, /a/, and /u/ with 80% accuracy in imitated speech tasks; produce final consonants in ≥50% of words during a spontaneous speech task
Psychosocial	Does not follow classroom rules	Demonstrate grade-appropriate classroom behavior	Receive positive reinforcement for adhering to classroom rules; accumulate 100 points in 3 mo
Educational	Reading delayed by 1 grade level; can read aloud but has reduced comprehension	Improve reading comprehension	Demonstrate comprehension on 85% of grade-appropriate reading samples

Reprinted from Tye-Murray N. Intervention plans for children. In Foundations of Aural Rehabilitation: Children, Adults and Their Family Members. San Diego: Singular, 1998.

programs should be developed for regular teachers, psychologists, administrators, and support personnel. Teachers of those with hearing loss whose previous experience was confined to the self-contained classroom are now being asked to service children with hearing loss either in a resource room or as an itinerant teacher. In addition, support personnel who previously only encountered children with mild to moderate hearing loss are now faced with the task of mainstreaming children with severe to profound hearing loss. Many educators find themselves needing to upgrade and broaden their skills to meet the demands of children with hearing loss and comply with the provisions of IDEIA 2004.

Teachers and support personnel say that they lack the knowledge to provide adequate programs for children with hearing loss. Even after special training, they often do not recognize basic malfunctions in equipment or programs. It is generally recognized that teachers of children with hearing loss receive little training in classroom amplification systems and other assistive devices. Other teachers have expressed concern about dealing with language and speech development and in training children with hearing loss to use their residual hearing.

In-service education for speech-language pathologists and teachers of children with hearing loss should concentrate on these general areas:

- The relationship between hearing loss and educational communicative skills;
- The behavior of children with hearing loss;
- Principles of personal and classroom amplification, including other assistive devices;
- The importance of the classroom environment and its effects on speech understanding;
- The use of audition in training children with hearing loss;
- The development of language skills in children with hearing loss; and
- The development of speech in children with hearing loss.

Provision of Rehabilitative Services

One other responsibility for educational audiologists may be the direct management of young children with hearing loss in need of rehabilitation. Typically, the audiologist works within a multidisciplinary team to identify the services that the child needs and to ensure sure that the services are provided. Some of the services that the audiologist might provide to a child with hearing loss in the schools may include development of communication strategies, auditory training, speech reading, hearing aid orientation, and development of psychosocial skills. Strategies for some of these services are outlined in Chapter 7.

SUMMARY

This chapter reviews various aspects of education for the child with hearing loss. It is clear that the changes in federal educational provisions for the child with hearing loss have challenged today's audiologists. The emphasis is now on the early identification and management of hearing loss, preferably before 2 years of age. Nevertheless, we find that hearing loss poses a significant threat to educational achievement. Even the milder forms of hearing loss have been shown to inhibit educational progress. These ever-increasing changes in the field of education for the hearing impaired result in expanding responsibilities for both the speech-language pathologist and the audiologist working in a school setting.

References and Suggested Readings

Alpiner JG, McCarthy PA, eds. Rehabilitative Audiology: Children and Adults. 2nd ed. Baltimore: Williams & Wilkins, 1993.

American Speech-Language-Hearing Association. Guidelines for audiology services in the schools by the American Speech-Language-Hearing Association, 1995. In ASHA Desk Reference for Audiology and Speech-Language Pathology, II. Rockville, MD: Author, 1995:71.

Commission on Education of the Deaf. Toward Equality: Education of the Deaf. A Report to the Congress of the United States. Washington: U.S. Department of Health, Education, and Welfare, 1988.

Bess FH, Dodd JD, Parker RA. Children with minimal sensorineural hearing loss: Prevalence, educational performance and functional health status. Ear Hear 19:339–354, 1998.

Bess FH. Unilateral sensorineural hearing loss in children. Ear Hear 7:1–54, 1986.

Bornstein H. Manual Communication: Implications for Deafness. Washington: Gallaudet University, 1990.

Davis J, Shephard N, Stelmachowicz P, Gorga M. Characteristics of hearing impaired children in the public schools: II. Psychoeducational data. J Speech Hear Dis 46:130–137, 1981.

Davis JM, Elfenbein J, Schum R, Bentler RA. Effects of mild and moderate hearing loss on language, educational and psychosocial behavior of children. J Speech Hear Dis 51:53–62, 1986.

DeConde Johnson C, Benson PV, Seaton JB. Educational Audiology Handbook. San Diego: Singular, 1997:17–25.

Feagans L. Otitis media: A model for long term effects with implications for intervention. In Kavanuagh JF, ed. Otitis Media and Child Development. Parkton, MD: York, 1986.

Katz J. Handbook of Clinical Audiology. 5th ed. Baltimore: Lippincott Williams & Wilkins, 2001.

Kurtzer-White E, Luterman D. Early Childhood Deafness. Baltimore: York, 2001.

Mitchell RE, Karchmer MA. More students in more places. Am Ann Deaf, 151(2):95–104, 2006.

Moeller MP. Intervention and outcomes for young children who are deaf and hard of hearing and their families. In Kurtzer-White, Luterman E, eds. Early Childhood Deafness. Baltimore: York, 2001:109–138.

Moores DF. Educating the Deaf: Psychology, Principles, and Practices. 5th ed. Boston: Houghton Mifflin, 2001.

Padden C, Humphries T. Deaf in America: Voices From a Culture. Cambridge, MA: Harvard University, 1988.

Quigley SP, Thomure FE. Some Effects of Hearing Loss Upon School Performance. Springfield, IL: Office of Education, 1968.

Regional and National Summary of Data from the 2001–2002 Annual Survey of Deaf and Hard of Hearing Children and Youth. Washington: Gallaudet Research Institute, Gallaudet University, 2003.

Schow RL, Nerbonne MA, eds. Introduction to Audiologic Rehabilitation. 5th ed, Boston: Pearson Education, 2007.

Seewald RC, Gravel JS, eds. A Sound Foundation Through Early Amplification 2001. Chicago: Phonak, 2002.

Tye-Murray N. Foundations of Aural Rehabilitation: Children, Adults and Their Family Members. San Diego: Singular, 2000.

United States House of Representatives 99th Congress, 2nd Session: Report 99-860. Report Accompanying the Education of the Handicapped Act Amendments of 1986.

Glossary

AAA See American Academy of Audiology.

ABR See Auditory brainstem response.

Acoustic neuroma A tumor that affects the eighth (auditory) nerve.

Acoustic reflex Reflexive contraction of the middle ear muscles caused by the presentation of a sound stimulus.

Acoustic reflex threshold Lowest possible intensity needed to elicit a middle ear muscle contraction.

Acquired hearing loss Hearing loss obtained sometime after birth.

Acute otitis media Middle ear disease of rapid onset and rapid resolution, characterized by a reddish or yellowish bulging tympanic membrane, obliteration of ossicular landmarks, and conductive hearing loss.

Adhesive otitis media Otitis media that results in adhesions between the tympanic membrane and the bony walls of the middle ear or the ossicles.

Admittance Ease of flow of energy through a system; reciprocal of impedance.

Afferent Centripetal; term pertaining to conduction of ascending nerve fibers from peripheral to central.

American Academy of Audiology Professional organization for audiologists.

American National Standards Institute Organization that develops standards for measuring devices (e.g., audiometers).

American Sign Language Sign language used in the United States to differentiate from some of the more recent modifications devised to make signs more like the English language.

American Speech-Language-Hearing Association Professional organization for audiologists and speech-language pathologists.

Anomaly A deviation from normal.

ANSI See American National Standards Institute.

Apex Term used to denote the top or near the top.

Apgar score A common assessment tool for describing the amount of depression exhibited by the infant at birth. Apgar scores consist of five criteria: (*a*) heart rate, (*b*) respiratory rate, (*c*) muscle tone, (*d*) response to stimulation, and (*e*) color. The highest possible score is 10.

ASHA See American Speech-Language-Hearing Association.

ASL See American Sign Language.

Assistive listening device Amplification system used to improve the signal-to-noise reaching an individual's ear.

Atresia Absence or closure of a normal body opening; in hearing, it most often refers to the external acoustic meatus.

Audiogram Graphic representation of a person's hearing. Intensity (in decibels) is plotted on the ordinate, and frequency is shown on the abscissa.

Audioscope Handheld otoscope with a built in audiometer.

Auditory brainstem response A series of five to seven waves in the electrical waveform that appear in the first 10 ms after the presentation of an auditory stimulus such as a click or a tone burst. The ABR is sensitive to dysfunction occurring from the auditory periphery to the upper auditory brainstem portions of the auditory central nervous system.

Auditory cortex Auditory area of the cerebral cortex in the region of the temporal lobe.

Auditory-oral approach Method used to teach children with significant hearing loss speech and language; emphasis is on hearing and speech reading with no manual communication.

Auditory-verbal approach Method used to teach children with significant hearing loss speech and language; emphasis is on listening and understanding the spoken message via the auditory system with no emphasis on vision for receiving information.

A-weighted scale A filtering network on the sound level meter that filters the low frequencies and approximates the response characteristics of the human ear.

Bandwidth Range of frequencies within a specific band.

Basal Term used to denote near the end.

Basilar membrane Membrane in the cochlear duct that supports the organ of Corti.

BC See Bone conduction.

Behavioral observation audiometry Evaluation of a child's hearing via observation of responses (e.g., head turn) to sound.

Bilateral Term used to denote both sides.

Bilirubin A red bile pigment, sometimes found in urine, that is present in the blood tissues during jaundice.

Binaural Pertaining to both ears.

BOA See Behavioral observation audiometry.

Bone conduction Transmission of sound to the inner ear via the skull.

Broadband (white) noise An acoustic signal that contains energy of equal intensity at all frequencies.

BTE Behind the ear.

Calibrate To set the parameters of an instrument such as an audiometer to an accepted standard (e.g., ANSI).

CANS Central auditory nervous system.

Carhart Father of the profession of audiology.

Cholesteatoma Accumulation of debris developed from perforations of the eardrum; sometimes referred to as a pseudotumor.

Chromosome One of several small rod-shaped bodies, easily stained, that appear in the nucleus of a cell at the time of cell division; they contain the genes, or hereditary factors, and are constant in number in each species.

Chronic otitis media Otitis media that is slow in onset, tends to be persistent, and often can produce other complications. The most common symptoms are hearing loss, perforation of the tympanic membrane, and fluid discharge.

Cilium (plural: cilia) Minute, vibratile, threadlike structures of cells that beat rhythmically.

CMV See cytomegalovirus.

Cochlea Auditory portion of the inner ear; sensory organ for hearing.

Collapsed canal A canal that collapses as the result of pressure caused by earphone placement.

COM See Chronic otitis media.

Compression Technique used to decrease or limit the wide range of sounds in the everyday world to match more closely the dynamic range of listeners with hearing loss.

Computed tomography Radiography in which a three-dimensional image of a body structure is constructed by computer from a series of cross-sectional images.

Concha Depression area of the auricle; serves to collect and direct sound to the external auditory meatus.

Congenital Before birth; usually before the 28th week of gestation.

Contralateral Pertaining to the opposite side.

CORFIG See Coupler response for flat insertion gain.

Cortex The outer layer of an organ such as the cerebellum.

Coupler Device that joins one part of an acoustic system to another.

Coupler response for flat insertion gain The difference between coupler gain and insertion gain, both measured with no venting and with the same sound bore.

CPS Cycles per second.

CT See Computed tomography.

Cytomegalovirus Congenital viral infection that in its severe forms produces symptoms similar to those of rubella and may cause hearing loss and other abnormalities.

Deaf culture Beliefs, traditions, customs, and attitudes of a subgroup of the deaf population.

Decibel The logarithm of the ratio between two sound intensities, powers, or sound pressures. The decibel (one-tenth of a bel) was named in honor of Alexander Graham Bell.

Deformity A deviation from the normal shape or size of a specific portion of the body.

Degeneration Decline, as in the nature or function, from a former or original state.

Delayed latency Abnormal time lapse between signal onset and primary peaks in the ABR response.

Dementia A breakdown or deterioration in cognitive function.

Deoxyribonucleic acid Molecules that carry genetic information.

Diagnosis The process of determining the nature of a disease.

Digital Numeric representation of a signal especially for use by a computer.

DNA See Deoxyribonucleic acid.

EAA See Educational Audiology Association.

Earmold Earpiece that is connected to the hearing aid for the purpose of directing sound into the external auditory meatus.

Earphone A transducer system that converts electrical energy from a signal generator, such as an audiometer, into acoustical energy, which is then delivered to the ear.

Educational audiology A subspecialty in audiology that focuses on providing audiologic services in the schools.

Educational Audiology Association Professional organization for audiologists interested in the provision of audiologic services in the schools.

EENT Eye, ear, nose, and throat.

Effusion Collection of fluid in the middle ear.

Electroacoustic Refers to the conversion of acoustic energy to electrical energy or vice versa to generate or measure sound.

Electromagnetic field Field of energy produced by electrical current flowing through a coil or wire.

Emission Acoustic emissions discharged from the cochlea.

Endogenous Hereditary, as in forms of hearing impairment; literally means *within the genes.*

Endolymphatic hydrops Ménière disease; buildup of endolymph within the cochlea and vestibular labyrinth; typical audiologic findings include vertigo, fullness, and fluctuating sensorineural hearing loss.

Epidemiology Branch of medical science that deals with incidence, distribution, and control of disease in a population.

Epithelium Tissue that forms the surfaces of the body.

ERP Event-related potentials.

Etiology The cause of a disorder or condition; also the study of causes.

Exogenous Acquired, as in forms of hearing impairment; literally means *outside the genes.*

Exudate discharge Usually secretion of fluid from the mucosal lining of the middle ear.

FAAA Fellow of the American Academy of Audiology.

Fetal alcohol syndrome Birth defects that may include facial abnormalities, growth deficiency, mental retardation, and other impairments; caused by the mother's abuse of alcohol during pregnancy.

Filter Device that rejects auditory signals while allowing others to pass.

Fistula A tubular passageway or duct formed by disease, surgery, injury, or congenital defect; usually connects two organs.

Flaccid Weak, such as a flaccid tympanic membrane.

FM Frequency modulation.

For- Door; opening.

Forensic audiology A subspecialty in audiology that focuses on litigation issues.

Format bands Regions of prominent energy distribution in a speech sound.

Fossa A pit or hollow.

Frequency response The output characteristics of hearing aids and other amplification devices; gain as a function of frequency.

Frequency The number of complete cycles per second for a vibrating system or other repetitive motion.

Functional hearing loss Audiometric evidence of hearing loss when there is no organic basis to explain the hearing loss.

Fundamental The harmonic component of a complex wave that has the lowest frequency and commonly the greatest amplitude.

Gain For hearing aids, the difference in decibels between the input level of an acoustic signal and the output level.

Gene The biologic unit of heredity, self-reproducing and in a definite position on a particular chromosome.

Genetic counseling Providing information to families with regard to the probability of an inherited disorder.

Genetic Related to heredity.

Genetics The study of heredity.

Genotype The genetic makeup of an individual.

Geriatric Related to aging.

Gestational age Time from mother's last menstrual period.

Glomus tumor A painful benign tumor that develops by hypertrophy of a glomus.

Habilitation Provision of intervention services designed to overcome the handicapping conditions associated with congenital hearing loss.

HAIC See Hearing aid industry conference.

Hair cells One of the sensory cells in the auditory epithelium of the organ of Corti.

Handicap Condition that affects psychosocial function; the consequence of a disability.

Hard of hearing Having residual hearing sufficient to enable successful processing of linguistic information through audition with the use of amplification.

Harmonic A component frequency of a complex wave that is an integral multiple of the fundamental frequency.

Hearing aid An electronic amplifying device designed to bring sound more effectively into the ear.

Hearing aid industry conference Organization of manufacturers of hearing instruments and devices.

Hearing aid performance inventory Communication scale that assesses the impact of hearing loss across several dimensions including speech comprehension, signal intensity, response to auditory failure, social effects of hearing loss, and occupational difficulties.

Hearing handicap inventory for the elderly Specific self-report communication scale made up of items dealing with social and emotional aspects of hearing loss.

Hearing impairment A generic term indicating disability that may range from slight to complete deafness.

Hearing loss A reduction in the ability to perceive sound; may range from slight to complete deafness.

Hearing sensitivity The ability of the ear to perceive sound.

Helicotrema Passage that connects the scala tympani and the scala vestibuli at the apex of the cochlea.

Hereditary deafness Genetically transmitted deafness.

Hereditary Genetically transmitted or transmittable from parent to offspring.

Hertz A unit of frequency equal to 1 cycle per second.

High-risk register Conditions for which children are at greater-than-average risk for hearing impairment.

HINT Hearing in noise test.

HL Hearing level (pertains to measurements in decibels).

HOH See Hard of hearing.

Hx History.

Hyperbilirubinemia An abnormally large amount of bilirubin in the circulating blood.

Hypertelorism An abnormally increased distance between two organs or parts.

Hypoxia Depletion of oxygen.

Hz Hertz.

IDEA See Individuals with Disabilities Education Act.

Identification audiometry Methods used to screen for hearing loss in a simple, quick, and cost-effective manner.

Idiopathic Pertaining to unknown causation.

IEP See Individualized education plan.

IHAFF See Independent Hearing Aid Fitting Forum.

Immittance A general term describing measurements made of tympanic membrane impedance, compliance, or admittance.

Impairment Abnormal or reduced function.

Impedance Opposition to the flow of energy through a system; reciprocal of admittance.

Implant An electronic device carried under the skin with electrodes in the middle ear on the promontory or cochlear window or in the inner ear in the cochlea to create sound sensation in total sensory deafness.

In situ In position.

Incidence Proportion of a group initially free of a given condition that develops the condition over time.

Inclusion Integration of hearing-impaired children into a regular classroom setting.

Incus The middle bone of the three ossicles in the middle ear; anvil.

Independent Hearing Aid Fitting Forum Working group of audiologists who promote specific recommendations for the selection and fitting of amplification.

Individualized education plan Plan developed by a multidisciplinary team for educating children with disabilities including hearing loss; mandated by IDEA 1997 and updated on an annual basis.

Individuals with Disabilities Education Act Legislation to ensure that children with disabilities over age 3 years receive a free and appropriate education; also encourages services for children under 3 years old.

Inertia The tendency of a body to remain in a state of rest.

Inner ear The organ of hearing and equilibrium in the temporal bone.

Insertion gain Real ear measurement of gain of a hearing aid.

Intensive care unit A separate, designated service area in a hospital that is used for the care and treatment of critically ill patients.

Inter- Between, among, together.

Ipsi- Self.

Ipsilateral On the same side.

ITC hearing aid In-the-ear hearing aid.

itis- Inflammation.

Jaundice A yellowish pigmentation of the skin, tissues, and body fluids caused by deposition of bile pigments.

JCIH See Joint Committee on Infant Hearing.

JND Just noticeable difference.

Joint Committee on Infant Hearing Organization of several groups including but not limited to the American Academy of Audiology, the American Academy of Otolaryngology, the American Academy of Pediatrics, and the American Speech-Language-Hearing Association.

Kanamycin An ototoxic antibiotic consisting of two amino sugars.

Keratoma A horny tumor.

Kernicterus A form of jaundice in the newborn; known to be associated with sensorineural hearing loss.

Labyrinth Inner ear.

Labyrinthitis Inflammation of the labyrinth.

Latency The period of apparent inactivity between the time a stimulus is presented and the moment a response occurs.

LCL See Loudness comfort level.

LDL See Loudness discomfort level.

Learning disability Generic term used to denote learning problems in young school-aged children.

Lesion Wound or injury; area of pathologic change in tissue.

Limen Threshold; boundary line.

Localization Identification of the origin of a sound in space (horizontal or vertical plane).

Loudness comfort level Intensity level needed to achieve a comfortable listening level.

Loudness discomfort level The intensity level that causes discomfort for an individual.

Mal- Defective, bad, wrong.

Malleus The largest auditory ossicle; the hammer.

Masking The ability of one acoustic signal to obscure the presence of another acoustic signal so that it cannot be detected.

Medial Toward the axis, near the midline.

Melotia A developmental anomaly characterized by displacement of the ear (auricle) on the side of the face.

Ménière disease See Endolymphatic hydrops disease.

Meningitis Inflammation of the meninges caused by bacterial or viral infection causing severe to profound sensorineural hearing loss in some cases (10%).

Meniscus A crescent-shaped structure.

Micrognathia An abnormally small mandible.

Microphone Transducer that converts acoustic energy into electrical energy.

Microtia A small deformed pinna (or auricle).

Mild hearing loss Hearing loss ranging from 25 to 40 dB HL.

Mixed hearing loss Type of hearing loss that includes both conductive and sensorineural impairments.

Moderate hearing loss Hearing loss ranging from 40 to 55 dB HL.

Monaural Pertaining to one ear.

Montage Placement configuration of electrodes in electrophysiologic measurements.

Mucus Viscous secretion of mucous glands.

Mumps A contagious viral disease occurring mainly in children; symptoms include parotitis, fever, headaches, and sudden profound unilateral sensorineural hearing loss.

Myelin The fatty sheath of the axon of a neuron.

Myringitis Inflammation of the tympanic membrane.

Myringotomy Surgical incision in the eardrum to release pressure, remove fluid, and restore hearing sensitivity.

Narrowband noise Band of noise limited to a restricted frequency region by filtering.

Nasopharynx The part of the pharynx (throat) behind and above the soft palate, continuous with the nasal passages.

Negative predictive value Probability that a person who has passed a hearing screening test truly has normal hearing.

Neomycin An ototoxic antibiotic administered orally or locally.

Neonate Young child, usually during the first 4 weeks.

Nephritis Inflammation of the kidney.

Nephrotoxic Toxic to the nephrons of the kidney.

Neuritis Inflammation of a nerve.

Neurologist An expert in neurology or in treatment of disorders of the nervous system.

Neurology Branch of medical science that deals with the nervous system, both normal and in disease.

Neuron Any of the conducting cells of the nervous system; a neuron consists of a cell body, containing the nucleus and the surrounding autoplasm, an axon and a dendrite.

NICU Neonatal intensive care unit.

NIHL See Noise-induced hearing loss.

NIPTS Noise-induced permanent threshold shift.

NITTS Noise-induced temporary threshold shift.

Noise-induced hearing loss Permanent sensorineural hearing loss as a result of exposure to high noise levels.

Nonorganic hearing loss See functional hearing loss.

Northwestern Auditory Test Number 6 Common open-set monosyllabic word test used in the audiologic assessment to determine word recognition ability at comfortable listening levels.

NST Nonsense syllable test.

OAE See Otoacoustic emission.

Ob- Against, in front of, toward.

Occlusion Blockage or obstruction, as of the ear canal.

Octave The interval between two sounds with a 2:1 ratio in frequency.

OHC See Outer hair cells.

Ohm Unit of resistance to the transference of other forms of energy.

OME See Otitis media with effusion.

Opacification The development of opacity (imperviousness to light rays), as of the cornea or lens.

Organ of Corti Organ of hearing on the basilar membrane.

Ossicles The three bones of the middle ear: malleus, incus, and stapes.

Otalgia Pertaining to the pain in the ear.

Otitic Pertaining to otitis.

Otitis Inflammation of the ear.

Otitis media Inflammation of the cleft or middle ear space.

Otitis media with effusion Inflammation of the middle ear cleft with a collection of fluid.

Otitis prone Having a predisposition for middle ear disease.

OTO Otolaryngology.

Otoacoustic emission Sounds produced by the cochlea; usually evoked by an auditory stimulus but can occur spontaneously; considered an outer hair cell phenomenon.

Otolaryngologist Physician who specializes in diseases of the ear, nose, and throat.

Otolaryngology Medical specialty associated with diagnosis and management of diseases of the ear, nose, and throat.

Otologist A physician who specializes in diseases of the ear.

Otorrhea Discharge from the ear.

Otosclerosis Formation of spongy bone in the labyrinthine capsule and the stapes footplate. The most common site of the formation is just in front of the oval window. The disease produces impaired stapedial mobility and a gradual conductive hearing loss. Also known as otospongiosis.

Otoscope Handheld device for visual inspection of the ear canal and eardrum.

Ototoxic Causing or pertaining to effects toxic to the ear.

Outer ear The auricle, external auditory meatus, and lateral portion of the tympanic membrane.

Outer hair cells Hair cells within the organ of Corti thought to be responsible for frequency resolution and energizing the inner hair cells.

Pa See Pascal.

Pascal Unit of sound pressure.

PB Max Intensity level at which maximum understanding for phonetically balanced words is achieved.

PB Phonetically balanced words.

PBK Word List Word recognition test used with children; words are within the receptive vocabulary of most school-age children.

Pediatric audiologist Audiologist who specializes in the assessment and management of young children.

Perforation Small hole; typically refers to perforation of the tympanic membrane.

Perilymph The fluid in the space separating the membranous from the osseous labyrinth of the inner ear.

Perinatal Occurring in the period shortly before or after birth (from 8 weeks before birth to 4 weeks after).

Periosteum Specialized connective tissue covering all bones of the body, consisting of a dense, fibrous outer layer and a more delicate inner layer capable of forming bone.

Peripheral Toward the outward surface or port.

Petrous Denoting or pertaining to the hard, dense portion of the temporal bone containing the internal auditory organs.

PHAB See Profiled hearing aid benefit self-assessment inventory.

PHAP See Profile of hearing aid performance.

Pneumatic otoscope Handheld instrument used to examine visually the external acoustic meatus and the tympanic membrane. A pneumatic bulb connected to the otoscope allows the examiner to vary air pressure in the canal while examining the mobility of the eardrum.

Positive predictive value Probability that a person who has failed a hearing screening test is truly hearing impaired.

Postnatal Acquired or occurring after the perinatal period.

Potential Electric tension or pressure; electric activity in a muscle or nerve cell during activity.

Prenatal Acquired or occurring before birth or before the perinatal period.

Presbycusis Hearing loss due to aging.

Prevalence The number of cases (of hearing impairment) in a given population at a given point in time.

Profile of hearing aid performance Scale to assess success of a hearing aid.

Profiled hearing aid benefit self-assessment inventory Scale to assess hearing aid benefit.

PSI Pediatric speech intelligibility test.

Psychogenic hearing loss See functional hearing loss.

PTA See Pure-tone average.

Pure-tone average Average of hearing thresholds at 500, 1000, and 2000 Hz.

Real-ear aided response Real-ear measurement with a probe microphone of sound pressure level as a function of frequency with the hearing aid turned on.

Real-ear coupler difference Measurement of difference in decibels between the output of the hearing aid measured with a probe microphone in the ear canal and the output obtained in a 2-cc coupler.

Real-ear insertion gain Probe microphone measurement of the difference between the unaided response and the real-ear aided response.

REAR See real-ear aided response.

RECD See real-ear coupler difference.

Recessive hereditary sensorineural hearing loss Form of hereditary deafness; both parents of a child with hearing loss are clinically normal. Appearance of the trait requires that the individual possess two similar abnormal genes, one from each parent. The recessive genes account for the transmission of hearing loss, which can skip several generations.

Recruitment An abnormal increase in loudness growth in an ear with sensorineural hearing loss once threshold has been reached.

Reflectometer Handheld instrument designed to detect middle ear disease with effusion.

Reflex An involuntary, relatively invariable adaptive response to a stimulus.

Rehabilitation Management strategies used to restore function following insult or injury.

REIG See real-ear insertion gain.

Renal Of or pertaining to the kidney.

Residual hearing Remaining hearing in individuals with hearing impairment.

Resonance A structure's absorption and emission of energy at the same frequency band.

Reticular lamina Netlike layer extending over the surface of the organ of Corti.

Retinitis Inflammation of the retina.

Retinitis pigmentosa A group of disorders, often hereditary, that show progressive loss of retinal response, retinal atrophy, and clumping of the pigment with contraction of the field of vision.

Retrocochlear Beyond the cochlea, especially nerve fibers along the auditory pathways from the internal auditory meatus to the cortex.

Reverberation Persistence of sound within an enclosed space; echo.

Rubella German measles; a mild viral infection characterized by a pinkish rash which occurs first on the face before spreading to other parts of the body. If contracted during pregnancy, especially during the first trimester, can result in mental retardation, hearing loss, visual complications, and mild heart problems in the baby.

Sagittal plane A vertical plane through the longitudinal axis dividing the body into left and right portions.

SAT See speech awareness threshold.

Saturation sound pressure level Maximum output of the receiver of a hearing aid.

Scala A subdivision of the cavity of the cochlea.

Scala media Middle cavity within the cochlea; filled with endolymph and contains the organ of Corti.

Scala tympani Perilymph-filled cavity below the scala media.

Scala vestibuli Perilymph-filled cavity above the scala media.

Secretion Production of a physiologically active substance and movement of the substance out of the cell or gland that produced it.

Senile Relating to or proceeding from old age.

Sensation level Intensity of a signal (in decibels) above the hearing threshold.

Sensitivity Proportion of affected persons in a population who give a positive test result for the condition in question; true positive results divided by number tested.

Serous otitis media Inflammation of the middle ear with a collection of serum.

Serum A clear fluid free of debris and bacteria.

Sickle cell anemia Hereditary disease of the blood that occurs almost exclusively in blacks.

Sickness impact profile Quality-of-life measure used to determine impact of chronic illness.

SIP See Sickness impact profile.

SL See Sensation level.

SNR Signal-to-noise ratio; usually refers to the relation between speech and ambient noise reaching an individual's ear.

SOA Spontaneous otoacoustic emission.

Sound field An area (usually a room) into which sound is introduced (usually by a loudspeaker).

Sound pressure level Magnitude of sound relative to a reference pressure (0.0002 dynes/cm^2).

Specificity Proportion of persons in a population correctly identified by a screening test as not having the condition; true negatives divided by the total number tested.

Spectrum (plural: spectra) Range of a sound's amplitude (amplitude spectrum) or phase (phase spectrum) as a function of frequency.

Speech awareness threshold Intensity level at which awareness of speech occurs.

Speech reading Visual recognition of speech by observing mouth movement.

Speech reception threshold Threshold for speech comprehension using spondaic words.

Spiral ganglion Group of nerve cell bodies in the modiolus of the cochlea, from which nerve fibers extend into the spiral organ.

SPL See Sound pressure level.

Spondee Two-syllable word with approximately equal stress on both syllables (e.g., baseball, cowboy).

SRT See Speech reception threshold.

SSPL See Saturation sound pressure level.

Stapes The innermost ossicle of the middle ear (stirrup).

Steno- Narrow or contracted.

Stigmata Findings or landmarks indicative of a specific disorder.

Streptomycin Ototoxic antibiotic.

Sub- Under, beneath, deficient.

Super- Above, excessive.

Suppurative Bearing or producing pus or fluid; often found in acute otitis media; characterized by white blood cells, cellular debris, and many bacteria.

Symmetrical hearing loss Hearing loss that is essentially equivalent in both ears.

Syn- With, together.

Synapse Region of contact between processes of two adjacent neurons where a nervous impulse is transmitted from one neuron to another.

Syncope A temporary suspension of consciousness caused by generalized cerebral ischemia.

Syndrome A group of symptoms that are characteristic of a specific condition or disease.

Synophrys A condition in which the eyebrows grow together.

Tactile Pertaining to touch.

Tangible Reinforcement Operant Conditioning Audiometry Management technique for difficult-to-test children; child receives reinforcement (candy, cereal, toys) for the correct identification of a signal.

TC See Total communication.

Tectorial membrane Membrane which projects like a roof over the organ of Corti; the edge of the outer hair cells are embedded within the tectorial membrane.

Temporary threshold shift Temporary elevation of an auditory threshold after exposure to noise. Frequently used to predict the potential danger of a noise environment.

TEOAE See Transient evoked otoacoustic emission.

Threshold Softest level at which a signal or change in signal can be detected.

Thyroid goiter An abnormally large thyroid.

Time compression Process whereby speech is recorded and then played back in less time than the original recording; commonly expressed as a percentage. For example, speech that originally was recorded in 1 second and played back in 0.5 second would be 50% time-compressed.

Tinnitus Sensation of ringing in the ear.

TM Tympanic membrane.

Tonotopic Refers to structures in the peripheral and central auditory nervous system that are spatially arranged according to frequency.

TORCH Acronym used to categorize major infections that may be contracted in utero: *to*xoplasmosis, *ru*bella, *c*ytomegalovirus, and *h*erpes simplex.

Total communication Intervention that incorporates a combination of auditory, oral, and manual communication techniques.

Toxoplasmosis Infection with *Toxoplasma gondii*, sometimes transmitted to a fetus via the placenta. Infection is typically contracted by eating uncooked meat or making contact with the feces of cats. Possible cause of hearing loss.

Transient evoked otoacoustic emission Echo emitted by the cochlea in response to a transient stimulus.

Treacher Collins syndrome Craniofacial anomaly characterized by poorly developed cheekbones, antimongoloid slant of the eyes, microtia, atresia, and micrognathia.

TROCA See Tangible Reinforcement Operant Conditioning Audiometry.

TTS See Temporary threshold shift.

Tympanogram Graphic representation of middle ear immittance as a function of air pressure presented to the ear canal.

Ultra- Excessive.

Uncomfortable loudness level Intensity level (in decibels) at which audio signals (pure tones, noise, or speech) become uncomfortably loud.

Uni- One.

Unilateral Refers to one side, as in unilateral hearing loss.

Utero Pertaining to the uterus; the womb.

Vertigo Dizziness; an illusionary sensation of movement such as spinning or whirling.

Vibrotactile Denotes the detection of vibrations via touch.

Viscosity The property of fluid which resists change in the shape or arrangement of its element during flow.

Visual reinforcement audiometry Technique for testing the hearing of young children; a head turn in response to an auditory stimulus is rewarded with a flashing lighted toy or a computer-animated character (e.g., SpongeBob SquarePants).

VRA See Visual reinforcement audiometry.

Waardenburg syndrome A group of genetic conditions that can cause hearing loss and changes in coloring (pigmentation) of the hair, skin, and eyes.

Warble tone Sound characterized by a continuous fluctuation in frequency of predetermined amount both above and below a central frequency.

Waveform Display of an acoustic (or electrical) signal with amplitude along the y-axis and time along the x-axis.

WIPI Word intelligibility by picture identification test.

Word recognition Ability to identify monosyllabic materials; typically expressed in percent correct.

Index

Page numbers in *italics* denote figures; those followed by t denote tables; those followed by n and number indicated note at bottom of page.